Communication in Nursing

Seventh Edition

Julia Balzer Riley,

RN, MN, AHN-BC, REACE

President
Constant Source Seminars
Adjunct Faculty
University of Tampa
Tampa, Florida

ELSEVIER
MOSBY

3251 Riverport Lane
St. Louis, Missouri 63043

COMMUNICATION IN NURSING

ISBN: 978-0-323-08334-8

Notices

Knowledge and best practice in this field are constantly changing. As new research and experience broaden our understanding, changes in research methods, professional practices, or medical treatment may become necessary.

Practitioners and researchers must always rely on their own experience and knowledge in evaluating and using any information, methods, compounds, or experiments described herein.
In using such information or methods they should be mindful of their own safety and the safety of others, including parties for whom they have a professional responsibility.

With respect to any drug or pharmaceutical products identified, readers are advised to check the most current information provided (i) on procedures featured or (ii) by the manufacturer of each product to be administered, to verify the recommended dose or formula, the method and duration of administration, and contraindications. It is the responsibility of practitioners, relying on their own experience and knowledge of their patients, to make diagnoses, to determine dosages and the best treatment for each individual patient, and to take all appropriate safety precautions.

To the fullest extent of the law, neither the Publisher nor the authors, contributors, or editors, assume any liability for any injury and/or damage to persons or property as a matter of products liability, negligence or otherwise, or from any use or operation of any methods, products, instructions, or ideas contained in the material herein.

Library of Congress Cataloging-in-Publication Data

Balzer-Riley, Julia W.
  Communication in nursing. -- 7th ed. / Julia Balzer Riley.
       p. ; cm.
  Includes bibliographical references and index.
  ISBN 978-0-323-08334-8 (pbk. : alk. paper)
  1. Nurse and patient. 2. Interpersonal communication. I. Title.
  [DNLM: 1. Nurse-Patient Relations--Nurses' Instruction. 2. Communication--Nurses' Instruction.
3. Interpersonal Relations--Nurses' Instruction. WY 88]
  RT86.3.B34 2012
  610.7306'99--dc23

                                                                      2011018918

Managing Editor: Michele D. Hayden
Developmental Editor: Heather Bays
Publishing Services Manager: Jeffrey Patterson
Project Manager: Anne Konopka
Design Direction: Amy Buxton

Printed in the United States of America

Last digit is the print number: 9   8   7   6   5   4   3   2   1

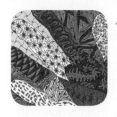

Preface

Communication is cited as a contributing factor in 70% of healthcare mistakes (Kohn, 2000), leading to many initiatives across all healthcare settings to improve the way healthcare professionals communicate. Maintaining quality and safe care depends on clear, concise, and accurate communication of observations, assessments, patient data, and instructions. Because nurses spend more time with patients than do members of other disciplines, it is imperative that they convey crucial information to other team members to make best practice decisions. This book is a basic resource for preparing nurses to apply communication skills to influence and guide care, and includes, in selected chapters, 10 exercises focused on application to quality and safety competencies.

In 2003, the Institute of Medicine delivered a road map for dramatic changes in how health professionals are educated if we are to improve healthcare outcomes. These changes were based on six essential competencies to achieve twenty-first century goals for quality and safety. Health professionals should be educated to *collaborate in interprofessional teams* to deliver *patient-centered care* based on the most current *evidence-based practice* guidelines and monitored for *quality improvement*. New *safety* science for preventing healthcare mistakes should form the framework for care provided. The work should be accomplished by applying skills in *informatics*. To apply these recommendations to prepare nurses to help lead improvements in our healthcare system, the Quality and Safety Education for Nurses (QSEN) project (www.qsen.org) has addressed how to implement these six competencies into nursing education and practice. The QSEN project goal is to transform nurses' education by integrating the knowledge, skills, and attitudes for these six competencies into nursing curricula (Cronenwett et al, 2007), including application in clinical learning experiences.

Cronenwett and colleagues (2007) describe each competency and the knowledge, skills, and attitudes that prelicensure nurses should master (www.qsen.org):

- *Patient-centered care* recognizes and respects the patient and family as full team members and includes

them as partners in providing compassionate and coordinated care guided by the patient's preferences, values, and needs. Understanding unique aspects of the patient's cultural background is important in planning care, assessing pain management and ethical considerations, and communicating care plans and outcomes honestly and accurately.

- *Teamwork and collaboration* are critical to quality and safe care by encouraging team members to work effectively within nursing and across other disciplines, using open communication, mutual respect, and shared decision-making. Team members must acknowledge the scope of practice for each discipline and recognize authority gradients that guide the hierarchy in making decisions. Transparent communication is important across the team as well as with patients and their families.

- Basing care on the most current *evidence base* requires skills in *informatics* to complete data-based searches and evaluate the evidence for applicability, yet allows the making of decisions, based on the values and beliefs of the patient and family, that may be different from the standard of care. Nurses should base their practice on inquiry by constantly asking questions about what they do, why they do it in a particular way, and whether other ways should be considered.

- *Quality improvement* (QI) monitors the outcomes of care delivered by collecting data on industry standard measures such as patient falls, hospital-acquired infection, and other aspects of care that nurses manage. The data are measured or benchmarked against data from other institutions to be able to discern whether there is a need to improve both the quality and safety outcomes.

- Healthcare has adapted *safety* science from other industries to focus on ways to minimize risk to patients and providers by examining system effectiveness as well as individual performance. New attitudes toward error mean errors are reported as always, but with the intent of learning from them through a systematic review, often root cause analysis. By tracing the pathway of an incident, we can learn where in the process different choices could have led to a different outcome. One example involves the misconnection of tubes for the multiple ports a single patient may have, that is, when the wrong tube is connected to the wrong device (e.g., when the nasogastric tube is connected to the IV bag). By collecting data about this error, nurses can learn ways to manage multiple tubes that prevent that mistake from happening.

• Informatics skills can help nurses achieve the goals of these six competencies by seeking information, using decision support tools, managing data for quality improvement, reporting errors, and documenting care in the electronic health record. Nurses should further be involved in the design of the informatics systems used in their facilities to ensure they address nursing issues as well as respect patient privacy and preferences.

Communication is the critical skill in delivering the complex care required for patients in the twenty-first century. Coordinating across disciplines such as physicians, pharmacists, and others involved in a patient's care requires nurses to both lead and participate in briefings (planning), huddles (problem solving), and debriefings (process improvement). The exercises in this book can help develop the emotional intelligence required to have the self-awareness and self-monitoring to be an effective team member. Communication really can make the difference in healthcare outcomes, reducing patient suffering, and improving the working environment for nurses.

Gwen Sherwood, PhD, RN, FAAN

References

Institute of Medicine: *Health professions education: a bridge to quality*, Washington D.C., 2003, National Academies Press. Retrieved from http://www.iom.edu/CMS/3809/4634/5914.aspx.

Kohn L, Corigan J, Donaldson M, editors: *To err is human: building a safer health system*, Committee on Quality of Health Care in America, Institute of Medicine. Washington D.C., 2000, National Academies Press.

Cronenwett L, Sherwood G, Barnsteiner J, et al: Quality and safety education for nurses, *Nurs Outlook* 55(3):122, 2007.

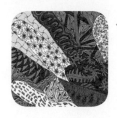

Contributors

Cindy Carter, MSN, BSN, RN, IBCLC, RLC

Clinical Faculty
University of Texas, Arlington;
Clinical Education Specialist
The Center for Learning
Texas Health Resources
Arlington, Texas

Margaret E. Erickson, PhD

Holistic Healing Consultants
Executive Director
American Holistic Nurses Certification Corporation
Cedar Park, Texas

Gwen Sherwood, PhD, RN, FAAN

Professor and Associate Dean for Academic Affairs
University of North Carolina at Chapel Hill School
of Nursing
Chapel Hill, North Carolina

Case Studies and PowerPoint Presentations

Robyn C. Leo, MS, RN

Associated Professor of Nursing
Worcester State University
Thompson, Connecticut

Testbank

Jo A. Voss, PhD, RN, CNS

Associate Professor
South Dakota State University
Rapid City, South Dakota

Writing Tutorial

Michele L. Deck, MEd, RN, BSN, LCCE, FACCE

CEO GAMES/Tool Thyme for Trainers
Baton Rouge, Louisiana

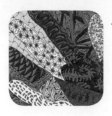

Reviewers

Maria Azpitarte, MS, RN

Director, Nursing Program
Seattle Central Community College
Seattle, Washington

Margaret E. Erickson, PhD

Holistic Healing Consultants
Executive Director
American Holistic Nurses Certification Corporation
Cedar Park, Texas

Mavra E. Kear, PhD, ARNP-BC

Professor, Department of Nursing
Polk State College
Winter Haven, Florida

Joyce A. Larson Presswalla, PhD, RN

Adjunct Professor
Hillsborough Community College
Tampa, Florida

Robyn C. Leo, MS, RN

Associate Professor Nursing
Worcester State University
Worcester, Massachusetts

Sharon L. Marquard, MS, CRRN

St. Ambrose University
Davenport, Iowa

Glenda Nickell, RN, MSN

Instructor of Clinical Nursing
MU Sinclair School of Nursing
University of Missouri
Columbia, Missouri

Roberta Rauer, RN, BSN

Senior Review Case Manager
St. Petersburg, Florida

Testbank Review

Christina D. Keller, RN, MSN

Instructor
School of Nursing
Clinical Simulation Center
Radford University
Radford, Virginia

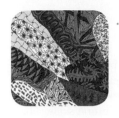

Introduction

Why Study Communication?

The gift of nursing is the intimate journey we take with the client and family from the miracle of birth to the mystery of death. Finely tuned communication skills are essential as nurses live their own life story and bear witness to the stories of those they serve. Nurses practice assertive communication for this journey. Nurses provide education that helps clients change lifelong habits. Nurses communicate with people under stress: clients, family, and colleagues. Nurses deal with anger and depression, with dementia and psychosis, with joy and despair. Nurses serve as client advocates and as parts of interdisciplinary teams whose members may have different ideas about priorities for care. Nurses return to school to specialize, write grants for research proposals, and become entrepreneurs. Nurses become administrators, leaders, case managers, infection control specialists, quality experts, and educators. Nurses blend their understanding of healthcare and technology to offer the skill of nursing informatics. Nurses combine their mission of faith and healthcaring in parish nursing. Nurses move into industry to work in occupational health and into schools and communities to improve the health of large populations and communities. Nurses create new positions where their voices can affect healthcare quality. Nurses cross international boundaries to share knowledge needed to promote worldwide health. Nurses must be assertive to ask the right questions and make their voices heard. Nurses must be assertive to communicate their own needs and be prepared to assert themselves to ensure balance in their own lives. Without such balance, the high-stress environment may diminish nurses' effectiveness.

Despite the complexity of technology and the multiple demands on nurses' time, the intimate moments of connection can make all the difference in the quality of care and meaning for the client and the nurse. As nurses refine their communication skills and build their confidence, they can move from being novices to

experts. Nurses honor, with humility, the differences in clients, and learn and grow in their ability to trust their intuition, to be open to what Martin Buber, a Jewish theologian, calls the I–Thou relationship—the sacred moment of connection when we acknowledge the divine presence in each of us, the essence of each person.

Notice the cover art on this seventh edition of the text, a circular design, a mandala. This piece of art, entitled "With These Hands," is created by the meditative art process called Zentangle, a kind of contemplative doodle. The expressive arts invitation of the same name is one the author uses at the bedside with clients, tracing the hand, and writing qualities clients identify that represent who they are, a kind of legacy. (To learn more about this art process, visit www.zentangle.com). The client is then invited to use art materials to decorate the hand; watercolors work well. In end-of-life care, these pieces could be framed in memory (Riley, 2010).

The *mandala*, a Sanskrit word meaning sacred circle, is a symbol for wholeness. Buddhist monks create intricate mandalas of sand with prayers of healing intention. On completion they are released in the wind to send forth their prayers. Carl Jung, a Swiss psychoanalyst, borrowed from this tradition, finding that patients who created mandalas, art within a circle, gained self-awareness and insight. He suggested that when we make art within a circle, it is as if we are addressing our whole self, our whole world (Marshall, 2003). Western therapists Kellog (2002) and Cornell (1994) used mandalas as therapeutic tools. Mandalas create a symbol of where we are at this moment. Holistic nursing teaches us that each of us is whole in each single moment, not needing to be fixed, but at the

---

Note: In this text we have chosen to use the word *client* rather than *patient* to emphasis the nature of the service that we render and to honor that people are whole persons, body, mind, and spirit, whose role at this time may be that of "patient," one role of many in life.

right place and time for our personal journey, that we make meaning from even the illness experience. Throughout this edition, the mandala is used to remind us that when we bring our whole selves to each interaction with clients, families, and colleagues, we demonstrate our caring. Wherever you see a mandala like the one here, you will find Moments of Connection, which are stories that seasoned nurses have shared to ease your journey along the sacred path of nursing.

References

Cornell J: *Mandala: Luminous symbols for healing*, Wheaton, Ill, 1994, Quest Books.

Kellog J: *Mandala: path of beauty*, Belleair, Fla, 2002, Association of Teachers of Mandala Assessment.

Marshall MC: Creative learning: the mandala as teaching exercise, *J Nurs Educ* 42(11):517, 2003.

Riley JB: *Art in small spaces: art at the bedside*, Ellenton, Fla, 2010, CSP. [This is an expressive arts guidebook for self-discovery and healing. For more information e-mail julia@constantsource.com]

What's New?

In this edition we emphasize the importance of assertive communication to promote quality, safe care for clients and include new exercises to support this process, as well as online case studies and a writing skills tutorial (see http://evolve.elsevier.com/BalzerRiley/communication/ and the preface by Gwen Sherwood, PhD, RN, FAAN, *Co-Investigator, Quality and Safety Education for Nurses Project*).

A press release, dated March 22, 2011, reported the results of "The Silent Treatment: Why Safety Tools and Checklists Aren't Enough to Save Lives," a national study of 6500 nurses and nurse managers, a follow-up to the study, "Silence Kills: The Seven Crucial Conversations for Health Care" (2005). The American Association of Critical Care Nurses (AACN) and the Association of periOperative Registered Nurses (AORN) partnered with VitalSmarts, a company providing evidence-based corporate communication consultation, to identify communication barriers that contribute to avoidable medical error, concluding that assertive communication is what saves lives. Participants cited dangerous shortcuts, incompetence, and disrespect as "undiscussable" topics that, when not addressed with clear communication, contribute to medical error. Compared with the earlier study in 2005, nurses now speak up at better rates; they are now

nearly three times more likely to have spoken directly to the person and shared their full concerns.

Assertive communication is an essential skill that can be learned and improved with practice.

Additional creative expression exercises have been added to give you alternative ways to grow in your own self-awareness to build your communication skills. These may include reflective writing, art-making, poem-making, creative movement, and cinema. Carper (1978) identified four patterns of knowing in nursing: empirical, personal, ethical, and aesthetic. Aesthetic knowing refers to the "art" of nursing, that is, the intangible quality that incorporates parts of the mind, the soul, and the imagination, identified by Florence Nightingale (Nightingale, 1852; Stockhausen, 2006). When nurses deal with not knowing, that is, the uncertainty in some situations, creativity can be a valuable force in coping. I teach a course, Expressive Arts in Healing: Health Promotion through the Arts, as an undergraduate course in the Department of Nursing at the University of Tampa. By the end of the semester, the students understand that the discomfort they feel at first as they try out art materials, still the voice of their inner critic, and explore their own emotions through art, is valuable and parallels the "not knowing" inherent in the practice of nursing.

References

Carper B: Fundamental patterns of knowing in nursing, *Adv Nurs Sci* 1(1):13, 1978.

Nightingale F: *Nightingale notes on nursing*, New York, 1852, Churchill Livingstone. [Reprinted 1980.]

Silence Kills: The Seven Crucial Conversations for Health Care, 2005. Retrieved at www.silencekills.com

Stockhausen L: Métier artistry: revealing reflection-in-action in everyday practice, *Nurse Educ Today* 26(1):54, 2006.

The Silent Treatment: Why Safety Tools and Checklists Aren't Enough to Save Lives, 2011. Retrieved at http://www.silenttreatmentstudy.com/media/Silent%20Treatment%20Release.pdf

What's Important?

To deepen your work in building communication skills through better understanding of yourself and your practice, begin a reflective journal. Some of the chapter exercises will refer to creating a reflective journal entry. Problem solving can be improved with reflection of experience over time. When you finish your course of study of communication, reviewing your journal will help you see how far you have come and give new insights for what's next in your nursing career.

Chapters on humor and spirituality help add perspective and support the practice of holistic nursing. Active reading skills promote the retention of content. The Reflections On . . . /Think About It . . . exercises in each chapter are designed to encourage the reader to reflect on how the content can be applied. Before reading each chapter, note these questions at the end of the chapter and read the objectives and boldface headings. As you read, think about what answers you will write. This will help you keep your attention focused as you read. Pay attention to the Wit & Wisdom sections and the proverbs and quotations at the beginning of each chapter, which add perspective to and involvement with the content. These added features help prevent the "where was I?" thoughts that come when your mind drifts with heavy reading assignments and multiple life commitments.

Honor the sacred nature of your work. Take time each day to connect with your own purpose in your work and set goals for your caring each day.

Remember:

Take time for your own spiritual practice
Honor your own body–mind–spirit connection.
Take your work seriously but yourself lightly
Laugh and play.
To be distracted from the person in front of you, is
to be otherwise attracted . . . and at this moment in
time, nothing is more important than this person.

Julia Balzer Riley, RN, MN, AHN-BC,
Registered Expressive Arts Consultant and Educator (REACE)

Author's note: As you continue your career in nursing, be open to unusual paths to meet new goals and find ways to embellish your practice with who you are. I have been curious about the therapeutic value of art since 1968, when I completed my psychiatric nursing affiliation at St. Elizabeth's Hospital in Washington, DC. This passion was rekindled as I began to offer expressive arts workshops to nurses as part of my work in holistic nursing. I worked with clients in private homes, hospice houses, nursing homes, and hospital rooms to facilitate art processes.

These expressive arts invitations provide an opportunity to explore emotions. They encourage conversation and reflection about the end-of-life experience and the illness experience. They add a bit of whimsy and fun at a difficult time and clients report they provide distraction from pain. As part of an elective course nursing students introduce the expressive arts to clients with poetry, simple collages, and mandala designs to color for relaxation. They report these brief interventions help them learn more about their clients. Students use these processes for their own stress relief and self-discovery through a creative expression journal they keep all semester.

Cover Art

The cover art is a mandala created by Julia Balzer Riley in her own practice of arts in healing. It is titled "With These Hands." The art, created by the Zentangle process, is referred to as a "tangle."

Acknowledgments

Thank you to Heather Bays, Developmental Editor, who responds so well to grandchildren pictures and offers support, encouragement, attention to detail, and additional resources and research when needed to smooth the writing process. Thank you to Michelle Hayden, Managing Editor, for holding the vision of this book's purpose and helping position it to serve more nurses and, thus, more clients.

And on a light note, thank you to Louie Louie, my feral kitten, whose energy and playfulness is a daily inspiration.

And to my husband, thank you for your unconditional love, for the balance you bring to my life, and for your support of my work and my play.

Dedication

This edition is dedicated to my twin grandchildren, Ben and Cate Balzer, born in December 2009, who bring me joy and delight beyond what words can express and recognize "This old man, he played one . . . " on treasured Skype visits . . . truly better living through technology.

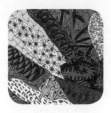

Framework

Part 1 *Getting Started: Basic Communication Competence*

CHAPTER	WILL HELP YOU
1 RESPONSIBLE, ASSERTIVE, CARING COMMUNICATION IN NURSING	Appreciate the significance of responsible, assertive, caring communication as fundamental approaches in nursing
2 THE CLIENT–NURSE RELATIONSHIP: A HELPING RELATIONSHIP	Develop a communication approach that has the interests of your clients at heart
3 SOLVING PROBLEMS TOGETHER	Collaborate and validate with your clients at each phase of the nursing process
4 UNDERSTANDING EACH OTHER: COMMUNICATION AND CULTURE	Understand others and recognize the need to incorporate differences in culture, gender, and age in nursing interventions
5 WORKING TOGETHER IN GROUPS	Understand the dynamics of communication in groups
6 THE CHANGING WORLD OF ELECTRONIC COMMUNICATION	Begin to use electronic communication skills and resources to enrich your work

Part 2 *Building Relationships*

CHAPTER	WILL HELP YOU
7 WARMTH	Demonstrate to your clients in concrete ways that you are concerned about and interested in them
8 RESPECT	Show your clients you consider them to be worthwhile and important
9 GENUINENESS	Say what you think and feel so that your clients receive honest communication from you
10 EMPATHY	Convince your clients and colleagues that you understand their feelings
11 SELF-DISCLOSURE	Relate your own feelings and experiences in a helpful way
12 SPECIFICITY	Be clear and to the point so that others understand your meaning
13 ASKING QUESTIONS	Streamline your interviewing techniques so that your clients understand what information you are seeking and why you are seeking it
14 EXPRESSING OPINIONS	Know when it is appropriate to state your views to your clients
15 HUMOR	Use humor to build relationships with clients
16 SPIRITUALITY	Explore the spiritual connection in nursing practice

Part 3 *Building Confidence*

CHAPTER	WILL HELP YOU
17 REQUESTING SUPPORT	Seek the support you need from your colleagues to deliver excellent care to patients
18 OVERCOMING EVALUATION ANXIETY	Use a rational approach to feel more confident in nursing situations that make you feel anxious
19 FEEDBACK	Be open to feedback from clients and colleagues about your performance as a helper and provide feedback to others in an assertive way
20 RELAXATION	Learn techniques for relieving tension and promoting the relaxation response so that you can remain calm in stressful interpersonal encounters
21 IMAGERY	Rehearse privately so that you can communicate effectively in real situations
22 POSITIVE SELF-TALK	Keep your internal dialogue supportive so that you can communicate with confidence

Part 4 *Meeting Challenges*

CHAPTER	WILL HELP YOU
23 CONFRONTATION	Invite your clients and colleagues to examine how their behavior is affecting others
24 REFUSING UNREASONABLE REQUESTS	Say no assertively to unreasonable requests from clients and colleagues
25 COMMUNICATING ASSERTIVELY AND RESPONSIBLY WITH DISTRESSED CLIENTS AND COLLEAGUES	Reverse your negative reactions to distressed behavior so that you can relate compassionately with clients and colleagues
26 COMMUNICATING ASSERTIVELY AND RESPONSIBLY WITH AGGRESSIVE CLIENTS AND COLLEAGUES	Overcome your reluctance to deal with aggression so that you can relate to aggressive clients and colleagues in useful ways
27 COMMUNICATING ASSERTIVELY AND RESPONSIBLY WITH UNPOPULAR CLIENTS	Become aware of your biases to clients and surmount them so you can provide nursing care to unpopular clients
28 MANAGING TEAM CONFLICT ASSERTIVELY AND RESPONSIBLY	Use a systematic problem-solving approach to deal effectively with conflict between colleagues
29 COMMUNICATING AT THE END OF LIFE	Reflect on the gifts and challenges of communicating with clients near the end of life, and with their families
30 CONTINUING THE COMMITMENT	Consider the commitments necessary to grow and embrace change

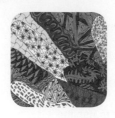

Contents

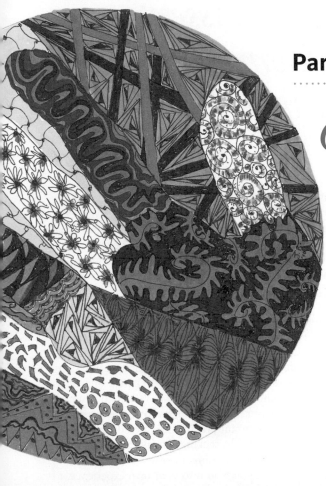

Part 1

Getting Started

Basic Communication Competence

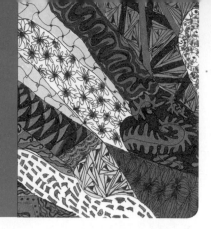

Chapter 1

Responsible, Assertive, Caring Communication in Nursing

> *Caring is the essence of nursing.*
> **Jean Watson**

Objectives

1. Identify the functions of interpersonal communication in nursing
2. Distinguish between assertive, nonassertive, and aggressive communication
3. Identify a three-step process to build assertiveness skills
4. Identify assertive rights
5. Identify irrational beliefs that impede assertive communication
6. Explain the DESC (describe, express, specify, consequences) script for developing an assertive response
7. Identify three types of assertions
8. Identify three essential criteria for presenting an assertive response
9. Describe the behavior of an assertive nurse
10. List the advantages of assertive communication
11. Describe responsible communication in nursing
12. Discuss the role of caring in nursing
13. Participate in exercises to build skills in responsible, assertive, caring communication

This book is designed to help you improve your ability to communicate assertively and responsibly with your clients and colleagues and to demonstrate caring, what Kleen (2004) calls a professional core belief, as you explore and respond to the uniqueness of each individual (Wilson, 2008). Nursing students can make use of this book as they begin their professional journey. Practicing nurses will also find this work useful as they come to understand that clear communication is an essential ingredient for success in a rapidly changing healthcare climate. Communication with clients, colleagues, administrative officials, and staff members of other community agencies is essential as nurses' roles change and more nurses move into the community to practice. If you have not read this book's introduction, do so now, and remember this as an important practice when reading a text, to be able to read actively, seeking to explore the intention of the book, posing questions to yourself as you read to help you fit what you read into your own experience, to retain content, and to be an adult learner, growing your own skills for health caring.

Next, you need to understand the meaning of four important concepts introduced in the opening sentence: communication, assertiveness, responsibility, and caring. These concepts are significant because they form the framework of this textbook.

> *Communication is the heart of nursing . . . your ability to use your growing knowledge and yourself as an instrument of care and caring and compassion*
> **JoEllen Goertz Koerner, 2010**
>
> **WIT&** *Wisdom*

The Meaning of Interpersonal Communication

Communication involves the reciprocal process in which messages are sent and received between two or more people. This book focuses on the communication exchange among you, the nurse, and your clients and colleagues. Communication can either facilitate the development of a therapeutic relationship or create barriers (Stuart, 2009).

In general, there are two parts of face-to-face communication: the verbal expression of the sender's thoughts and feelings and the nonverbal expression. Verbally, cognitive and affective messages are sent through words, voice inflection, and rate of speech; nonverbally, messages are conveyed by eye movements, facial expressions, and body language. Communication by telephone or other electronic media loses the impact of gestures and other nonverbal communication. Powerful nonverbal messages can stand alone: a suspicious glance, for example, or a warm smile or eyes widened with fear.

Senders determine what message they want to transmit to the receiver and encode their thoughts and feelings into words and gestures. Senders' messages are transmitted to the receiver through sound, sight, touch, and, occasionally, smell and taste.

Receivers of the messages have to decode the verbal and nonverbal transmission to make sense of the thoughts and feelings communicated by senders. After decoding the senders' words, speech patterns, and facial and body movements, the receivers encode return messages, either verbally through words or nonverbally through gestures.

In an interaction between two people (e.g., a nurse and a client), each person is both a sender and a receiver and alternates between these two roles. When senders are speaking, they are also receiving messages from the person who is listening. Listeners not only are receiving speakers' messages but also are simultaneously sending messages. Figure 1-1 illustrates this reciprocal nature of the communication process.

At any point in an interpersonal communication, verbal and nonverbal messages about thoughts and feelings are sent and received. With little prompting you know that the complex process of interpersonal communication is influenced by many variables that affect how messages are sent and received. Take a few minutes to think of the variety of factors that can affect the exchange of messages between people. Add your own ideas to those in the following list:

- Environmental factors: formality, warmth, privacy, familiarity, freedom or constraint, physical distance

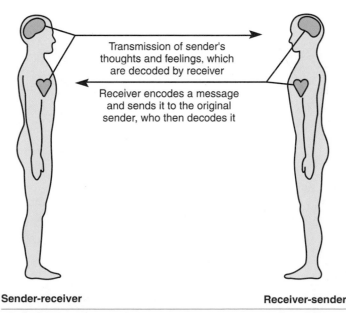

Sender-receiver   **Receiver-sender**

FIGURE 1-1 Reciprocal nature of interpersonal communication.

between people, climate, mood, architecture, arrangement of furniture

- Territory and personal space: crowding, seating arrangements, roles, status, position, physical characteristics (size, height)
- Physical appearance and dress: body shape, race, body smell, hair, gender, body movements, body adornments, posture, age
- Nonverbal cues: facial expressions, eye movements, vocal cues
- Intrapersonal factors: developmental stage, language mastery, differences in perception, differences in decision-making processes, differences in values, self-concept
- The use of "I" messages to own one's responses, such as, "I don't agree with you," instead of "you" messages, which sound blaming, such as, "You are wrong"

Note that any of the preceding factors has the potential to facilitate communication or to act as a barrier to effective communication, depending on the situation. When these factors are considered, the interpersonal communication process looks something like the diagram shown in Figure 1-2.

An important function of communication is to transmit messages from one person to another. The real purpose of communication is to create meaning. Senders of messages wish to convey meaning to receivers, and vice versa. With this intent, senders choose certain words and gestures in a manner that they believe is congruent with their intended messages. The sender's objective is to transmit a message to receivers that is clear and understandable.

The purpose of communication does not stop there, however. The real purpose of creating understanding in another person is to influence the other person to effect some change. The sender attempts to persuade the receiver to respond to the sender's requests. Requests from clients and colleagues may be for the following:

- Understanding
- Action
- Information
- Comfort

Requests may be stated in obvious or indirect ways. The following examples illustrate both direct and indirect requests.

A client has postoperative pain. His physiological need is for pain relief. He asks you, "When was the last time I had my painkiller?" (He winces and

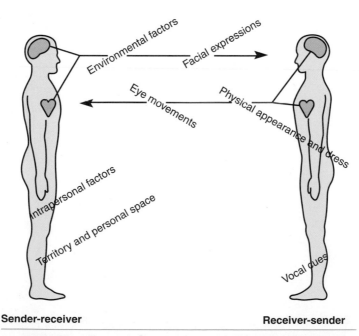

Sender-receiver   **Receiver-sender**

FIGURE 1-2 Factors influencing interpersonal communication.

holds his wrist.) His direct request is for information about the time of his last analgesic. His indirect request is for information about when he can have more. He is anticipating action (you giving him the medication) so that he will be comforted.

A nursing assistant says at the beginning of the shift: "I have a terrible headache. I was up for 3 hours last night with my sick daughter. Do you have an aspirin?" Her physiological need is for rest and pain relief. Her obvious requests are for understanding (for you to empathize with her pain) and action (for you to give her an aspirin). She is possibly hoping that you will comfort her by making allowances for the fact that she is not at her best.

A nurse, newly hired to a unit, needs to feel that he belongs to and fits in with the group. When he asks you to show him around the unit, he is indirectly asking you to understand that he feels alone and unsure. He is directly asking you to take action to orient him and provide him with information about procedures and policy. He is likely hoping that you will make him feel welcome (comforted).

In your interpersonal relationships as a nurse, you will act as both sender and receiver. The purpose of this book is to help you develop your clarity as a sender and your comprehension as a receiver of messages. You will learn how to deliver assertive and responsible messages and to accurately decode messages from your clients and colleagues. You will be able to confidently interpret both direct and indirect requests and make responsible decisions about how to respond assertively (Box 1-1).

Box 1-1	*Important Functions of Interpersonal Communication in Nursing*

- Communication is the vehicle for establishing a therapeutic relationship.
- Communication is the means by which people influence the behavior of others, and thus it is critical to the successful outcome of nursing intervention.
- Communication is the relationship itself, because without it, a therapeutic nurse–client relationship is impossible.

From Stuart GW: *Principles and practice of psychiatric nursing*, ed 9, St. Louis, 2009, Mosby.

The Meaning of Assertive Communication

Moments of Connection...
A Student Nurse Reflects

The woman was lying in her hospital bed. She had remained distant in conversation. She had no family members visiting her and no one could get to know her. It wasn't until I suggested a bath that she began to warm up. She began to talk and her stories flowed one to another. At the end of her morning washing-up, she said thank you. It was as if she was a different person. As I turned to leave, she grabbed my hand, looked into my eyes, and said, "You made me feel human again." I smiled and said it was my pleasure. I never realized the impact of what to me seemed a small part of my day. This was my second semester in nursing school . . . I felt a real connection.

Assertiveness is the key to successful relationships for the client, the family, the nurse, and other colleagues. It is the ability to express your thoughts, your ideas, and your feelings without undue anxiety without any expense to others. Assertiveness means being clear about what you need and respectful in your language and behavior.

The assertive nurse appears confident and comfortable. Assertive behavior, an active behavior, is contrasted with nonassertive or passive behavior, in which individuals disregard their own needs and rights, and aggressive behavior, in which individuals disregard the needs and rights of others. The assertive nurse is positive, caring, nonjudgmental, clear, and direct without threatening or attacking (Table 1-1).

Assertive communication is a lifelong learning skill that requires time and practice. Be willing to accept the fact that you will make mistakes. Be patient. When a person accustomed to behaving passively tries on this new behavior, the results may seem abrupt and abrasive, or shy and tenuous. The goal is not to be continually confrontational. When learning this new skill, you must be assertive all the time or you will be seen as nonassertive. When you practice techniques to learn to become more assertive, it is helpful to begin in a supportive environment with people who are accepting of you. Consider sharing your reading material on assertiveness with a roommate, spouse, or friend with whom you can begin practicing your assertive behavior. Start

Table 1-1 *Assertive and Nonassertive Styles of Communication*

CHARACTERISTIC	ASSERTIVE	NONASSERTIVE	AGGRESSIVE
Attitude toward self and others	I'm OK You're OK	I'm OK You're not OK	I'm OK You're not OK
Decision-making	Makes his or her own decisions	Lets others choose for him or her	Chooses for others
Behavior in problem situations	Engages in direct, fair confrontation	Flees, gives in	Is outright assaultive
Verbal behaviors	Clear, direct statement of wants; objective words; honest statement of feelings	Apologetic words; hedging, rambling; failure to say what is meant	Loaded words; accusations; superior haughty words; labeling of other person
Nonverbal behaviors	Confident, congruent messages	Actions instead of words (not saying is what is felt); incongruence between words and behaviors	Air of superiority; flippant, sarcastic style
Voice	Firm, warm, confident	Weak, distant, soft, wavering	Tense, shrill, loud, cold, demanding, authoritarian, coldly silent
Eyes	Warm, in contact, frank	Averted, downcast, teary, pleading	Expressionless, cold, narrowed, staring
Stance	Relaxed	Stooped; excessive leaning for support	Hands on hips; feet apart
Hands	Gestures at appropriate times	Fidgety, clammy	Fists pounding or clenched
Pattern of relating	Puts himself or herself up without putting others down	Puts himself or herself down	Puts himself or herself up by putting others down
Response of others	Mutual respect	Disrespect, guilt, anger, frustration	Hurt, defensiveness, humiliation
Consequences of style	I win, you win; strives for "win-win" or "no-lose" solutions	I lose, you lose; succeeds only by luck or charity of others	I win, you lose; beats out others at any cost

Modified from Piaget G: Characterological lifechart of three fellows we all know. In Phelps S, Austin N: *The assertive woman*, San Luis Obispo, Calif, 1975, Impact Publishers; and Gerrard B, Boniface W, Love B: *Interpersonal skills for health professionals*, Reston, Va, 1980, Reston Publishing.

with small issues such as returning a damaged product to a store or offering a compliment.

Assertiveness is a matter of choice. It is important to feel confident that you can speak up for yourself, yet it is not necessary or even wise to speak your mind in every situation. With each person you encounter in any situation, you have the choice of communicating in an assertive or nonassertive style. The words you choose and the way you express them can be assertive, nonassertive, or aggressive. Realistically, you may not always have the energy or desire to assert your rights or express yourself fully. There are times when people cannot respond rationally, such as when they are experiencing high levels of anxiety or panic. A person might fear retaliation from a manager or fear the loss of a job. You must choose the issues for which your assertive behavior is appropriate as well as when, where, and with whom to express your assertiveness. The goal in this text is to help you develop the skills that will enable you to choose to act in the best interests of yourself and your clients. Remember, assertiveness helps you give or receive immediate feedback about a behavior that might have serious consequences if ignored (Grover, 2005). This "positive pushback" might be live saving (Gaddis, 2008).

How Do You Get Started?

As you read and think about assertive communication, begin to analyze situations in your life in which you think you would like to respond assertively. Think about what is happening, what your response to it is, what you want to do or have happen, and what the consequences are of action versus no action. Use this three-step process:

1. Review the list of assertive rights (Box 1-2) to see which right or rights you are giving up by not asserting yourself.
2. Review the irrational beliefs that interfere with acting in your own best interest (Box 1-3).
3. Review the DESC script to formulate an assertive response (Box 1-4).

To build your assertive skills, you will need further study and application. Be patient with yourself and remember that becoming assertive is a lifelong journey (Box 1-5).

Box 1-2　　*Assertive Rights*

1. You have the right to be treated with respect.
2. You have the right to a reasonable workload.
3. You have the right to an equitable wage.
4. You have the right to determine your own priorities.
5. You have the right to ask for what you want.
6. You have the right to refuse without making excuses or feeling guilty.
7. You have the right to make mistakes and be responsible for them.
8. You have the right to give and receive information as a professional.
9. You have the right to act in the best interest of the patient.
10. You have the right to be human.

From Chenevert M: *Mosby's tour guide to nursing school: a student's road survival kit*, ed 6, St. Louis, 2011, Mosby.

Box 1-3　　*Irrational Beliefs*

Irrational beliefs arise when we are anxious about being assertive and focus on possible negative outcomes. The rational counterparts focus on possible positive outcomes.

IRRATIONAL BELIEF

- If I am assertive, other people will be upset, hurt by it, or angry with me.
- If someone gets angry with me, I will be devastated.
- Assertive people are seen as cold and self-serving.
- It is wrong for me to turn down legitimate requests.

RATIONAL COUNTERPART

- The other person may not be hurt or angry. This person might prefer being open and honest, too. This person might feel closer to me and help me solve the problem.
- I will not fall apart in the face of anger. The anger is not my responsibility. An angry response is a choice.
- Assertive responses are honest and demonstrate respect for the other person's point of view. Assertion builds healthy relationships.
- It is acceptable for me to turn down even reasonable requests. I can consider my own needs first, and it is not possible to please all of the people all of the time!

Modified from Ellis A: *Overcoming destructive beliefs, feelings, and behaviors: new directions for rational emotive therapy*, Amherst, NY, 2001, Prometheus Books.

Box 1-4　　*Anatomy of an Assertive Response*

A framework for developing assertive responses is known as the DESC script. Although not all steps are used in every situation, it is a useful tool.

　Describe the situation
　Express what you think and feel
　Specify your request
　Consequences

Developed by Bower SA, Bower GH: *Asserting yourself*, Reading, Mass, 1991, Addison-Wesley.

1. Basic—simply expresses an idea, belief, or opinion; stands up for your rights or the rights of others, for example: "I want to . . ." "I don't want you to . . ." "Would you . . .?" "I liked it when you . . ." "I have a different opinion. I think that . . ." "I have mixed reactions. I agree with these aspects for these reasons, but I am disturbed by these aspects for these reasons" (University of Illinois, Counseling Center, 1984).
   - To buy time to consider: "I can give you an answer tomorrow after I have had time to think about it."
   - To deal with an interruption: "Excuse me, I am almost through. I'd like to finish my thought."
   - To return merchandise: "I am not satisfied with this product and I would like a refund."
   - To say no: "I cannot loan you any money."
2. Empathic—conveys sensitivity to the situation while taking an assertive position.
   - "I know the unit is short-staffed, but I have a pressing personal commitment and cannot work a second shift."
   - "I know you cannot tell me the exact time the computer technician will arrive, but I have a full day and would appreciate knowing if it will be in the morning or afternoon."
3. Escalating—expresses your needs more emphatically when a simple assertion did not accomplish your goals and your rights are still being violated.
   - "I told you that as a nurse I cannot have a social relationship with you. I must insist that you refrain from asking me personal questions."
   - "I asked you not to use my computer without my permission. You have turned it off improperly and some files have been damaged. Please do not use it again."

Developed by Bower SA, Bower GH: *Asserting yourself*, Reading, Mass, 1991, Addison-Wesley. Modified from Lange JA, Jakubowski P: *Responsible assertive behavior*, Champaign, Ill, 1978, Research Press.

When you decide to use an assertive response, remember to consider three essential criteria for success:

- Timing
- Content
- Receptivity

Is the person able to hear your concerns at this time, or is this an extremely busy time? Have you gotten the person's attention by calling the person by name (Adubato, 2004)? Are you phrasing your intervention in a way that demonstrates respect for yourself and for others? Is the person receptive now, or is a cooling-off period necessary? Consider this: Sometimes the assertive response is to be quiet and listen for more information (Box 1-6 through Box 1-8).

Remember: Assertive behavior does not guarantee that you will get what you want, but it does increases the probability that you will. If you want to change shifts with another nurse to be able to go to a family gathering, try asking assertively. Which of the following statements is assertive?

A. "Jim, I was wondering if you would mind . . . it is probably an imposition, but . . . well, uh, if you could switch this Saturday for next so I could go to a family party?"

- Being skilled in a variety of communication strategies for expressing your thoughts and feelings in a way that simultaneously protects your rights and those of others.
- Having a positive attitude about communicating directly and honestly.
- Feeling comfortable and in control of anxiety, tenseness, shyness, or fear.
- Feeling confident that you can conduct yourself in a self-respecting way while still respecting others.
- Honoring the fact that you and the other person both have rights.

- Appears self-confident and composed
- Maintains eye contact
- Uses clear, concise speech
- Speaks firmly and positively
- Speaks genuinely, without sarcasm
- Is nonapologetic
- Takes the initiative to guide situations
- Gives the same message verbally and nonverbally

Box 1-8	*Advantages of Assertive Behavior*

- It is more likely you will get what you want when you ask for it clearly.
- People respect clear, open, honest communication.
- You stand up for your own rights and feel self-respect.
- You avoid the invitation of aggression when the rights of others are violated.
- You are more independent.
- You become a decision-maker.
- You feel more peaceful and comfortable with yourself.

B. "Jim, how many times have I traded with you and you never think of my social life? I insist you trade weekends with me so I can finally have a life, too."

C. "Jim, my family is having a special party this Saturday that I would really like to attend. I would appreciate it if you could trade with me. I would be glad to return the favor."

Did you select C? If so, you understood that this request honored the nurse's right to make a request and the colleague's right to refuse. The language was clear, nonapologetic, and respectful. Refer back to Box 1-4.

Describe: "My family is having a party."
Express: "I would really like to attend."
Specify: "Trade with me?"
Consequence: "I would return the favor."

Notice that response A is hesitant and apologetic, not straightforward. The wording denies the right of the request. Response B is aggressive and blaming and even a bit whiny.

Nonassertive communication is a failure to stand up for our legitimate rights and possibly for those of others. It means communicating in an uncertain or uncomfortable way. Our nonassertive behavior may be based on thinking that we are inferior to others in some way. When we are passive or do not speak up to share our views, others may interpret our behavior as a sign of lack of interest or knowledge (Sully and Dallas, 2005). Sometimes being nonassertive gets us off the hook for the moment. We may agree to run an errand for someone because it is uncomfortable to say it is not convenient. Consider the phrase "short-term gain, long-term pain" the next time you consider not speaking up for your own needs. When we are nonassertive, we lose

because we fail to show respect for ourselves, which lowers our self-esteem. We begin to feel like doormats. Our needs are not met, and we invite others to take advantage of us via aggressive behavior. We may find that our anger and frustration build up and we may become aggressive ourselves (Gaddis, 2008). An outburst of anger resulting from such frustration can serve to reinforce passivity due to embarrassment at a side of ourselves we do not like.

Aggressiveness is that loud, forceful, often confrontational way of trying to get what we want, even at the expense of others. When we act aggressively, our rights are responded to out of proportion to those of others. Although we may temporarily gloat at our achievement, the experience is short-lived when we realize how we may have embarrassed ourselves or, worse, hurt other people in our determination to get what we wanted. Aggressive behavior frequently provokes anger or resentfulness and may lead to retaliation or passive–aggressive behavior. When an aggressive approach is taken, mutual respect is lacking; others are treated as objects standing in our way. Table 1-1 differentiates among assertive, nonassertive, and aggressive styles of communication.

When you are assertive, you feel better about yourself. It may take a while, however, for nurses who have been socialized to put others first to understand that there is a healthy balance between meeting personal needs and responding in a caring way to others. Nurses who have been more aggressive in their style may soon learn that this behavior distances people. It does get easier when you learn you can choose when to speak up and when to remain silent. You can choose lovingly to do something extra for someone, to inconvenience yourself by choice, not because you feel helpless. A good test of whether you have acted assertively is how you feel after the interaction. If you feel good, it is likely you have been assertive. Remember that if you have been passive most of the time, you may still feel guilty for setting your own priorities first, but the resentment that builds if you do not do so will erode the relationship.

Remember: Assertive communication skills make interactions more equal. All parties have a right to express their thoughts, feelings, and beliefs. The next time you feel irritated with a "demanding" client, consider that today's clients are not passive recipients of care but consumers with the expectation of good customer service (Box 1-9). Assertiveness refers to a style of communicating that has positive benefits for you and for others. It builds your self-confidence to know that you can treat others fairly while taking care of your

Box 1-9	*An Assertive Consumer . . .*

- Wants convenience
- Is informed and better educated
- Wants what he or she wants when he or she wants it
- Wants to be heard and to be involved in the problem-solving process
- Does not want to depend on the "expert"

Modified from Herzlinger R: *Market driven health care: who wins, who loses in the transformation of America's largest service industry,* Reading, Mass, 1997, Addison-Wesley.

own needs. This experience creates a healthy attitude of mutual respect. Speaking out about your thoughts and feelings provides others with clear, direct messages that are easier to receive than passive–aggressive ones. Assertiveness helps build trust between people. Adubato (2004) reports that nearly 90% of healthcare errors involve communication and suggests assertiveness is an important strategy to minimize microcommunication. Trust is built when nurses have the courage to acknowledge when things go wrong, right the wrong, express regret, and work to find out how to avoid the mistake in the future.

The Meaning of Responsible Communication

Responsible means "liable to be called on to answer for one's conduct and obligations . . . called on to account as the primary cause" (Merriam-Webster Online Dictionary, 2011). For nurses, this accountability may be described as being personally responsible for the outcome of their own professional actions, which are based on knowledge.

Sometimes, responsible communication is a simple statement of caring: "The pain medication will make you feel more comfortable." Other times, responsible communication may be the art of listening. If you don't know what to say, you can just sit quietly with a client.

To communicate responsibly when a problem must be solved means to communicate in a logical way based on your nursing knowledge and on the facts presented in the situation. Responsible communication demonstrates accurate problem-solving behavior

for the particular situation. The nursing process is a systematic means for nurses to demonstrate accountability and responsibility to clients. It is organized into five phases: assessment, diagnosis, planning, implementation, and evaluation (Iyer et al, 1995):

Assess—Collect information about the client, family, and community to identify the client's needs, problems, concerns, and responses.

Diagnose—Critically analyze and interpret the data collected and draw conclusions to identify nursing diagnoses that provide a focus for the rest of the process.

Plan—Establish priorities in the problems identified in the nursing diagnosis. Include the client and at times the family to create a plan of care that prescribes interventions to attain expected outcomes. Organize your communication strategy: what the care plan will contain and when, how, and where you will present it.

Implement—Implement the interventions identified in the plan of care. At this point, you respond to your client or colleague. This book encourages you to respond assertively and responsibly.

Evaluate—Conduct an ongoing evaluation of the client's progress toward attainment of outcomes. This is the phase in which you check whether your response was assertive and responsible, and whether your objectives (expected outcomes) were achieved.

A problem-solving process becomes a way of examining every client–nurse (or nurse–colleague) interaction. It becomes a natural part of your day. While you are receiving a message, you are trying to determine its meaning. You decide whether you will meet the sender's request, and then you transmit an assertive and responsible message that conveys your decision. As you send your message, you observe the effects of your words and gestures on the receiver. During the course of your day, you are sending and receiving messages continuously (Box 1-10). Building communication skills supports your contribution to delivery of safe care by the healthcare team in complex and critical care situations (Swinny, 2010).

Even your silence holds a sort of prayer.
Apache proverb

WIT&*Wisdom*

Box 1-10	*A Nurse Who Communicates Responsibly . . .*

- Is naturally focused on the nursing process and problem-solving process
- Considers the world of the client and the client's family
- Performs the role of client advocate
- Appreciates the sacred role of intimate care of the sick
- Maintains a sense of wonder at the human experience and treats each person as an individual
- Is open to learning to trust intuition as another way of knowing about the client

Moments of Connection . . .
Daring to Care

A nurse worked with a client who was unable to communicate because of a brain tumor. He sat up in bed, rocking back and forth and crying out in pain. His distress was not alleviated by pain medication. The nurse reported that she climbed up into the bed, rocked him, and sang lullabies to him the way she sang to her son. He relaxed, became quiet, and "nestled" into the nurse's arms. He was able to go to sleep a bit later and died in his sleep that night. The nurse said that never before or since had she been moved to do this and talked about the importance of trusting your intuition. "I guess God must have directed my actions that day. He put me in the right place and time and gave me the courage to step outside the practice . . . to care in a special way" (Riley, 1999).

The Meaning of Caring

Caring is the basis of the nursing profession. Your communication may be technically responsible and assertive, but without caring you still may not be able to facilitate a change in behavior. It is important to examine what caring means.

Caring is not an abstract concept. There are explicit ways we as nurses can communicate to show that we care. Encompassed by caring is a commitment to the preservation of our shared humanity and respect for the uniqueness and dignity of each individual we encounter. Caring is an essential ingredient in life and must characterize the nurse–client relationship. Nurses at St. Luke's Medical Center in Milwaukee have created a clinical practice development model that delineates novice, advanced beginner, competent, proficient, and expert behaviors in what they call the domain of caring. Nurses used their own stories to provide a qualitative, narrative approach to defining caring behaviors. The expert level is evidenced by the following (Haag-Heitman and Kramer, 1998):

- Trusting relationships based on "being with," not "doing to," the client
- Understanding of the meaning of the experience to the client and the family
- Creation of an environment of hope and trust

Reflecting on times when we are clear our caring makes a difference helps nurses balance the demands of a working environment with complex technology, financial restraints, and clients who are acutely ill with multiple diagnoses (Adamski et al, 2009; Iranmanesh et al, 2009).

Nurses are demonstrating their caring globally in volunteer organizations to bring better healthcare services and quality of life to underserved populations. One nurse says, "Since we live in such difficult times, the best we can do is wage peace one person at a time" (Justin, 2002).

Caring is the moral ideal that guides nurses through the caregiving process and knowledgeable caring is the highest form of commitment (Watson, 1995). Nurses can have an extensive command of scientific facts and theories and be technically expert without being caring professionals. In addition, nurses can be technically and scientifically correct but still make moral errors. Although there is satisfaction in being technologically competent, that satisfaction is not as lasting as the satisfaction derived from meaningful moments of connection with clients, family, and colleagues. These are moments that focus on the relationship with and support of the client rather than on illness and pathology (Hunter, 2006). Caring communication is holistic, taking into account the entire person and demonstrating respect for clients as people, not just as bodies requiring nursing interventions. Take a moment to consider that at times a client's family may need to be cared for as a unit, with care delivery organized around its needs instead of the needs of an individual (Guilianeli et al, 2005). How can you ensure that your communication is caring? Although we as nurses may consciously desire to generate the feeling of being cared for in our clients and intend our behavior to convey this desire, we must remember that not all intended caring on our part is perceived as caring by our clients. A nurse may believe caring is being demonstrated by careful drug administration from a computerized cart taken to the bedside. The client may see the nurse paying more attention to scanning the bar code on an identification armband than to giving eye contact or inquiring about how the client is feeling. Caring is situation specific. Caring includes an ongoing commitment to sharpening knowledge and skills to identify care needs and nursing actions that will bring about positive change while protecting and enhancing human dignity.

> *Give me knowledge so I may have kindness for all.*
>
> **Plains Indian proverb**
>
> **WIT&***Wisdom*

The implications are clear. We must find out what is perceived to be important to our clients in their return to health, validate the effect our caring actions are having on them, and adjust our actions in keeping with their needs. Taking these steps is a necessary component of responsible nursing. Consider these challenges. It is easier to be offended by a client's anger than to gently explore its source. It is easier to tell an abused wife to leave her husband than to listen to her pain. It is easier to instruct an adolescent to make sure her partner uses condoms than to listen to her story of a mother who is an addict, a father who is absent, and her 22-year-old boyfriend who says he will marry her if she gets pregnant (Carpenito, 2000). In a study to understand clients' experience of caring, caring meant that the clients could unburden their heart to express their suffering and discomfort. The experience of not being cared for communicated that clients were of no importance, that they were troublesome. It meant that nurses listened to their wishes and showed evidence of thinking of them. A nurse saved lunch for a patient after a procedure that required no drinking or eating (Karlsson et al, 2004). The next time you feel pressured and anxious in your caregiving, stop and take a deep breath and ask yourself how your nonverbal behavior might be interpreted. Consider something as simple as smiling, which conveys approval, encouragement, and acceptance (Hader, 2006).

Caring communication is as important with colleagues as with clients. If caring exists between co-workers, that sense of well-being will likely be passed on to clients. Conversely, if there is little caring between colleagues, then nurses will be unlikely to feel complete and satisfied enough to demonstrate a sense of caring with their clients. Caring involves being assertive and responsible. If you let others control you because you are nonassertive, or if you invade others' rights by being aggressive, you cannot act in a caring way. If you care enough for yourself to be assertive, you will know how to care for others. Watson (2007) states that nurses need to love, respect, and care for ourselves, and treat ourselves with dignity, before we can respect, love, and care for others and treat them with dignity.

How Can You Learn to Communicate Assertively and Responsibly?

This book is based on the belief that effective and caring nurse communicators are not born, they are made. You can learn to communicate in competent, caring, and confident ways. You can replace ineffective and nontherapeutic communication habits with helpful interventions. You can continually add to your communication repertoire so that you develop confidence in your ability to communicate effectively in a variety of situations. When you lack confidence, remember that being assertive is more about valuing yourself and nursing and your confidence will increase with success (Sudha, 2005).

Educational psychologists have proposed that learning involves three domains (Woodruff, 1961; Meichenbaum, 1977; McCroskey, 1984). This book attends to the cognitive aspects (understanding and meaning), affective aspects (feelings, values, and attitudes), and psychomotor aspects (physical capability) of your communication learning process.

By following the guidelines in this text, you will learn basic communication skills (cognitive domain), you will build confidence through a belief in the value and impact of positive communication (affective domain), and you will meet the challenge, putting skills into action in the real world (psychomotor domain).

Cognitive Domain: Basic Communication Competencies

Communication competence is your ability to demonstrate knowledge of the appropriate communicative behavior in any situation. Communication competence is demonstrated by the identification of behaviors that would be appropriate or inappropriate in an observed interpersonal situation.

Affective Domain: Belief in the Value and Impact of Positive Communication

A belief in the value and impact of positive communication motivates the nurse to seek feedback and practice self-care strategies that build confidence.

Psychomotor Domain: Putting It All Together

Communication skill is your ability to perform appropriate communication behaviors in any given situation. To be considered a skilled nurse communicator, you must be able to successfully implement communication strategies that are assertive and responsible.

Figure 1-3 illustrates how to become a caring nurse communicator by developing skills in all three

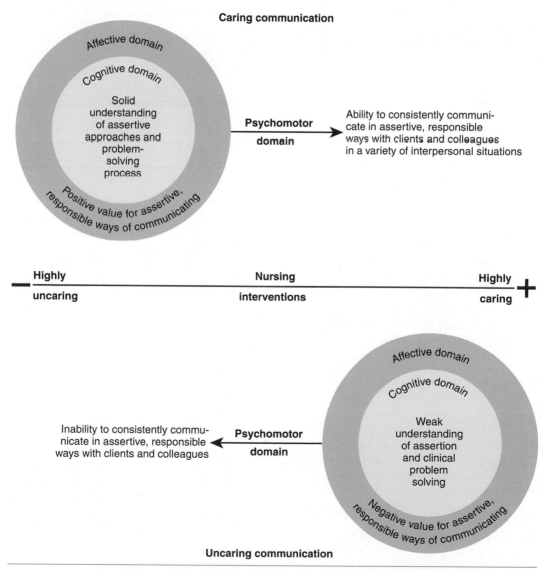

FIGURE 1-3 Differences between caring and uncaring communication.

domains. The negative consequences of incomplete development in all three aspects are also illustrated.

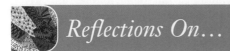

Reflections On…

Responsible, Assertive, Caring Communication in Nursing

We know that reading comprehension is improved when the reader is actively asking and answering questions while reading. To build your communication skills, answer the questions in this section in each chapter. Be thinking about how you will write your answers as you read each chapter.

What? . . .
Write one thing you learned from this chapter.

So what? . . .
How will this affect your nursing practice?

Now what? . . .
How will you implement this new knowledge or skill?

Think about it . . .

Practicing Assertiveness

Exercise 1
Think about what the statement, "Communication is the heart of nursing" means to you. Identify a time in your nursing experience in which you truly came to understand this. Write a brief reflection of this experience. Consider other stories you can write about your own nurse wisdom . . . a time in which you knew you made a difference.

Exercise 2
Consider how you see yourself as a caring nurse. Try your hand at a poetic approach to embellishing your image of yourself. Write responses to one of the following:

Your caring is like a tree . . . its branches reach out to others . . .

Or perhaps

My caring is like a flower . . . its petals are rich in color and vibrant.

Now you try sentences to continue.

Or close your eyes and evoke an image of your own, "What is the image of my caring?" Write lines in response to your image. The *American Journal of Nursing* has a section called "Art of Nursing" and offers a monthly podcast of a poet or artist reading or discussing his or her 's submission. Consider submitting your poem or another for publication. Notice other journals that welcome such submissions.

Exercise 3
Now, to build your assertive skills, review Box 1-2. List any rights you have relinquished.

Review Box 1-3. For each right you listed, identify which irrational beliefs you held that interfered with your acting in your own best interest.

Exercise 4
Keep a journal for a week to examine your behavior to build assertive communication skills. Record items in the following format:

In what event was I not assertive? Was my behavior nonassertive or aggressive? How would I prefer to have handled this situation?

Exercise 5
Observe other students, faculty, and staff in your clinical area as well as colleagues and family members. Identify one person who could be a role model for assertive communication. Identify one situation in your professional life and one situation in your personal life in which you would have preferred to be assertive. Close your eyes and envision the role model. Ask yourself how this person would have handled the situation and pretend you can see what the person is saying and doing. Write what you imagined and examine the lessons you learn from this to build your own assertive communication skills.

References

Adamski M, Parsons V, Hooper C: Internalizing the concept of caring: an examination of student perceptions when nurses share their stories, *Nurse Educ Perspect* 30(6):358, November–December 2009.

Adubato S: Making the communication connection, *Nurs Manage* 35(9):33, 2004.

Carpenito LJ: Nurse, always there for you, *Nurs Forum* 35(2):3, 2000.

Gaddis, S: Positive, assertive, "pushback" for nurses, *New Hampshire Nursing News* July, August, September: 17, 2008.

Grover SM: Shaping effective communication skills and therapeutic relationships at work: the foundation of collaboration, *AAOHN J* 53(4):177, 2005.

Guilianeli S, Kelly R, Skelsky J, et al: The critical care nurse manager's perspective: the critical care family assistance program, *Chest* 128(3):118S, 2005.

Haag-Heitman B, Kramer A: Creating a clinical practice development model, *Am J Nurs* 98(8):39, 1998.

Hader R: If you're happy and you know it . . ., *Nurs Manage* 37(2):6, 2006.

Hunter LP: Women give birth and pizzas are delivered: language and Western childbirth paradigms, *J Midwifery Womens Health* 51(2):119–124, March–April 2006.

Iranmanesh S, Axelsson K, Savenstedt S, et al: A caring relationship with people who have cancer, *J Adv Nurs* 65(6):1300, 2009.

Iyer PW, Taptich BJ, Bernocchi-Losey D: *Nursing process and nursing diagnosis*, Philadelphia, 1995, WB Saunders.

Justin F: Acting globally, *Adv Nurs* 4(13):21, 2002.

Karlsson M, Bergbom I, von Post I, et al: Patient experiences when the nurse cares for and does not care for, *International Journal for Human Caring* 8(3):30, 2004.

Kleen K: To care or not to care, *Nurs Manage* 35(17):13, 2004.

Koerner JG: Reflections on transformational leadership, *J Holist Nurs* 28(1):68, March 2010.

McCroskey JC: The communication apprehension perspective. In Daly JA, McCroskey JC, editors: *Avoiding communication: shyness, reticence and communication apprehension*, Beverly Hills, Calif, 1984, Sage Publications.

Meichenbaum D: *Cognitive-behavior modification: an integrative approach*, New York, 1977, Plenum Press.

Merriam-Webster Online Dictionary: Definition of *responsible*. http://www.merriam-webster.com/dictionary/responsible. Accessed February 17, 2011.

Riley JB: *From the heart to the hands . . . keys to successful healthcaring connections*, Ellicott City, Md, 1999, Integrated Management Publishing Systems.

Stuart GW: *Principles and practice of psychiatric nursing*, ed 9, St. Louis, 2009, Mosby.

Sudha R: How to be an assertive nurse, *Nurs J India* 96(8):182, August 2005.

Sully P, Dallas J: *Essential communication skills for nursing*, Edinburgh, 2005, Mosby.

Swinny B: Assessing and developing critical-thinking skills in the intensive care unit, *Crit Care Nurse Q* 33(1):2, January–March 2010.

Watson J: *Nursing: human science and human care: a theory of nursing*, Sudbury, Mass, 2007, Jones and Bartlett Publishers.

Watson J: Postmodernism and knowledge development in nursing, *Nurs Sci Q* 8(2):60, 1995.

Wilson MH: "There's just something about Ron": one nurse's healing presence amidst failing hearts, *J Holist Nurs* 26(4):303, December 2008.

Woodruff AD: *Basic concepts of teaching*, Scranton, Pa, 1961, Chandler.

Suggestion for Further Reading

Alberti RE, Emmons M: *Your perfect right: assertiveness and equality in your life and relationships*, San Luis Obispo, Calif, 2008, Impact Publishers.

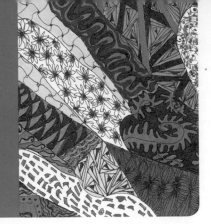

Chapter 2

The Client–Nurse Relationship: A Helping Relationship*

This is the true joy in life—being used for a purpose recognized by yourself as a mighty one; being thoroughly worn out before you are thrown on the trash heap; being a force of nature instead of a feverish selfish little clod of ailments and grievances complaining that the world will not devote itself to making you happy.

George Bernard Shaw

Objectives

1. Identify the purpose of the client–nurse relationship
2. Describe the cognitive, affective, and psychomotor abilities that nurses and clients bring to the therapeutic encounter
3. Discuss clients' rights as consumers of healthcare service
4. Identify characteristics of a successful client–nurse relationship
5. Identify therapeutic communication techniques
6. Identify nontherapeutic communication techniques
7. List do's and don'ts in the client–nurse relationship
8. Identify behavioral dimensions indicative of bonding in the client–nurse relationship
9. Identify qualities of a storycatcher
10. Discuss listening skills
11. Participate in exercises to build skills in the client–nurse relationship

"Friendly nurses seem like they know everything" is a telling quote from a participant in a study to examine clients' perceptions of nurses' competencies. Qualities such as cheerful, happy, and smiling created the impression that nurses were skilled (Wysong and Driver, 2009). Have you ever been in the patient role, vulnerable, unsure, frightened? A friendly word, a smile, a question about how you are feeling can reassure and calm you. Clients value interpersonal skills in nurses as highly as technical skills and want to be treated like a "real person" (Geanellos, 2004). Encounters we have with our clients can be caring and helpful or unfeeling and even harmful. As a compassionate and caring nurse, you will want your interactions with your clients to be helpful and pleasant. In this chapter you will learn how to build effective relationships with your clients.

You will learn about the professional client–nurse relationships so that you can understand how they differ from social, collegial, and kinship relationships. The responsibilities of nurses in client–nurse relationships have also been outlined so that you will be able to articulate your roles and interventions at each stage of the helping relationship. As you read, reflect upon the extent to which you foster a helping relationship in your interactions with clients.

*Portions of this chapter were contributed by Margaret E. Erickson, PhD.

Self-assessment Tool

In the heathcare profession we are beginning to understand that our clients have a choice of care providers. Clearly, we need to understand the business of healthcare provision and the importance of being sensitive to good customer service. If you think back to your own experiences as a customer in any industry, you will understand that customer service is not common sense; rather, it is a set of skills and attitudes that needs to be central to our work. Your ability to communicate clearly and with compassion, to meet and even exceed your clients' expectations, is the essence of customer service. Many complaints are not about clinical issues but about perceived rudeness or lack of caring. Remember that you also have internal customers, your colleagues and staff from other departments and disciplines. Let us combine a look at communication skills and attention to customer service. Complete this self-assessment not only as a quick check of your skills but also as a tool to teach the basics of customer service. Just as when you read course or clinical evaluation objectives at the beginning of a class, knowing what is expected of you sets you up to be successful.

Self-assessment Tool: Communication—The Key to Customer Service

Instructions: Rate yourself from 4 (very skilled) to 1 (not skilled).

	4	3	2	1
1. I feel good about my communication skills.	4	3	2	1
2. I smile at clients, families, and staff.	4	3	2	1
3. I make eye contact.	4	3	2	1
4. I introduce myself and wear my name badge.	4	3	2	1
5. I learn names and use the correct pronunciations.	4	3	2	1
6. If I don't understand, I seek clarification.	4	3	2	1
7. I take a moment to calm myself before interacting with clients.	4	3	2	1
8. I take responsibility for finding answers to questions.	4	3	2	1
9. I answer the telephone promptly and with a smile (that helps!).	4	3	2	1
10. I explain procedures clearly.	4	3	2	1
11. I encourage clients and their families to ask questions.	4	3	2	1
12. I encourage feedback about my work.	4	3	2	1
13. I receive positive feedback about my work.	4	3	2	1
14. I thank a colleague who helps me.	4	3	2	1
15. I offer to help my colleagues.	4	3	2	1
16. I listen, knowing it is OK to be quiet and not have all the answers.	4	3	2	1
17. I respect the client's confidentiality.	4	3	2	1
18. I apologize for delays.	4	3	2	1
19. When I touch a client, I do it gently.	4	3	2	1
20. I dress professionally and pay attention to my grooming.	4	3	2	1
21. I try to do something extra for clients, families, and colleagues.	4	3	2	1
22. I am learning to deal with multiple demands on my time.	4	3	2	1
23. I give compliments to clients, family, and colleagues (yes, doctors, too!).	4	3	2	1
24. I understand that I am still learning and that it is impossible to be perfect.	4	3	2	1
25. I try to be myself, bringing my own special gifts to my nursing practice.	4	3	2	1

Scoring: Add the numbers you have selected. Remember that this is a self-assessment, and feedback from your instructor, peers, and clients adds more data. 77-100, High awareness of necessary skills. 53-76, Average awareness of skills. Review your lower scores and select areas for growth. 25-52, Low awareness of necessary skills. Pay more attention to skill development.

Nature of the Helping Relationship

A set of preestablished rules and expectations directs the course of client–nurse interactions. There may be some overlap between these interactions and those involving friends and family, but one factor in particular differentiates helping relationships from social relationships. A helping relationship is established for the benefit of the client, whereas kinship and friendship relationships are designed to meet mutual needs.

In particular, the client–nurse relationship is established to help the client achieve and maintain optimal health.

A successful helping relationship between nurse and client represents an order of interaction different from what occurs in a friendship. This is not because of any superiority in the nurse but because of the mutual trust and the responsibilities for assisting others that characterize true professional relationships.

Nursing care is planned to meet an individual client's unique needs and situation with respect for the patient's and family's goals and preferences. Nurses provide patient education so that clients have the information necessary to make informed decisions about their healthcare, health promotion, disease prevention, and attainment of a peaceful death. Nurses establish a partnership with the client and family and with other healthcare providers. Professional practitioners of nursing bear a responsibility for the nursing care that clients–patients receive as sanctioned by state nurse practice acts (American Nurses Association, 2004). Client–nurse relationships are entered for the benefit of the client, but such a relationship is more effective if it is mutually satisfying. Clients are satisfied when their healthcare needs have been met and they sense that they have been treated in a caring manner. Nurses feel a sense of accomplishment when their interventions have had a positive influence on their clients' health status and when their conduct has been competent and caring. Client–nurse relationships may be a mutual learning experience, but in general the goals of therapeutic relationships are directed toward the growth of clients (Stuart and Laraia, 2005).

Never assume that in client–nurse relationships clients play the role of passive receiver awaiting the soothing ministrations of influential nurses. Both clients and nurses bring their respective knowledge, attitudes, feelings, skills, and patterns of behaving to the relationship. Indeed, referring to their interaction as a relationship indicates a sense of affiliation that bonds clients and nurses as well as an interdependency and reciprocity between them.

Clients and nurses alike come to the relationship with unique cognitive, affective, and psychomotor abilities that they use in their joint endeavor of enhancing the clients' well-being. Nurses are responsible for encouraging this interchange of ideas, values, and skills. In an effective helping relationship a definite and guaranteed interchange occurs between clients and nurses in all three dimensions.

Cognitive, Affective, and Psychomotor Abilities in the Therapeutic Encounter

Following are some of the cognitive, affective, and psychomotor abilities that clients and nurses bring to their therapeutic encounter. Table 2-1 further illustrates that both clients and nurses start with notions and expectations that will influence the course and outcome of their relationship.

Cognitive

Clients and nurses both know something about health and illness in general, and about the individual client's health concerns in particular. Clients bring their model or world view; "the way they perceive life, events, people, and situations . . . communicate, think, feel, act, and react" (Erickson et al, 1983, p. 84) to the relationship. Clients have definite knowledge about what has made them ill and interfered with their growth and fulfillment. They also know "what will make them well, optimize their fulfillment and or promote their growth." This knowledge is called *self-care knowledge* (Erickson et al, 1983). As nurses we want to help our clients access and use their self-care knowledge to achieve a greater state of health and well-being. Nurses have their own views, based on their knowledge and beliefs about what will help their clients. To prevent clients and nurses from operating in isolation or at cross-purposes, they must exchange essential information.

In addition to having different ideas, clients and nurses also have preferred ways of observing their worlds and making decisions about what they see. Each of us has a preferred mental process—the one we have developed most highly, the one we use best—that forms the core of our personalities (Myers, 1998). Clients and nurses have different ways in which they prefer to use their minds, specifically, the ways they choose to perceive and to make judgments (Myers, 1998). Perceiving includes becoming aware of things, people, occurrences, and ideas. Judging includes reaching conclusions about what has been observed.

Some clients and nurses, for example, are primarily practical. They are attuned to immediate experiences, literal facts at hand, and concrete realities. Myers used the word sensing to describe this preferred way of collecting data in problem solving. Other clients and nurses prefer to think about what could be, rather than what is. Their intuitive imaginations fill their minds with ideas and explanations that do not always depend

Table 2-1 *Interchange of Knowledge, Attitudes, and Skills between the Client and Nurse in the Helping Relationship*

WHAT CLIENTS BRING TO THE CLIENT–NURSE RELATIONSHIP	WHAT NURSES BRING TO THE CLIENT–NURSE RELATIONSHIP
COGNITIVE	
Preferred ways of perceiving and judging	Preferred ways of perceiving and judging
Knowledge and beliefs about illness in general and their illness in particular	Knowledge and beliefs about illness in general
Knowledge and beliefs about health promotion and maintenance in general and information about their own healthcare activities	Knowledge about their clinical specialty and knowledge and beliefs about health behaviors that prevent illness and promote, regain, and maintain health
Ability to problem solve	Ability to problem solve
Ability to learn	Knowledge about factors that increase client compliance with the treatment regimen
AFFECTIVE	
Cultural values	Cultural values
Feelings about seeking help from a nurse	Feelings about being a nurse-helper
Attitudes toward nurses in general	Attitudes about clients in general
Attitudes toward treatment regimen	Biases about nursing treatment regimen
Values about preventing illness	Value placed on being healthy
	Value placed on people's active prevention of illness or enhancement of well-being
Willingness to take positive action about own health status at this time with this particular nurse	Willingness to help clients take positive action to improve their well-being
PSYCHOMOTOR	
Ability to relate to and communicate with others	Ability to relate to and communicate with others
Ability to carry out own healthcare management	Proficiency in administering effective nursing interventions
Ability to learn new methods of self-care	Ability to teach nursing interventions to the client

on the senses for verification. Myers called this preferred way of collecting data intuitive.

Consider the following situation to understand what the differences are in these two ways of perceiving and how they affect the client–nurse relationship.

Mr. Zabrick is an 80-year-old resident of a senior citizens' apartment complex where he lives with his retired, 70-year-old widowed sister. In the past 9 months, Mr. Zabrick has had chemotherapy and radiation treatments for lung cancer. His tumor has vanished and his blood levels are stabilized; yet, to his disappointment, he feels lethargic and anorexic.

Eight days ago his sister awoke in the night and found Mr. Zabrick in the bathtub, where he had fallen after mistaking it for the toilet. She noticed that her brother is unsteady on his feet and is losing weight.

Clients (or family members) and nurses who prefer concrete details, or sensing, would evaluate Mr. Zabrick's situation by focusing on the visible evidence that might account for his deterioration. They would observe the lack of saliva under the tongue and its brown furry appearance, and note his report of an unpleasant taste and odor in the mouth. They would see the small, hard stools and the abdominal distention. They would feel the decreased turgor of his skin and notice the muscle weakness. They would count the amount of fluids and quantity of food consumed by Mr. Zabrick.

Clients or nurses who prefer detailed information would put these pieces together and likely come to the conclusion that Mr. Zabrick is dehydrated. Those who use this way of perceiving prefer information that is measurable, and the thinking process is systematic, with one step taken at a time.

Clients (or family members) and nurses who prefer a more intuitive perceiving process might not gather all these data before jumping to a conclusion about what is happening to Mr. Zabrick. They are likely to look for patterns in the data (as opposed to discrete pieces of information). They would start thinking about possible explanations and then work backward to obtain the facts. They might notice, for example, that Mr. Zabrick has said, "Why bother with trying anymore? If I had a chance to do it again, I'm not sure I'd take the treatments," and wonder if his fatigue and grief are consuming him. They might remember that Mr. Zabrick's daughter-in-law died despite rigorous chemotherapy and that his lifelong friend was diagnosed with brain cancer 3 weeks earlier, and wonder if Mr. Zabrick's symptoms reflect his doubt about living with such losses. Another theme on which intuitive individuals might focus is the relationship between the assault on Mr. Zabrick's body from treatments, changes in diet and exercise, and sleep deprivation, and the impact of the severe heat and humidity of the previous 7 weeks.

These two perceiving processes, sensing and intuitive, are quite different. It is important for nurses to understand their preferred way of perceiving and try to discover which process their clients prefer. Both ways of seeing the world are valuable—one is not better than the other; each simply selects different information on which to focus.

Judging—the process of making decisions about the information collected through perception—is the other mental process in which clients and nurses may differ. Some persons have logical, orderly, analytical decision-making processes and treat the world objectively (Myers, 1995). Decision makers such as these prefer to fit all experience into logical mental systems. Myers called this preference thinking and said that these people make decisions based on critical analysis of facts, valuing fairness. Other clients and nurses prefer to tune into the subjective world of feelings and values. Myers called this preference

feeling and said that these individuals make decisions by analyzing how they will affect people, valuing harmony.

Each of us prefers one of these decision-making processes to the other (Myers, 1995). Consider the following situation to better understand the two judging processes.

> Jossie is a 19-year-old first-year university student who is 8 weeks pregnant and unmarried. She is receiving counseling about her options. She sees three choices and will soon decide whether to have an abortion, continue with the pregnancy and give up her baby for adoption, or carry her baby to term and raise the child herself.

Clients and nurses who prefer a rational, objective way of making decisions would invite Jossie to consider all the facts and then make a logical decision based on them. They would look at the consequences of any decision Jossie might make and judge it using their head rather than their heart. They would be able to remain emotionally uninvolved. They have the ability to see the "long view" and would likely encourage Jossie to consider her future pragmatically and act on the most sensible choice (Myers, 1995).

Clients, family members, and nurses who prefer to consider effects on the people in the situation would likely explore how Jossie feels about each of the choices and how each fits her values. Such people would probably emphasize the benefits of any plan Jossie considers rather than criticizing it; they would also likely support Jossie's personal convictions.

This glimpse at two different methods for using our minds alerts us to the misunderstandings that can arise in helping relationships. We cannot assume that clients' minds are guided by the same principles as our own. Clients, their family members, and professional colleagues may reason in the same way that you do, or they may prefer using different ways of perceiving and judging. They may not value the things you value or show interest in the same things you do (Myers, 1998).

We all use different combinations of perceiving and judging, and colleagues and clients with the same preferences are likely to be the easiest to like and understand. They will tend to have similar interests (because they share the same kinds of perceptions) and consider the same matters important (because they share the same kinds of judgment) (Myers, 1998).

On the other hand, it will be harder to understand and predict the behavior of colleagues and clients whose perception and judgment preferences differ from our own. We are likely to take opposite stands on any issue with colleagues and clients who prefer different thinking processes (Myers, 1998). "The therapeutic nurse–patient relationship is a mutual learning experience and a corrective emotional experience for the patient. It is based on the underlying humanity of nurse and patient, with mutual respect and acceptance of ethnocultural differences" (Stuart and Laraia, 2005).

If you would like to learn more about your preferences for perceiving and making decisions, as well as about other personality preferences, arrange with your school's counseling or guidance department to take the Myers–Briggs Type Indicator (MBTI). The aim of the MBTI is to identify, from self-reporting of easily recognized reactions, the basic preferences of people in regard to perception and judgment (Myers, 1998). Learning about your own preferences will make you more aware of how your way of thinking influences your behavior in client–nurse helping relationships. The Keirsey Temperament Sorter provides similar content and is available online at www.keirsey.com or in his book (Keirsey, 1998).

Affective

All clients and nurses have positive and negative feelings about helping relationships; each also has biases about the other. Each has different priorities for working on particular health concerns. The attitudes of both clients and nurses greatly affect whether they work in harmony or discord, whether their respective knowledge surfaces or is submerged, and whether they carry out the commitment of improving the health of individual clients. In addition, people's "Model" or "Worldview" (Erickson et al, 1983) includes their definition or perception of what constitutes health. Smith (1981) discovered that people view health from four different models: the Clinical Model, which means that there is an absence of disease; the Role-Performance Model, in which the person is able to carry out his or her role in life; the Adaptive Model, in which health is determined by a person's ability to cope with stress; and the Eudemonistic Model, in which health is perceived as a quality of life, a person's ability to enjoy life, have meaningful relationships, and have a state of well being. Understanding how a nurse and client define health is very important as it affects the plan of care, the desired goals, and the outcomes. As noted earlier, when nurses listen to their client's story they gain greater insight and knowledge into how a person defines "health."

The major source of our value system is our culture. In America today, the culture is heterogeneous (with a variety of cultural groups), so that nurses and clients are likely to encounter different beliefs and values, particularly as the United States is home to people from all parts of the world. Modern medical and nursing practices become two of the external forces with which immigrants come in contact. This encounter with the American healthcare system is loaded with choices for immigrants to make in deciding how much of their culture's traditional medical practices they wish to maintain. Cultural patterns are one of the important means by which people adapt to recurrent change in their environments (see Chapter 4).

Psychomotor

The client needs to know what skills the nurse has, and the nurse needs to determine the client's ability to participate in his or her own treatment plan. Both parties must come to an agreement about what their respective tasks will be in their effort to improve the client's health status. Consider a scenario in which a client is more proficient at finding information via the World Wide Web than is the nurse. Can you envision a partnering to share information? The client can find the information and the nurse can help the client determine which sources are most reliable (see Chapter 6).

Clients' Rights in the Helping Relationship

Together nurses and clients share their energy and resources and commit to healing. Together they confront issues regarding the meaning of illness to the client and family and work toward self-realization and personal growth. As consumers of our healthcare services, clients have the following rights:

- To expect a systematic and accurate investigation of their health concerns by thorough and well-organized nurses
- To be informed about their health status and have all their questions answered so that they clearly understand what nurses mean
- To receive healthcare from nurses who have current knowledge about their diagnosis and are capable of providing safe and efficient care

- To feel confident that they will be treated courteously and that their nurses show genuine interest in them
- To trust that the confidentiality of any personal information will be respected
- To be informed about any plans of action to be carried out for their benefit
- To refuse or consent to nursing treatments without jeopardizing their relationship with their nurses
- To secure help conveniently, without hassles or roadblocks
- To receive consistent quality of care from all nurses

Characteristics of Client–Nurse Helping Relationships

Client–nurse relationships are special helping relationships that are characterized by the following features:

- A partnership between clients and nurses, both working together to improve the client's health status.
- A philosophy about human nature and what motivates humans in health and illness: As nurses, we should know our beliefs and values and be able to articulate them clearly.
- A purposeful and productive objective: Together clients and nurses agree about the nature of the health problem in question, and they develop and implement a plan designed to reach agreed-upon objectives. Clients and nurses together evaluate the outcomes and decide whether the desired and expected outcomes have been achieved.
- Preservation of the client's present level of health and protection from future health threats because of the increased knowledge gleaned from the helping relationship.
- Palliation of clients' worries and fears through nurses' reassurances, and easing of pain through soothing comfort measures.
- A psychic or morale boost: Clients perk up from the positive attention and interest they receive from nurses.
- Practicality: Efficacious, effective, and efficient ways of handling health concerns are offered.
- Portability: The helping relationship is present wherever and whenever clients and nurses come together.

- A series of phases, with a beginning (initiation), middle (maintenance), and end (termination), to each encounter.
- A personally tailored interaction designed to meet the needs of each particular client.
- Platonic and not passionate expressions of caring: Even though nurses may have strong feelings for their clients, it is expected that they can maintain adequate objectivity and perspective to provide therapeutic assistance.
- A sense of privacy so that clients may disclose intimate details about their life: Nurses are responsible for protecting their clients' confidentiality.
- Powerful emotions: Clients and nurses can develop attachments for each other, which makes the relationship special for each.

Nurses use therapeutic communication techniques (Table 2-2), as contrasted with nontherapeutic communication techniques (Table 2-3), to implement the nursing process.

Pointers to Guide You in Your Client–Nurse Helping Relationships

This section offers do's and don'ts for conducting yourself in client–nurse helping relationships.

Do

- Be prepared mentally, emotionally, and physically to assist your clients in resolving their healthcare problems
- Be punctual and polite in your manner of relating to clients
- Promote clients' well-being, comfort, and increased health status
- Be philanthropic in your approach to clients by putting their needs and concerns first
- Be plucky in planning and generating creative solutions to your clients' health concerns
- Be proficient in the nursing skills required to safely and successfully care for your clients
- Praise and encourage clients in their efforts to take better care of themselves
- Be patient and understanding about clients' reactions to their particular health situations
- Persevere in pursuing your pledge to help clients preserve their health

Table 2-2 *Summary of Therapeutic Communication Techniques*

TECHNIQUE	DEFINITION	THERAPEUTIC VALUE
Listening	An active process of receiving information and examining one's reactions to the messages received	Nonverbally communicates the nurse's interest in the client
Remaining silent	Periods of no verbal communication among participants	Nonverbally communicates the nurse's acceptance of the client
Establishing guidelines	Statements regarding roles, purposes, and limitations for a particular interaction	Helps the client to know what is expected of him or her
Making open-ended comments	General comments asking the client to determine the direction the interaction should take	Allows the client to decide what material is most relevant and encourages the client to continue
Reducing distance	Diminishing of physical space between the nurse and client	Nonverbally communicates that the nurse wants to be involved with the client
Acknowledging	Recognition given to a client for contribution to an interaction	Demonstrates the importance of a client's role within the relationship
Restating	Repetition to the client of what the nurse believes is the main thought or idea expressed	Asks for validation of the nurse's interpretation of the message
Reflecting	Direction back to the client of his or her ideas, feelings, questions, or content	Attempts to show the client the importance of his or her own ideas, feelings, and interpretations
Seeking clarification	Request for additional input to understand the message received	Demonstrates the nurse's desire to understand the client's communication
Seeking consensual validation	Attempts to reach a mutual denotative and connotative meaning of specific words	Demonstrates the nurse's desire to understand the client's communication
Focusing	Questions or statements to help the client develop or expand an idea	Directs conversation toward topics of importance
Summarizing	Statement of the main areas discussed during an interaction	Helps the client to separate relevant from irrelevant material; serves as a review and closing for the interaction
Planning	Mutual decision making regarding the goals, direction, and so forth, of future interactions	Reiterates the client's role within the relationship

From Sundeen SJ, DeSalvo Rankin EA, Stuart GW, et al: *Nurse–client interaction: implementing the nursing process*, St. Louis, 1998, Mosby, p 113.

Don't

- Patronize clients
- Preach at them or pressure them to change
- Pigeonhole clients with labels such as "good," "lazy," or "uncooperative," which prevent you from seeing clients as they really are
- Procrastinate in following through on clients' reasonable requests
- Put down clients by using medical jargon or in any way making them feel inadequate or estranged
- Punish clients for acts of omission or commission that have negatively affected their health
- Reveal prejudices against the race, religion, or creed of clients
- Be pleasure seeking or try to meet your own needs through the client–nurse relationship
- Pretend to have knowledge that you do not have, to avoid looking uninformed. It is the client's health with which you are dealing, and clients have the right to receive honest, forthright communication

Table 2-3 *Summary of Nontherapeutic Communication Techniques*

TECHNIQUE	DEFINITION	THERAPEUTIC THREAT
Failing to listen	Failure to receive the client's intended message	Places the needs of the nurse above those of the client
Failing to probe	Inadequate data collection represented by eliciting vague descriptions, getting inadequate answers, following standard forms too closely, and not exploring the client's interpretation	Generates an inadequate database on which to make decisions; leads to lack of individualization of client care
Parroting	Continual repetition of the client's phrases	Projects the meta-communication that "I am not listening" or "I am not a competent communicator"
Being judgmental	Approving or disapproving statements	Implies that the nurse has the right to a dependency relationship
Reassuring	Attempts to do magic with words	Negates fears, feelings, and other communications of the client
Rejecting	Refusal to discuss topics with the client	The client may feel that not only communication but also the self was rejected
Defending	Attempts to protect someone or something from negative feedback	Negates the client's right to express an opinion
Getting advice	Declaration to the client of what the nurse thinks should be done	Negates the worth of the client as a mutual partner in decision making
Making stereotyped responses	Use of trite, meaningless verbal expressions	Negates the significance of the client's communication
Changing topics	Nurse's direction of the interaction into areas of self-interest rather than areas of concern to the client	Nonverbally communicates that the nurse is in charge of deciding what will be discussed; may cause topics important to the client to be missed
Patronizing	Style of communication that displays a condescending attitude toward the client	Implies that the client–nurse relationship is not based on equality; places the nurse in a superior position

From Sundeen SJ, DeSalvo Rankin EA, Stuart GW, et al: *Nurse–client interaction: implementing the nursing process*, St. Louis, 1998, Mosby, p 117.

As a nurse, it is your responsibility to ensure that a thorough assessment is made of your clients' health concerns, that suitable nursing actions are chosen and implemented to help your clients, and that an evaluation of the results is carried out. Assuming this leadership does not mean that you take over and do for, or to, your clients. The quality of your nursing care is determined by the completeness of the interchange of knowledge, attitudes, and skills between you and your clients.

> *Good silence is called holiness.*
> **Panamanian proverb**
>
> **WIT&***Wisdom*

To be most helpful to all your clients, make sure that you solicit their knowledge, become aware of their feelings and attitudes, and take into account their strengths and limitations in caring for themselves. You must use this information to tailor your nursing care to suit your clients. In addition, you need to be aware of how your knowledge, attitude, and skills affect your ability to be helpful.

Effective nursing requires being assertive and responsible. Your goal is to help your clients achieve their best possible health status and to do so in a way that allows expression of your professional competence. It is expected that you will attempt to meet both of these desired outcomes.

You must act responsibly to achieve your nursing goals. You need to collect pertinent information from your clients and make an accurate assessment on which you will base your nursing care. The interpersonal communication behaviors in this book will help you develop your skills in these areas. The next chapter will show you how to make problem solving a mutual process between you and your clients. Using this approach, you will be an assertive and responsible nurse-helper.

Bonding in the Client–Nurse Relationship

The client and nurse both contribute to the success of the relationship. Bonding is the shared experience between the client and the nurse that occurs when each feels connected to the other. Research has developed instruments to measure the caring behavior of the nurse and others to measure client satisfaction. Tejero (2010) developed an instrument to determine the degree of bonding between the nurse and the client. The instrument was developed using qualitative data from observations and interviews and was corroborated from literature and validated in a bedside setting. The study identified two indicators of bonding, openness and engagement, and delineated behavioral dimensions for each. The bonding scores for nurses and patients were higher in relationships of longer duration and in relationships in which there was more frequency of contact. Reflect on these dimensions to provide you with clues as to the development of bonds with your clients. Box 2-1 lists dimensions that indicate the patient's and nurse's openness or engagement, or the lack thereof.

How to Listen

How does it feel when someone really listens to you? How does it feel when someone smiles and nods with a vacant look? How does it feel when the person looks poised to jump into the conversation without fully hearing you? Nichols tells us that "few motives in human experience are as powerful as the yearning to be understood. Being listened to means that we are taken seriously, that our ideas and feelings are known and ultimately, that what we have to say matters" (1995, p. 9).

Box 2-1	*Bonding between Nurse and Patient: Openness and Engagement*

Reflect on the following behaviors as indicators of openness and engagement or the lack thereof on the part of the client/patient and the nurse as indicators of bonding. These dimensions were generated from qualitative research observations and interviews with collaboration from literature validated in the bedside setting.

OPEN

THE PATIENT	THE NURSE
Looks at the approaching nurse in seeming anticipation of the nurse's arrival	Greets patient, or returns a greeting verbally or nonverbally
Greets the nurse first/initiates greeting	Pauses to visually check on the patient, seemingly trying to validate the assessment or data
Greets the nurse back in a verbal or nonverbal way, e.g., smiles	Touches the patient for further assessment
Acknowledges the nurse's statements by replying, smiling, nodding, and similar behaviors	Exchanges friendly/light comments or jokes, showing ease with the patient
Manifests at-ease behaviors such as light comments, friendly remarks/jokes	Makes clarifications, asks follow-up questions for further assessment

Continued

Box 2-1   *Bonding between Nurse and Patient: Openness and Engagement—cont'd*

Volunteers information and elaborates on the patient's physical condition and past and present health status even when not prompted to do so

Verbalizes feelings, psychosocial implication of disease in his or her life

Talks about support persons and other resources

Talks about other personal concerns

Inquires about what the patient already knows, e.g., medications, procedures, hospitalization, etc., or what the patient would like to know more about

Listens attentively to the verbalization of the patient's feelings, health condition, personal/family information

Asks the patient/family about other pertinent information that may not be in the record but is needed for the care of the patient

NOT OPEN

The Patient	The Nurse
Shows avoidance of the nurse as he or she approaches	Ignores patient's questions or comments
Interrupts the nurse in mid-sentence	Discourages inquiries from the patient by cutting the patient off in mid-sentence, or makes remarks suggesting that the patient not make more comments or ask questions
Shows cold treatment toward the nurse, e.g., not looking at the nurse, turning his or her back, focusing on something else during the conversation	
	Has a stern or aloof facial expression
Demonstrates irritation through facial expression, e.g., pouting, curt replies, high-pitched tone of voice, impatient gestures	Focuses on tasks, not maintaining eye contact with the patient
Converses in an angry tone	Projects irritable behavior through facial expression, voice tone, and body language
	Shows hurried behavior through terse replies, brisk movements, and fleeting presence
	Converses in an angry tone

ENGAGED

The Patient	The Nurse
Accepts nursing care without reluctance	Implements needed interventions/procedures promptly and competently
"Prepares" for a procedure by voluntarily assuming the needed position	Completes routine tasks with friendly comments or other manifestations of high regard/caring for the patient
Seeks clarification for proper implementation of care	
Demonstrates an understanding/agreement with what the nurse tells him or her and readily follows the nurse's instructions	Acknowledges and addresses inquiries of the patient about care
Provides data asked for by the nurse	Volunteers needed information without being asked by the patient or family
Asks about other anticipated procedures or interventions	Touches the patient for reassurance when appropriate
Takes time to respond to questions or asks that questions or instructions be repeated	Provides verbal reassurance

BOX 2-1	*Bonding between Nurse and Patient: Openness and Engagement—cont'd*

NOT ENGAGED

THE PATIENT	THE NURSE
Demonstrates verbal or nonverbal cues of reluctance/refusal to comply with what the nurse says	Attends only to the intravenous line and other routine procedures and ignores the patient Scorns the patient's questions by laughing with sarcasm or getting irritated Sternly demands that the patient comply with instructions, demonstrating irritation

Adapted from Tejero LM: Development and validation of an instrument to measure nurse–patient bonding, *Int J Nurs Stud* 47:608–615, 2009.

Consider the difference it would make if you listen to someone as if you have something to learn (Mlyniec, 2006). Seek first to understand and then to be understood (Covey, 2004).

To listen: Use open body language, arms open not crossed; make eye contact without staring; echo words or paraphrase facts and feelings; lean toward the person speaking; do not interrupt; pay attention; try to relax. You might use these words to keep the person speaking: "I see. I understand. Good point. I can see that you feel strongly about that. I understand how you could see it like that." Keep your mind from wandering by focusing your attention on what the person is saying, repeat it in your mind, and reflect upon what it might be like to be in the person's situation. The term mindful listening means to be still and listen, to be fully present moment to moment, without trying to change anything (Shafir, 2000). Take a breath and relax. Consciously set aside your own distractions knowing that if you are distracted, you are otherwise attracted: something else is more important than the other person. This distraction can be communicated nonverbally and undermine your being seen as an authentic, caring nurse.

In a data analysis of a study to explore how undergraduate nursing students experience making a difference in practice settings, a pattern emerged. The pattern is concernful practice. Students experienced knowing and connecting with clients to make a difference. The things they learned by staying with clients and listening helped the students negotiate with staff to make changes in the client's care and contributed to one student's first experience with feeling a responsibility toward the client and the client's care (Ironside et al, 2005). In hospice care, it has been suggested that quality of care improves when the care is client centered, as evidenced by "caring conversations." The connections between clients and nurses are made by presence, touch, and listening (Olthuis et al, 2006).

Finally, it is important to be aware that human beings are always communicating. According to Watzlawick (1967), when two people are within each other's visual field they cannot *not* communicate. What does this mean? It means that communication is always occurring whether we are communicating verbally or nonverbally. Communication experts believe that 60% to 75% of our communication is actually done nonverbally. As mentioned earlier, how we hold our body, are our arms opened or crossed, are we leaning in toward the person or leaning away from them, are we giving direct eye contact or staring vacantly all communicate a message. How that communication is received is dependent on the person's perceptions and worldview (Erickson, 2006). As nurses it is extremely important that we be aware of what we are communicating nonverbally to our clients and in turn what their nonverbal language is telling us. "The bottom line is, we are communicating any time someone else is attending to us directly or indirectly" (Erickson, 2006, p. 308).

> *Suppose we were able to share meanings freely without a compulsive urge to impose our view or to conform to those of others and without distortion and self-deception. Would this not constitute a real revolution in culture?*
>
> **David Bohm**
>
> **WIT&***Wisdom*

True Presence

And what about technology? What does it mean to be a competent nurse? Remember that the dazzling technology that seems to create miraculous recovery is a means to an end, not an end in itself. Nursing care is person focused, not technology focused (Bernardo, 1998). To be truly present is to bear witness to the client's experience, understand the client's perspective, and respect the client's dignity and rights to self-determination. "Intention to nurse is the dynamic that is expressed through being authentically present with the other in the moment"; it is understanding that the person is complete in this moment and does not need to be fixed or made whole again (Locsin, 2002). Presence, "being with" in contrast to "doing to," is a central role for hospice nurses (Krisman-Scott and McCorkle, 2002).

> *You may light another's candle at your own without loss.*
>
> **Danish proverb**
>
> **WIT&***Wisdom*

In a study of the "technologically induced vulnerability and the inherent uncertainty" of clients undergoing bone marrow transplantation, one participant said, "Care was the nurse just being there" (Cooper and Powell, 1998). When clients did not feel like banter or small talk, they could be "certain of the presence of the nurse" (Cooper and Powell, 1998). The research "depicts a caring presence that appears to transcend the distractions of technology and acknowledged a kinship with patients that derived from an acknowledgment of their shared human experience" (Younger, 1995).

The nurse implements the nursing process based on the client's experience and clarifies the client's and nurse's "responsibilities, expectations, opportunities, and accountabilities" (Bernardo, 1998). "True presence is grounded in nursing science, the essence of nursing as a scholarly discipline" (Lynaugh and Fagin, 1988). Presence, at the very core of nursing practice, is the art of nursing. Moments of "intense presencing, although they may be physiologically driven in our highly technological environment of healthcare today, are 'moments of truth' for both the patient and the nurse the unique opportunity, with artful caring and expert practice, for

nurses to use their hearts and their hands to create a moment in which healing can begin" (Wendler, 2002).

Competence in the advanced technology of critical care nursing has been described as a component of caring, and this view is supported by nurse theorists (Orem, 1985; Rogers, 1985; Newman, 1986; Parse, 1992). The suggestion is made that technological competence is another way of knowing more about the client. The helping relationship uses this information to deliver nursing care that focuses on this person in this moment, a person with a desire to live fully as a human being with his or her own hopes and dreams and vision of himself or herself. The challenge then is to be competent in many ways—to be able to use technology and follow critical pathways to deliver nursing care to a unique person. Building your skills in communication in the helping relationship helps you and the client find meaning in moments of connection.

> **WIT&***Wisdom*
>
> In the novel *Please Remember This*, K.G. Seidel writes about a young woman who has opened a coffee bar. Read this very clear description of being present. "But serving coffee—she was very good at serving coffee. Her therapist training helped. She knew how to be warm and engaged, but without issues of her own, how to let the moment be about the other person. And this manner didn't feel false, or as if she were denying herself. She was interested in other people; she wanted to hear them talk about themselves."
>
> Seidel KG: *Please remember this*, New York, 2002, Avon Books, p 183.

Becoming a Storycatcher

Baldwin (2005) says that a storycatcher is a practitioner of the heart of language. Story creates context, context highlights relationships and leads to holistic and connected action, and connected action becomes a force for restoring/restorying the world. She says that we have lost the space for story and may have lost the understanding of how essential storytelling is to who we are.

Consider these qualities of a storycatcher and see how attention to these might deepen your understanding of clients' experiences as reflected in their stories. Story-catchers are intrigued by human experience; inquisitive about meaning and insight; curious not judgmental; more in love with questions than answers; able to hold personal boundaries in relationships; present while others experience emotions and have insight; able to hold the sacred space for listening; able to invite forgiveness, release, and grace; and aware of the power of story and use it consciously.

Hearing the client's story is an important assessment tool that allows nurses to access a client's self-care knowledge and gain greater understanding of their world view (Erickson, 2011). By listening to a person's story the nurse is able to learn what is important to the client and begin to create a personalized plan of care.

Moments of Connection . . .

Erickson (2011) shared the following story. Upon entering the room she introduced herself to the older gentleman who had been admitted for angina to rule out myocardial infarction. She asked why he thought he was in the hospital. He replied "you can check my chart. It is all in there." She replied: "I want to hear your story and why you think you are here." He replied: "My wife and I were married for 61 years. She was my other half and best friend. She died 6 months ago and I am heartbroken." Based on his story she developed a holistic plan of care that helped him deal with his loss and grief. His angina disappeared.

Reflections On . . .

The Client–Nurse Relationship

Consider what you read about clients' rights and other issues in the client–nurse relationship to answer these questions.

What? . . .
Write one thing you learned from this chapter.

So what? . . .
How will this affect your nursing practice?

Now what? . . .
How will you implement this new knowledge or skill?

Think about it . . .

Practicing the Client–Nurse Relationship

Exercise 1

Read the following poetic journal entry, written by a nurse after a surgical admission. Identify which of the therapeutic communications techniques in Table 2-2 might not have been used by the nurses assigned to this nurse patient. Do you think these nurses did not "care" for this patient? If you learned a patient had written such comments, what could the nurses on this unit do, given time constraints, to help this patient feel more cared for?

> I came to you . . . patient.
> You scurried, in all directions
> Returning only to scan a wrist band,
> Give a pill, check lung sounds.
> I leave you . . . in-patient.
> Transforming from in-patient
> To person healing . . .
> Little thanks to you.
> The leavings of your time,
> Too "well" to deserve
> your full attention
> Too "sick" to be totally ignored.
> Did you have a
> Calling to nursing?
> If so, when did you
> Stop listening?
> Heart of nursing, weakened
> Barely beating . . . I pray
> For your resuscitation now
> And at every remaining moment of your career.

Exercise 2   **QSEN**

Student Nurse Jane is checking her patient's medication to be sure she is applying the five rights of medication administration: right patient, right medication, right dosage, right delivery method, and right time. She enters the patient's room, checks his armband identifier, calls his name, and offers him his two oral medications. The patient looks at the pills and asks, "Why am I getting a blue pill today? I usually get a green pill?" How should Jane respond? In developing the client–nurse relationship, how can patients and their families be included as part of the team so that they become safety allies?

QSEN Competencies: Patient-centered Care and Safety

Exercise 3

The following questions have been designed to help you think about yourself as a nurse-helper. They are not easy questions, because they focus on your basic beliefs and values about being a helper. To begin, answer the questions on your own. Later, get together with your classmates and discuss your responses. You will learn a lot from each other.

- What does *health* mean to you?
- What factors positively influence clients to take care of their health?
- Do you think health is a right or a privilege?
- To what extent do you think clients are responsible for the development of their health problems?
- What can you do, as a nurse, to increase the likelihood that your clients will take better care of themselves?
- To be an effective helper, you must know how your feelings about this role influence the way you relate to your clients.
- To what extent do you think clients are responsible for solving their own healthcare problems?
- What degree of dependence (independence) are you comfortable with in your clients?
- What do you like most about helping clients?
- What do you like least?
- Nurses are expected to be proficient in carrying out a range of nursing treatments.
- How competent do you feel in implementing the most essential nursing interventions in your clinical area?
- How would you rate your ability to teach clients how to take care of their own health?

Exercise 4

Try free writing in a journal to help build your skills of understanding yourself and your responses to clients and colleagues. Take a few minutes to write your thoughts and feelings continuously without correction . . . just write anything that comes to mind. Write without spaces between words. Reflection on the writing may bring clarity to a confusing or ambiguous issue or help you organize your thoughts. You can write free hand or at the keyboard (Shellenbarger et al, 2005).

Exercise 5

Interview someone who has recently been hospitalized or had contact with a nurse or nurses in any medical setting. Using open-ended questions, encourage the person to relate the personal story of experiencing the care of a nurse. Look for what this person saw as positive and supportive or negative and nonsupportive. Reflect on this anecdotal evidence and write a paragraph about what you learned and how it can relate to your journey of healthcaring as a nurse. Include this in your journal. Consider how others you know can benefit from sharing their healthcare experiences and continue to record thoughts that support your own growth in relationship building and tending in healthcare.

References

American Nurses Association: *Standards of clinical nursing practice*, Atlanta, 2004, American Nurses Association.

Baldwin C: *Storycatcher: making sense of our lives through the power and practice of story*, Novato, Calif, 2005, New World Library.

Bernardo A: Technology and true presence in nursing, *Holistic Nurs Pract* 12(4):40, 1998.

Cooper MC, Powell E: Technology and care in a bone marrow transplant unit: creating and assuaging vulnerability, *Holistic Nurs Pract* 12(4):57, 1998.

Covey SR: *The 7 habits of highly effective people*, New York, 2004, Free Press.

Erickson H, editor. *Modeling and role-modeling: a view from the clients' world*, Cedar Park, Tex, 2006, Unicorns Unlimited.

Erickson H, Tomlin E, Swain MA: *Modeling and role-modeling: a theory and paradigm for nursing*. Englewood Cliffs, NJ, 1983–2010, Prentice-Hall; second–ninth printing, Cedar Park, Tex, 1988–2009, EST Co; tenth printing, Cedar Park, Tex, 2010, Unicorns Unlimited.

Erickson, M: Personal communication, 2011.

Geanellos R: Patients value friendly nurses, *Aust Nurs J* 11(11):38, 2004.

Ironside P, Diekelmann N, Hirschmann M: Learning the practices of knowing and connecting: the voices of students, *J Nurs Educ* 44(4):153, 2005.

Keirsey D: *Please understand me, II: temperament, character, intelligence*, Del Mar, Calif, 1998, Prometheus Nemesis Book Company.

Krisman-Scott MA, McCorkle R: The tapestry of hospice, *Holistic Nurs Pract* 16(2):32, 2002.

Locsin RC: Culture of nursing, preoccupation with prediction, and nursing intention, *Holistic Nurs Pract* 16(4):1, 2002.

Lynaugh J, Fagin C: Nursing comes of age, *Image* 20:184, 1988.

Mlyniec V: How to talk so your teen will listen, *Family Circle* January:20, 2006.

Myers IB: *Gifts differing*, Palo Alto, Calif, 1995, Consulting Psychologists Press.

Myers IB: *Introduction to type*, Palo Alto, Calif, 1998, Consulting Psychologists Press.

Newman M: *Health as expanding consciousness*, St. Louis, 1986, Mosby.

Nichols MP: *The lost art of listening: how learning to listen can improve a relationship*, New York, 1995, The Guildford Press.

Olthuis G, Dekkers W, Leget C, et al: The caring relationship in hospice care: an analysis based on the ethics of the caring conversation, *Nurs Ethics* 13(1):29, 2006.

Orem D: *Nursing: concepts of practice*, New York, 1985, McGraw-Hill.

Parse RR: Human becoming: Parse's theory of nursing, *Nurs Sci Q* 5:35, 1992.

Rogers M: Science of unitary human beings: a paradigm for nursing. In Wood R, Kekahbah J, editors: *Examining the cultural implications of Martha Rogers' science of unitary human beings*, Lecompton, Kans, 1985, Wood-Kekahbah Associates.

Shafir R: *The Zen of listening: mindful communication in the age of distraction*, Adyar, India, 2000, Quest Books.

Shellenbarger T, Palmer EA, Labant AL, et al: Use of faculty reflection to improve teaching, *Annu Rev Nurs Educ* 3:343, 2005.

Smith, JA: The idea of health: A philosophical inquiry, *Adv Nurs Sci* 3(3):45–50, 1981.

Stuart GW, Laraia M: *Principles and practice of psychiatric nursing*, ed 8, St. Louis, 2005, Mosby.

Tejero LM: Development and validation of an instrument to measure nurse–patient bonding, *Int J Nurs Stud* 47:608–615, 2009.

Younger JB: The alienation of the sufferer, *Adv Nurs Sci* 17:53, 1995.

Watzlawick, P: *Pragmatics of human communication: a study of interactional patterns, pathologies, and paradoxes*, New York, 1967, W. W. Norton and Company.

Wendler MC: *The art of nursing*, Indianapolis, Ind, 2002, Sigma Theta Tau International Honor Society of Nursing.

Wysong PR, Driver E: Patient perceptions of nurses' skill, *Crit Care Nurse* 29(4): August 2009.

Suggestions for Further Reading

Balzer Riley J: *Customer service from A to Z: making the connection*, Albuquerque, 2003, Hartman Publishing. Offers training modules and exercises to build relationships in health care.

Balzer Riley J: *From the heart to the hands: key to healthcaring connections*, Ellicott, Md, 1999, Integrated Management Publishing Systems. Features more than 100 stories and tips on nurse–client relationships; order at 800-368-7675.

Fox J: *Finding what you didn't lose: expressing your truth and creativity through poem-making*, New York, 1995, Jeremy P. Tacher.

Fox J: *Poetic medicine: the healing art of poem-making*, New York, 1997, Jeremy P. Tacher.

Watson J: Intentionality and caring-healing consciousness: a practice of transpersonal healing, *Holist Nurs Pract* 16(4):12, 2002.

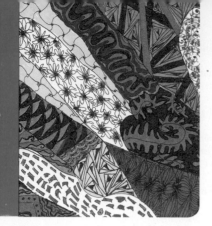

Chapter 3

Solving Problems Together

> *We must not talk to them, or at them, but with them.*
>
> **Florence Nightingale [on partnership with clients] (Atwell, 2010)**

Objectives

1. Define mutuality in nurse–client relationships
2. Discuss the use of face work and politeness theory in approaching clients
3. Discuss mutual problem solving to involve the client in the implementation of the nursing process
4. Complete exercises to practice a mutual problem-solving approach to the nursing process
5. Examine the steps in making contracts with clients
6. Participate in exercises to build skills in solving problems with clients

Moments of Connection . . .
Setting Goals Together

A nurse was called to a client's room to discuss her therapy options for cancer treatment. As they talked, the client began to clearly understand that this disease was going to be what claimed her life. The client cried the most deep, painful, gut-level crying the nurse had ever experienced with an adult. The nurse held her hand and cried with her. They began to talk when the client relaxed. They set goals of her leaving the hospital and experiencing her next Christmas. The nurse said she felt good that she was able to take the time to let the client cry.

Mutuality in Nurse–Client Relationships

Mutuality, a concept grounded in research, is an essential element in building relationships with the client, although it is not always easy to achieve (Berg, 2005; Chalmers, 2005; Geanellos, 2005; Jack, 2005; Porr, 2005; Zoffmann, 2005). Mutuality is characterized by empathy, collaboration, equality, and interdependency (Jeon, 2004). Mutuality is "the experience of real or symbolic commonalities of visions, goals, sentiments, or characteristics, including shared acceptance of difference that validates the person's world-view" (Hagerty et al, 1993, p. 294). Responsive relationships between the nurse and client are based on respect, trust, and mutuality that reflect both personal moral knowledge and ethical nursing knowledge (Tarlier, 2004). Mutuality is a sharing of collective knowledge (McCance et al, 2008). An ongoing sharing of knowledge between healthcare professionals and shared decision making help ensure patient satisfaction (Cerda et al, 2010).

Face Work and Politeness Theory

The outcome of the client–nurse interaction depends on the nurse's ability to engage the client in decision making and share the control and power in the relationship (Roberts et al, 1995; Spiers, 1998). Nurses build their communication skills by study and practice of techniques, trial and error, observation of role models, experience, and achievement of comfort with the use of their own intuition. Face work and politeness theory point to the need to consider the client's and nurse's "sense of self-esteem, autonomy, and solidarity in conversation" (Spiers, 1998). We speak of "saving face" or helping the other "save face" and mean the preservation of dignity so that each party continues to be willing to invest in the interaction without experiencing any threat. Consider a patient stepping up on the scale to be weighed. Clients want to preserve or manage their image of self or "face." How the nurse handles this situation can influence the client's willingness to problem solve if the weight is "face threatening," that is, not what the person wanted or expected (Pillet-Shore, 2006). If the client is discouraged, the nurse might offer, "We all have things to work on. If your weight is not what you desire just now, we can work together to meet your goals."

In the complex process of problem solving with the client to promote health, many factors can present barriers, including perceptions and negotiations about the rules, norms, expectations, and boundaries that can distort both information and interpersonal intent (Cauce and Srebnik, 1990). Nurses must "negotiate a mutually acceptable and satisfying level of distance or intimacy, self-disclosure, privacy, and information exchange with a context of power differences, a need for help, and a right to act" (Spiers, 1998). Each party wants to maintain a sense of personal competency and control. Attacks on these or on the person's poise or sense of belonging or being liked are called face threats.

Consider the actions of the nurse in assessment: questioning about the client's behavior, a physical assessment, and assessment of and intervention in spiritual needs. These actions are invasive. Polite behavior, which is more than just our notion of the conduct traditionally required by mothers and is a part of the consideration of face theory, refers to ways in which nurses ease the interaction to help decrease fear, embarrassment, and anger. Polite behaviors lessen the threat of the intimate nature of nursing interventions. Nurses may gently and indirectly encourage the client's participation in problem solving, whereas a direct order in such a situation would be considered impolite and inappropriate. When discussing a potentially embarrassing situation such as safe sex, the nurse is careful about the language used and asks questions gently to help the client save face. Because of the complicated balance between considerations of face work and politeness and the necessity for client involvement, further research is required to identify methods to supplement successful intuitive strategies, which are difficult to teach. Nurses understand the importance of tact in engaging the client's participation. Nursing research validates the concept that treating the client as a unique individual and actively engaging the client in problem solving are associated with increased client satisfaction, an important quality indicator (Roberts et al, 1995).

Defining the Difference between Problem Solving and Mutual Problem Solving in Nursing

Problem Solving: The Nursing Process

In Chapter 1 we identified a five-step model of the nursing process, the problem-solving process:

1. Assessment
2. Diagnosis
3. Planning
4. Implementation
5. Evaluation

The Mutual Problem-solving Process in Nursing

Validation

Validation signifies the difference between problem solving for clients and mutual problem solving with clients. Incorporating validation keeps us focused on the rights and obligations of clients to make their own decisions about their health.

The important activity of validation must be incorporated at each step of the problem-solving process in nursing. Validation means consciously seeking out our clients' opinions and feelings at each phase of the nursing process. Validation means unearthing any questions or concerns our clients have about plans for their healthcare and securing their understanding and willingness to proceed to the next step. Incorporating validation into our problem solving stops us from moving too quickly and alienating our clients. It ensures that we obtain complete agreement and commitment from our clients about the plans for nursing care being considered for their particular health problems.

A mutual problem-solving process in nursing looks like this (Iyer et al, 1995):

I. Assessment
   A. Collecting data regarding the client, client–family system, or community
   B. Identifying needs, problems, concerns, or human responses
II. Diagnosis
   A. Analyzing data
   B. Validating the interpretation of data with the client
   C. Identifying nursing diagnoses
   D. Validating the nursing diagnoses with the client
III. Planning
   A. Setting priorities for resolution of identified problems with the client
   B. Determining expected and desired outcomes of nursing actions in collaboration with the client
   C. Writing nursing interventions to achieve these outcomes in collaboration with the client
IV. Implementation
   A. Implementing nursing actions with assistance from the client
   B. Encouraging client participation in carrying out nursing actions to achieve the outcomes
   C. Continuing to collect data about the client's condition and interaction with the environment
V. Evaluation
   A. Evaluating the outcomes of nursing care in consultation with the client
   B. Ongoing evaluation to revise the nursing care plan

Including validation in the nursing process does not necessarily increase the time or energy required to carry out nursing care. Much of the checking can be done quickly and naturally while interacting with clients. Ensuring that clients understand and agree with each step of the nursing process increases the probability that they will do their part to comply with treatment. Clients who have a clear understanding of their health problems, as well as what they and their nurses can do about them, expend less energy worrying and more energy doing something constructive.

Clearly understanding their nursing diagnoses and having a say in how best to respond to them enable clients to maintain a sense of control.

Validation invites the collaboration that is essential for successful client change. The trust developed from working together is likely to increase the accuracy and validity of the database and thus enrich the foundation for the rest of the nursing process. The trust growing out of mutuality provides the clients with an anchor, giving them the support they need to risk changing health behaviors. Collaboration ensures the benefits of two heads working on a health problem; this is essential because nursing cannot exist in a vacuum. We cannot strive for excellence without including the full participation of our clients. Nurse researchers report that "recognition of the client as a unique person and encouragement of active client participation in the nursing encounter are highly associated with client satisfaction, one important indicator of quality care" (Roberts et al, 1995). "Nursing interactions characterized as task oriented and that disregard the client as an equal participant have been related to acts of resistance" by clients (Hallberg et al, 1995).

Many of today's healthcare customers are speaking up, asking questions, seeking second opinions, demanding alternative healthcare options, and forming their own self-help groups to take action. Their assertiveness and independence reflect the true meaning of the label "client," designating those who claim the rights and privileges of partnership in healthcare.

The client contracts for services with a qualified healthcare provider. This relationship is a negotiated partnership in which the client implicitly agrees to comply with the plan they generate together. The proliferation of advanced nurse practitioners in response to the demands for cost-effective care in a managed care environment demonstrates such a partnership from a holistic perspective. Advanced nurse practitioners identify collaboration with clients and other healthcare professionals as part of their nursing philosophy (Grando, 1998). C. Everett Koop, former U.S. surgeon general, emphasized that clear communication between clients and physicians could prevent serious medical problems. He reported results from a Louis Harris poll indicating that of 1000 clients questioned, 25% admitted a hesitancy to talk with their physicians because the physician seemed rushed or distracted or because the client was embarrassed (Koop, 1998). Nurses can build working relationships among nurses, clients, and physicians by assisting with collaborative communication.

Not all healthcare customers think of themselves as active, responsible partners in their care. Some do what healthcare professionals tell them, living out the definition of the label "patient." The passive nature of this role creates an imbalance between the power of the nurse and that of the client. The passivity of this stance creates an inequitable relationship between nurses and others. As nurses, we can help reverse this apathy and listlessness by encouraging our clients to be partners in their own healthcare (Cooper and Powell, 1998). This means appreciating the worth of our clients and calling on their strengths. We can transform our nursing care into a mutual problem-solving process when we invite, even request, the full participation of our partners, the clients.

Earlier in this century patients were more satisfied with a system of illness care that focused on disease eradication. As the influence of science and technology on healthcare has increased, discontent has emerged, along with resentment of chauvinistic, "all-knowing," healthcare professionals. Clients have begun demanding more influence in their healthcare and requesting more individualized care. Evidence of this movement was seen as early as 1972, with the publication of the Patient's Bill of Rights (presented by the American Hospital Association). This document describes the expectations for respect, knowledge, privacy, and confidentiality, and access to any information essential for adequate treatment. Nurses need to focus on the individual's responsibility for healthcare along with his or her rights. It is important to emphasize what clients can do to take care of themselves, as well as to safeguard their right to quality, informed care. The notion of clients as consumers of healthcare that arose in the 1970s has evolved into the idea of clients and their families as customers. In addition to providing informed care, nurses must now give attention to customers' expectations of service. Decreased hospital stays, outpatient surgery, and the movement toward home healthcare make the need for problem solving even more essential because clients and their families and significant others play a more active role. Because clients are frequently discharged from the hospital before they are able to care for themselves, much client education and care must be done in the home. Clients need to be able to make informed decisions about their choices for insurance. Nurses need to be informed about the differences in the choices of providers and services covered by managed care organizations to assist clients in the selection of and in the proper procedures for reimbursement.

The standards set forth in *Standards of Clinical Nursing Practice* by the American Nurses Association (2004)—quality of care, diagnosis, outcome identification, planning, implementation, and evaluation—provide support for a mutual problem-solving approach with clients. The following statements are taken from two of the standards of nursing practice.

Standard IV: Planning. Within the measurement criteria for standard IV we find: "The plan is developed with the patient, family, and health care providers, as appropriate." This standard demands that clients, family, and significant others be kept informed about the patient's current health status, changes in health status, total health care plan, nursing care plan, roles of healthcare personnel, and healthcare resources. Clients, family, and significant others must be provided with the information needed to make decisions and choices about promoting, maintaining, and restoring health; seeking and utilizing appropriate healthcare personnel; and maintaining and using healthcare resources.

Standard VI: Evaluation. Within the measurement criteria for standard VI we find: "The patient, family, and other health care providers are involved in the evaluation process, as appropriate." Clients are an essential part of the comprehensive and intelligent determination of the impact of nursing on the patient's health status. Clients, family, significant others, and healthcare providers evaluate nursing actions and goal achievement.

Incorporation of Validation into the Nursing Process

The example given in the following subsections illustrates suggested methods for ensuring maximum client participation in a mutual problem-solving approach.

Validating the Interpretation of Collected Data. From the time clients enter our nursing care, we start asking them questions about their health problems. As we receive information about their situations from the answers they give us, the way they answer our questions, and objective data from laboratory tests and physical assessment, we start to piece together a meaningful picture. That picture is our interpretation of the data. It starts off as fuzzy and develops into a clear explanation of our clients' health problem(s).

Nurses are not the only ones who crave a clear picture of what is going on—clients are usually eager to know as well. Put yourself in the following clinical nursing situation:

Mrs. Cook is 48 years old and has been referred to a home healthcare agency by her family physician to help establish control of her adult-onset diabetes. She has been on oral hypoglycemic agents for the past 2 years. Her most recent blood glucose level was 350 mg/dl.

> *Mrs. Cook:* "Oh, don't worry about me. I'll be fine. You won't need to visit me. I can't be worrying my husband. He wants a healthy wife!"

As you talk, you learn that Mrs. Cook has little knowledge about what special care she must take, how to monitor her nutritional intake, how to pay careful attention to skin care, and how to check her urine daily for glucose. You learn that sickness is "unacceptable" in her family. She has two sisters who are "perfectly healthy" and a husband she calls a "fitness fanatic."

All her life Mrs. Cook has received verbal and nonverbal messages from her parents and husband that she must be a perfect wife and homemaker and that sickness is not tolerated. When the symptoms of hyperglycemia first occurred, Mrs. Cook tried to ignore them and pretend nothing was wrong. Her neighbor insisted that Mrs. Cook see a doctor when her symptoms of increased thirst and appetite were accompanied by diminished strength and weight loss.

You want to share with Mrs. Cook your assessment that she appears to have little knowledge about how to manage her diabetes to prevent complications. You suspect she has never really learned much about diabetes in an attempt to be "healthy" so as to live up to her parents' and husband's expectations. It was easier to pretend she was healthy than to admit she had a chronic illness. You sense that she may mistakenly assume that she will not be able to live an active and full life as a diabetic. You validate this interpretation of the information with the following statements:

> *You:* "Mrs. Cook, I know you are eager to feel better, and I have some concerns about your ability to continue to feel healthy without learning more about taking care of yourself and managing your diabetes. From what you've told me, I know it is important to you and your husband that you be healthy. It is my experience that if people exercise proper self-care, diabetes doesn't have to stop them from doing anything they want, but to accomplish this you must accept the fact that you have diabetes. You can do things to be healthy. Tell me what you think about that."

This validation respectfully lets your client know your assessment of her health situation. Your ending allows Mrs. Cook to argue, disagree, or ask questions about your interpretation of her situation.

Identifying Actual or Potential Problems with the Client. When Mrs. Cook has either agreed with or amended your assessment, you can then formulate and validate the nursing diagnosis.

> *Mrs. Cook might say:* "What else is there to learn? The nurse practitioner in Dr. Wood's office taught me to give myself insulin. I am fine with that."

Her response presents an opportunity to teach her about potential problems people with diabetes need to avoid. You could respond as follows:

> *You:* "You have mastered taking your insulin; however, there is more to learn. You need to understand the signs of low blood sugar and have a plan for emergencies. Since diabetes affects the circulation, you would benefit from learning about skin care. Taking care to regulate your calories to adjust to your changing levels of energy is also essential to keep you feeling well. Learning how to manage your daily activities can help you stay healthy and active like your family."

This identification of some of the potential problems of diabetes empowers Mrs. Cook to take charge of her own health. You offer hope that she can live normally.

> *She might respond:* "I thought all I had to do was give myself this insulin every day and I'd be OK. I guess there's more to it. My husband wants me to be healthy, and you have to be to keep up with him. He worries about me but doesn't want me to know. He's due home from work early today. Will you talk with him, too? Will you help him understand that I'm OK?"

Validating the Nursing Diagnoses with the Client.

You respond: "I'd be glad to talk with him. You and I have some work to do, too. The three main areas you need to learn about are adjusting your caloric intake to match your activity level, taking special precautions with your skin care—especially care of your feet—and having a plan to cope with low blood sugar, should that occur. Does that about cover it for you?"

Mrs. Cook: "That sounds like a lot to learn. The thing that surprises me is this talk about skin care. I've always had good skin, and I can't imagine having problems with it."

Setting Priorities with the Client for the Resolution of Identified Problems. In this case, it is appropriate to start with the problem of interest to the client because there is no current crisis.

You: "OK, let's start with skin care."

This validation gives Mrs. Cook some control of the teaching session.

Determining Expected and Desired Outcomes of Nursing Actions in Collaboration with the Client. You and your client are concerned about outcomes. It is important for each of you to reveal your goals so that you can work together. To begin the negotiation of the plan, you can clarify expectations:

You: "We both need to have some idea where we are headed in our work together so we know when we have met our goals. I would expect you to be able to have a plan to prevent skin breakdown and low blood sugar and to have a plan to deal with them if they do occur. As for nutrition, it is my hope you will be able to figure out the number of calories you need to have the energy required for your active lifestyle. This sounds like a lot, but I think it's manageable. I'd like to hear what you think."

These suggestions make it clear what you want to accomplish. Now Mrs. Cook needs to indicate her goals.

Mrs. Cook: "It does seem like a lot to learn, but I guess I don't have much choice. I don't want to feel that sick again. I don't think either my husband or I would want to go through that again. What you say makes sense. I'll give it a try."

You: "We can start with these goals. I believe you'll feel more in control of your body, and that will make it easier for you to accept the differences in your body that diabetes causes. Just knowing there are things you can do can take away much of the fear. It will get easier, and these things will become a part of your routine. If you have questions and can't reach me, there is a 24-hour hotline number for the American Diabetes Association."

With this reply you have given Mrs. Cook another good reason for learning about her condition—to be less fearful.

Deciding on Nursing Strategies to Achieve These Outcomes in Collaboration with the Client. You and Mrs. Cook agree on your goals, and you have access to the knowledge, people, and material resources to help this client achieve the expected and desired outcomes.

You: "You indicated you would like to start with learning about skin care. I see you have a DVD player. We have a DVD I can bring that has examples of how to ensure that your skin does not break down. We also have booklets on skin care. And I can answer any questions you have. Which would you prefer?"

Mrs. Cook: "Booklets sound too much like school. I'd like to start with the DVD and then look at the booklets just to make sure I understand."

You have now made a plan with Mrs. Cook's help to start work on the first goal. When she is ready, you can introduce resources for the other goals and supply her with the 24-hour hotline number for the American Diabetes Association. Later on, you can recommend a support group that might be useful as well.

Implementing Nursing Actions with Assistance from the Client and Encouraging Client Participation in Carrying out Nursing Actions to Meet the Outcomes. In Mrs. Cook's case, your main focus is to encourage her participation in the various forms of learning how to manage the diabetes. One way to show your interest and involvement is to ask open-ended questions about her progress. For example:

"What are your thoughts about the tape?"
"What questions do you have about skin care after seeing the tape and reading the booklets?"

The answers reveal areas in which additional teaching is needed and provide an opportunity to offer praise and reinforcement.

Evaluating the Outcomes of Nursing Care in Consultation with the Client. After Mrs. Cook uses the resources, you might adopt a light, humorous approach for evaluation.

You: "Just like being back in school . . . it's time for a quiz! Are you ready to tell me what you have learned and how you are working on meeting our goals?"

Mrs. Cook: "I feel like I've had a home correspondence course like they advertise on television. Ask me anything!"

You: "I know you've been working hard. Tell me what you are doing to prevent skin problems."

Mrs. Cook: "Sure. First, no more tight shoes. They may interfere with the circulation. I threw out my knee-highs. My husband always teases me about those anyway. He says they just aren't sexy. With the rings they leave on my legs, I can see how bad they are for me. The DVD showed me how to cut my toenails straight across. I bought toenail clippers. Oh, yes, I remember to pat dry with the towel instead of rubbing hard. OK, teacher, what grade do I get on skin care 101?"

You: "I'd say an A, and I just happen to be carrying gold stickers. You are a star. You can use them or share them with your children. I want to add that it's important to stay warm enough in this cold weather and to use body lotion to keep your skin from getting dry and irritated. Rubbing the lotion in will improve your circulation."

Mrs. Cook: "I love those stickers and I feel like I've earned an A. My daughter gave me some fancy lotion for my birthday. I'll use that and thank her for making a good choice."

You can continue to review with Mrs. Cook the other expected outcomes on which you both agreed and discuss her progress. You can encourage her to share what she has learned with her husband and how good she feels about her ability to manage the diabetes. Mr. Cook may need help adjusting to the idea that his wife has a chronic illness. Think of ways to involve the entire family: perhaps a conference during your next home visit. The family context is where the notion of health and illness is learned and fostered. Any support the family can give will likely enhance Mrs. Cook's health and motivate her to continue with preventive care. Joining a support group might also be useful for Mrs. Cook. Seeing that other people lead productive lives, even if their health is not perfect, may alter the idea that Mrs. Cook's diabetes will set her apart as different and unhealthy.

Benefits of Mutuality That Go Beyond the Client–Nurse Dyad

March (1990) believed that the benefits of the collaborative client–nurse relationship (which she terms therapeutic reciprocity) go beyond any isolated meeting and contribute to growth and development for both clients and nurses. The shared meanings about clients' experiences are a natural precursor to the shared control and responsibility for the outcomes of their relationship. Nurses and clients gain trust in each other as human beings and in their own ability to relate effectively in the helping relationship. This discovery, although of primary value in the healthcare context, may transfer to other interpersonal relationships as the worth of interdependence is demonstrated.

Matheis-Kraft and colleagues (1990) claimed that clients who take more active roles in their treatments recover faster. This benefits hospitals, which are struggling to contain costs of healthcare. They reported how one American hospital instituted patient-driven healthcare. The goal of the hospital's patient-centered approach is to create a caring, dignified, and empowering environment in which their clients truly direct the course of their care and call on their inner resources to speed the healing process. The staff encourages client awareness of how their own physical, mental, and spiritual resources can promote healing.

In addition to the endorsement by clients and their families, nurses working in an environment with this philosophy report a number of spin-offs that have boosted their morale (Matheis-Kraft et al, 1990):

- The opportunity to bring more nurturing and caring into their profession
- The enjoyment of expanded autonomy and authority, which allows them to make a real difference
- The experience of a more equal relationship with physicians who listen to their recommendations and even seek their counsel
- The satisfaction of being client advocates as they were educated to be

Schwertel-Kyle and Pitzer (1990) described their implementation of Orem's self-care model for nursing in a critical nursing care unit as a way of providing optimal care to clients within concise time frames. Originally spurred by the financial constraints of prospective payment systems with set reimbursement rates (which led to shorter hospital stays, more acute illness in those admitted, and decreased caregiving resources), the plan enhanced clients' self-confidence and feelings of accomplishment. The transformation from passive, dependent patient to active partner is one way for America's nursing clients to start taking responsibility for their healthcare, in addition to securing their healthcare rights.

Ways to Make Clinical Problem Solving a Mutual Affair

1. Explore what you believe about the issue of clients having an active part in their healthcare. The extent to which you uphold clients' responsibility for their health mirrors how you involve them in the nursing process. Remember to step back, listen, openly discuss the issue, and focus on collaboration (Grover, 2005).

2. Be aware that an environment in which "questioning, curiosity, risk taking and scepticism" are tolerated and even encouraged supports critical thinking skills (Seifert, 2010, p 198).

3. Watch for "teachable moments," times when events or circumstances may lead to positive behavior change (Lawson and Flocke, 2009). Clients who have had coronary artery bypass surgery may pay more attention to smoking cessation when this risk factor is linked to the possibility of further coronary artery disease and future surgery.

4. Practice revealing your opinions to clients. Increase your confidence in telling clients about your assessment of their particular situations.

5. Avoid giving nursing care without checking with your clients to see where they would like to start. Do not assume you know best because you are the nurse. Clients usually have personal preferences for where to begin working on their healthcare problems. Whereas you might go from easiest to most difficult, your client may want to work on the most complex problem first.

6. Do not negotiate nursing strategy if there is in fact no choice for your client. Occasionally the philosophy of the institution in which you work, technical policies, time, and/or staff shortages dictate the prioritization and methodology. Most clients resent being given the false impression that they have some choice.

7. Before you do something for your clients, ask yourself: Could my clients be doing this (turning, transferring, making a telephone call, speaking to a relative, making a bed, changing a dressing) for themselves? By doing for our clients we rob them of the opportunity to discover their own power to take care of themselves. Every time we provide clients with the wherewithal (information, equipment, contacts) to do something for themselves, we save ourselves time and energy, two precious commodities in this time of tight restraint on health dollars, and we empower clients.

8. Remember to evaluate with your clients. If you have been successful in collaborating through all the steps of the nursing process, then continue your good performance through this last phase. The only way to know if your clients are satisfied with the outcomes of your nursing care is to ask for, and listen to, their opinions.

9. Keep in mind that validating is an assertive act. We are not effective when we hesitate to express our points of view or shy away from seeking those of our clients. Validation does not mean commanding or coercing clients. Mutual problem solving is a two-way street; open communication is exchanged between clients and nurses.

Client–Nurse Contracts

Once you have mastered the skills of validation and mutual problem solving, you have the basic ingredients for making a contract with your client. This agreement involves formalizing many of the steps you already carry out in your nursing practice.

Moments of Connection . . .
Partners in Life and Death

A neonatal intensive care unit (NICU) was caring for a premature infant who was near death. The parents were concerned that their baby had never experienced anything but the NICU environment in 7 months of life. The nurse and family decided to take the baby outside to feel the sun on his face and to see the flowers. The nurse bagged the baby while the family introduced him to the family dog. There was a brief rain shower that washed the baby's face. It was a beautiful experience to see their final moments with their baby.

A contract is an agreement between you and your client outlining the activities and responsibilities for each party (Box 3-1). The contract is often a motivator for learning for both client and staff (Rankin and Stallings, 1990). Contracts should be realistic, spell out measurable behaviors, have dates of expected completion, be worded positively, and build in rewards for success. In a formal contract both parties indicate their availability, the time and skills they will contribute, the commitments they will make, and the areas for which they will assume responsibility to improve the health status of the client. This negotiation can usually be covered in a verbal agreement. In some situations you may wish to create a written, signed agreement.

Under the terms of a contract both parties must fulfill their complementary obligations. Nurses have the right to make their clients aware of any occasion on which they have not carried out those tasks to which they have agreed, and clients can indicate to their nurses any occasion on which the nurse has reneged on his or her part of the bargain. Similarly both parties are eligible for praise when they have successfully accomplished their respective tasks.

When nurses and clients have both done their parts to perform the agreed on activities, they can evaluate the effectiveness of their efforts and determine if their contract has been completed. A contract provides standards for evaluation because the expected outcomes are clearly delineated (Rankin and Stallings, 1990). If both parties are satisfied with the results, the contract can be terminated. If clients want more treatment, they must negotiate with their nurses, who may or may not be willing to continue. Conversely, it may be nurses who want their clients to do more for themselves or to reach a higher level of health. If so, they must entice their clients to pursue further treatment and make clear their own part in the extended contract.

Sometimes clients try to extract a promise from their nurses to hold certain information in confidence. This should be a red flag. Nurses can say that they are obligated to share any information that is important to their clients' well-being. Such a request may precede the revealing of information that clients are planning to harm themselves or others. Such a contract of confidentiality cannot be made before or after such information is disclosed. If you must reveal something your clients have told you in confidence, explain that you cannot withhold potentially harmful information.

Through participation in a contract, clients can take personal control of their health rather than becoming passive recipients of healthcare directed by the provider. As clients become more assertive about taking an active part in their healthcare planning, nurses are forced to respond by renegotiating the terms of their mutual commitment. As nurses become more vocal about their contribution to healthcare, they become more accountable. Whether for legal, ethical, or philosophical reasons, nurses are likely to become much more explicit about the terms of contracts with their clients in the years to come.

It is important to remember that life's problems sometimes require the healing power of time for resolution. Sometimes simply assisting your client to set a goal for the day can start the day on a positive note. Take time to review progress with the client to assess whether the goal has been achieved and if modification is needed (Yetter, 2010). Nurses, clients, family members, and colleagues all share in common their own humanity, working to solve problems—this is the beauty and the challenge of the situation!

| **Box 3-1** | *Elements of a Client–Nurse Contract* |

The following is a list of components of a client–nurse contract for you to adapt to your workplace:
- Names of client and nurse
- Purpose of the client–nurse relationship
- Roles of client and nurse
- Responsibilities of client and nurse
- Expectations of client and nurse
- Specific details such as meeting times and structure for confidentiality
- Conditions for termination

Modified from Stuart GW: *Principles and practice of psychiatric nursing,* ed 9, St. Louis, 2009, Mosby.

If you can't solve the problem, at least have a good laugh together!

Author Unknown

WIT&_Wisdom_

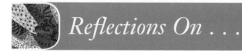

Reflections On . . .

Solving Problems Together

Consider what you read about mutual problem solving in nursing and how you can involve clients in the implementation of the nursing process.

What? . . .

Write one thing you learned from this chapter.

So what? . . .

How will this affect your nursing practice?

Now what? . . .

How will you implement this new knowledge or skill?

Think about it . . .

Practicing Solving Problems Together

Exercise 1

For each of the following client situations, describe what you would say to these clients to encourage them to take a more active part in their healthcare.

1. Mr. Bane is a 33-year-old client newly diagnosed with epilepsy. He has to take medication every 4 hours.
2. Mrs. McNeil is a 63-year-old client with arthritis. She has been urged by her physician to do wrist and finger range-of-motion exercises three times a day.
3. Johnny is a 17-year-old client who has been advised to use specially prepared soap for his facial acne.
4. Beth is a tense young client who has been urged to meditate twice a day to promote relaxation.
5. Mr. Jameson has a high cholesterol level. He has been taught how to reduce the cholesterol in his diet. He selects his own menu daily.

Compare your strategies for approaching each client situation with the suggestions of your colleagues.

Exercise 2

For each of the following case studies write down how you would discuss the fact that your client has broken your mutual agreement about what actions he or she would take to improve his or her health status.

Write out specifically what you would say when you approached the topic with your client.

1. Miss Marson is a 19-year-old client admitted to the hospital for investigation of severe, debilitating headaches. She has agreed not to consume any of her own over-the-counter drugs to alleviate her pain while tests are being done to discover the source of her headaches. On your night rounds you find Miss Marson in the washroom swallowing one extra-strength pain reliever tablet and about to take another.
2. Mrs. Dodds is a 22-year-old client admitted for investigation of severe and rapid weight loss. She has agreed to stick to a bland diet while the reasons for her weight loss are being unearthed. On the evening shift you discover her eating spicy chili her visitor brought her from the local deli.
3. Mr. Jones is a 45-year-old patient who had surgery 5 hours earlier. Preoperatively he agreed to do his deep breathing and coughing after surgery, yet now he is adamant that he has no intention of letting you support his incision so that he can cough. He only wants to sleep peacefully.
4. You are completing a health history on a client who has had chest pain in the past few weeks. She agreed to bring the pertinent information about her family's cardiac health history to you at her appointment today. She comes in without the information, telling you that she was too busy with her friends this week to get the information from her aunt.

After you have done this exercise on your own, compare your responses with those of your colleagues in your class. Be aware of the many ways to assertively inform your clients that they are not completing part of the nursing care plan to which they agreed.

Exercise 3

In the following situation you and your client disagree about the priority of the client's health problem. Think about how you would assertively handle such a situation and be prepared to discuss your suggested strategies with your classmates.

Mrs. Boyd is a 30-year-old woman admitted for a cholecystectomy. She is 2 months postpartum and is eager to continue breast-feeding even though she is about to undergo surgery. You are concerned about

Continued

her physical health because Mrs. Boyd is lethargic and jaundiced and has dry, itchy skin and severe abdominal pain. She wishes to have her baby brought in to be nursed at his regular feeding periods. You would prefer that she get as much rest as possible and start her baby on formula feedings.

Mrs. Boyd believes strongly that breast-feeding is essential to the health of her baby. She acknowledges that it may be difficult to continue breast-feeding at this time, but she fears that if she stops she will not be able to restart, and then her baby will suffer. In addition, breast-feeding is a special part of being a nurturing mother for Mrs. Boyd, and she does not want to miss the experience.

Compare your strategy for working out this difference in priorities with Mrs. Boyd to the suggestions of your colleagues.

Exercise 4

The next time you are on the nursing unit on which you are doing your clinical course work, attempt to practice a mutual problem-solving approach with your assigned clients. Use the following questions to evaluate your ability to perform validation with your clients:

I. Assessment
  A. Assessing
    1. Do you provide clients with the opportunity to tell you what they know and believe about their health concerns?
    2. In what ways are your views about health congruent with your clients' views and in what ways are they divergent?
    3. What client knowledge gaps surfaced?
    4. What have you learned about your clients' health beliefs, healthcare habits, and problem-solving abilities?
  B. Validating the nursing diagnosis with your clients
    1. Do you determine what your clients think their problems are and what they think might be causing them?
    2. Do you inform your clients about your assessment of their health problem?
    3. Do you and your clients agree on the assessment?

    4. How do you handle the situation when you and your clients' views are disparate?
    5. Do you explore how your clients feel about their nursing diagnoses?
    6. How comfortable are you with sharing your views about the nursing diagnoses with your clients?

II. Planning
  A. Determining desired outcomes for your clients
    1. Are you and your clients in agreement about the desired outcomes?
    2. Are you realistic in your hopes and expectations for your clients' health?
    3. Are you and your clients able to agree on mutually acceptable outcomes?
  B. Choosing nursing strategies to help your clients achieve their expected and desired outcomes
    1. Do you take into account how your clients feel about the options?
    2. Do you take into account your clients' personal and cultural preferences, schedules, finances, and abilities?
    3. Are you able to inform your clients about the efficacy of the various options?
    4. Are you willing to express your opinions about the various treatment choices?

III. Implementation
  A. Implementing a plan of action to help meet your clients' needs
    1. How much consideration do you give to your clients' ability to carry out the action plans themselves?
    2. Do you do for your clients when they could be doing for themselves? Conversely, do you expect too much from your clients without adequately training them?
    3. Do you take the opportunity to find out how your clients feel about carrying out the action plans?
    4. Do you make certain your clients are ready and willing to continue with the plans?
    5. Do you make clear what your role is and what the role of your clients is?

IV. Evaluation

    A. Evaluating the outcomes together

        1. How extensively do you ask your clients their opinions and feelings about the outcomes of treatment to date?

        2. To what extent do you share your views about progress with your clients?

        3. How do you handle situations in which you and your clients disagree (they are pleased with the outcomes whereas you wish to persevere for greater excellence, or vice versa)?

        4. How well do you prepare your clients for terminating the client–nurse relationship?

Answering the questions posed previously will crystallize your awareness of how you may already be encouraging mutual problem solving with your clients and can stimulate your anticipation of ways in which you can facilitate even more interchange.

Exercise 5

The next time you are a client (of a lawyer, nurse, pastor, priest, rabbi, physician, or dentist), make note of how much this professional engages you in mutual problem solving. Notice exactly what the professional does to make you feel included in the planning.

- In what ways does the professional make you feel that your opinions are important?
- In what ways could this professional include you more in the problem-solving process?
- How do your feelings differ in a situation in which you are included and in one in which the professional takes over and does not consult you?

Compare your experiences with those of your classmates. What has this exercise taught you about mutual problem solving?

Exercise 6

Reflect upon what it means to allow someone to "save face." Consider ways in which a nurse can help elderly clients "save face" considering some of the limitations they encounter.

Exercise 7

Generate a list of topics you would find embarrassing in a conversation or assessment with clients and families. With other students or nurses, make a list of topics and discuss potential strategies to approach these topics and manage embarrassment for clients, family, and nurses.

Exercise 8

Begin a reflective journal of your clinical experiences to build your communication skills. Watch for examples of situations in which you had to communicate with clients and families about potentially embarrassing content and how you handled it. Begin now to think about publishing in your nursing career. Perhaps the content of your journal might make a good article for the Reflections section of *Imprint*, the publication of the National Student Nurses Association, www.nsna.org. For guidelines for publication, visit http://www.nsna.org/pubs/authorgd.asp.

Exercise 9

Consider the use of a collage, creating a picture from images and words cut from magazines and glued together onto paper or mat board, to help a client envision success and strategies for success for a health challenge such as losing weight. Try it yourself. Create a collage with the intention to see yourself as an expert nurse with a balanced life. Or, choose another intention for the collage. Take time to reflect on your art and write your thoughts and feelings about it. This will help you to facilitate the client's ability to process and learn from expressive art; see the article by Walsh and colleagues (2004) in the Suggestions for Further Reading.

> *It is good to be reminded that each of us has a different dream.*
>
> **Crow Indian proverb**
>
> **WIT&** *Wisdom*

References

American Nurses Association: *Standards of clinical nursing practice*, Atlanta, 2004, American Nurses Association.

Atwell A: Florence Nightingale's relevance to nurses, *J Holist Nurs* 28(1):101, March 2010.

Berg M: A midwifery model of care for childbearing women at high risk: genuine caring in caring for the genuine, *J Perinat Educ* 14(1):9, 2005.

Cauce AM, Srebnik DS: Returning to social support systems: a morphological analysis of social networks, *Am J Commun Psychol* 18:609, 1990.

Cerda JC, Rodriguez MAP, Corril OP, et al: Quality of internal communication in health care and the professional–patient relationship, *Health Care Manag* 29(2):179, 2010.

Chalmers KI: Mothers of children at risk described engaging with home visitors in terms of limiting family vulnerability, *Evid Based Nurs* 8(4):123, 2005.

Cooper MC, Powell E: Technology and care in a bone marrow transplant unit: creating and assuaging vulnerability, *Holist Nurs Pract* 12(4):57, 1998.

Geanellos R: Sustaining well-being and enabling recovery: the therapeutic effect of nurse friendliness on clients and nursing environments, *Contemp Nurse* 19(1–2):242, 2005.

Grando V: Articulating nursing for advanced nursing practice. In Sullivan T, editor: *Collaboration: a health care imperative*, New York, 1998, McGraw-Hill.

Grover SM: Shaping effective communication skills and therapeutic relationships at work: the foundation of collaboration, *AAOHN J* 53(4):177, 2005.

Hagerty BMK, Lynch-Sauer J, Patusky KL, et al: An emerging theory of human relatedness, *Image J Nurs Sch* 25(4):291, 1993.

Hallberg IR, Holst G, Nordmark A, et al: Cooperation during morning care between nurses and severely demented institutionalized patients, *Clin Nurs Res* 4(1):78, 1995.

Iyer PW, Taptich BJ, Bernocchi-Losey D: *Nursing process and nursing diagnosis*, Philadelphia, 1995, Saunders.

Jack SM: A theory of maternal engagement with public health nurses and family visitors, *J Adv Nurs* 49(2):182, 2005.

Jeon Y: Shaping mutuality: nurse-family caregiver interactions in caring for older people with depression, *Int J Ment Health Nurs* 13(2):126, 2004.

Koop CE: Patient–provider communication and managed care, *Med Pract Communicator* 5(4):1, 1998.

Lawson PJ, Flocke SA: Teachable moments for health behaviour change: a concept analysis, *Patient Educ Couns*, 76:25, 2009.

March P: Therapeutic reciprocity: a caring phenomenon, *Adv Nurs Sci* 13(1):49, 1990.

Matheis-Kraft C, George S, Olinger MJ, et al: Patient-driven healthcare works! *Nurs Manage* 21(9):124, 1990.

McCance T, Slater P, McCormack B: Using the caring dimensions inventory as an indicator of person-centered nursing, *J Clin Nurs*, 18:409, 2008.

Pillet-Shore D: Weighing in primary-care nurse-patient interactions, *Soc Sci Med* 62(2):407, 2006.

Porr C: Shifting from preconceptions to pure wonderment, *Nurs Philos* 6(3):189, 2005.

Rankin SH, Stallings KD: *Patient education: issues, principles, and practices*, ed 2, Philadelphia, 1990, Lippincott.

Roberts SJ, Krouse HJ, Michaud E: Negotiated and nonnegotiated nurse-patient interactions: enhancing perceptions of empowerment, *Clin Nurs Res* 4(1):67, 1995.

Schwertel-Kyle BA, Pitzer SA: A self-care approach to today's challenges, *Nurs Manage* 21(3):37, 1990.

Seifert, PC: Thinking critically, *AORN J* 91(2):197, 2010.

Spiers JA: The use of face work and politeness theory, *Qual Health Res* 8(1):25, 1998.

Tarlier DA: Beyond caring: the moral and ethical bases of responsive nurse–patient relationships, *Nurs Philos* 5(3):230, 2004.

Yetter D: Preserving a positive image of nursing in a complicated healthcare environment, *Nursing Made Incredibly Easy* 8(2):5–7, March/April 2010. www.NursingMadeincrediblyEasy.com.

Zoffmann V: Life versus disease in difficult diabetes care: conflicting perspectives disempower patients and professionals in problem solving, *Qual Health Res* 15(6):750, 2005.

Suggestions for Further Reading

Benson H: *The breakout principle: how to activate the natural trigger that maximizes creativity, productivity and personal well-being*, New York, 2004, Scribner. (Science-based path to breakthrough to solutions to blocks to problem-solving, creativity.)

Walsh S, Martin SC, Schmidt LA: Testing the efficacy of a creative-arts intervention with family caregivers of patients with cancer, *J Nurs Sch* 36(3):214, 2004.

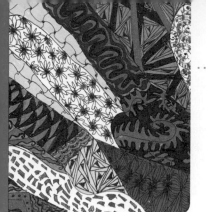

Chapter 4

Understanding Each Other: Communication and Culture

| CONTRIBUTED BY LOIS O. GONZALEZ, PhD, ARNP, BC, AND JULIA BALZER RILEY, RN, MN, AHN-BC |

> *The tongue slow and the eyes quick.*
> **Mexican proverb**

Objectives

1. Define culture, ethnicity, and ethnocentrism
2. Discuss reasons why nurses need to become informed about the healthcare beliefs and behaviors of diverse cultures
3. Discuss two common American values that may interfere with nurses' recognition and appreciation of the healthcare beliefs and behaviors of diverse cultures
4. Describe your own cultural background and its influence on your healthcare beliefs and behaviors
5. Identify the components of communication suggested for assessment in Purnell's model for cultural competence
6. Discuss techniques that enhance communication with clients from diverse cultures
7. Apply communication techniques to improve the care of clients from diverse cultures
8. Discuss how the variables of age and gender relate to culture and communication
9. Participate in exercises to build skills in understanding each other

Cultural competence is a major component in the quality and safety of care (Larson et al, 2010; Frohlich and Potvin, 2008). According to the Quality and Safety Education for Nurses (QSEN) Initiative, an understanding of how diverse cultural, ethnic, and social backgrounds function as sources of patient, family, and community values, is vital for today's future nurses (QSEN, 2010a). QSEN calls patient-centered care, which includes diversity, one of the six pillars of safe and effective nursing care, recognizing this competency as a required Knowledge, Skills, and Attitudes (KSAs) needed to promote patient safety (QSEN, 2010a). According to their definition, nurses should be able to

> "Provide patient-centered care with sensitivity and respect for the diversity of human experience. Seek learning opportunities with patients who represent all aspects of human diversity. Recognize personally held attitudes about working with patients from different ethnic, cultural and social backgrounds. Willingly support patient-centered care for individuals and groups whose values differ from own" (QSEN, 2010b).

Being culturally aware takes a great deal of commitment and effort on the part of the nurse. Merely talking about culture does not necessarily mean that you have translated knowledge into action. Individuals are not likely to translate cultural knowledge into behavior until they experience direct contact with people from other cultures. This exposure is becoming more and more inevitable in the United States.

Data from the 2010 census provide evidence that America is becoming even more racially and ethnically heterogeneous. Considerable growth among the Hispanic and Asian populations due to increased immigration and the decline of growth in the non-Hispanic White alone population are indications that America is becoming a nation with no ethnic majority (Humes et al, 2011). Recent projections indicate that by 2020 the white population will decrease by 53%, while the number of African Americans will double, and the number of Hispanic and Asian Americans will triple (Giger and Davidhizar, 1999). By 2050, no group will constitute more than 50% of the population (RAND, 2006). This multiracial, ethnically complex population will challenge U.S. healthcare providers who are attempting to offer culturally driven client care. Changing demographic trends indicate that America is making progress in efforts to reduce inequalities and barriers to opportunities. Unfortunately, despite improvements in access to healthcare across U.S. ethnic populations, disparities between the majority population and most ethnic groups still exist. Intercultural knowledge, communication, and competence will become necessities in almost every occupation (Weaver, 2000).

Eliminating racial and ethnic healthcare disparities is urgent, and our efforts must focus on social, cultural, and environmental factors that reach far beyond the traditional medical model. Effective communication between and among cultures is essential because it is the way that we interact globally. In the American healthcare setting, nurses indicate an understanding of the importance of communication and demonstrate awareness of the need for cultural awareness, but many have not operationalized into their practice the significance of culture. Because nurses spend more time with clients than do most other healthcare professionals, it is particularly important that nurses realize that both communication and culture are inextricably connected to healthcare. Nurses need to know about culture—their own and their clients'—because it influences both nurses' and clients' healthcare perceptions and behaviors.

The impact of culture and communication-related issues can be life threatening, particularly in cases in which there are differing perceptions and descriptions of pain. For example, an assessment of the quality of chest pain is a critical piece of data so that an acute myocardial infarction can be distinguished from other conditions causing pain in the chest or epigastric area. Missed diagnoses and delayed treatments occur when responses to pain are culturally dictated and an individual may delay coming for treatment because of fear, stoicism, or meanings attributed to pain. Such delays can be life threatening (Sobralske and Katz, 2005).

Negotiating a larger, white-dominated culture can be painful for minorities, particularly when people in the majority are not aware of cultural differences. After living for an extended period of time in a majority culture, a minority person can choose one of two paths. He or she can either become acculturated or live apart in isolation or within the safe boundaries of a familiar cultural neighborhood. The latter prevents participation in and enrichment of the larger culture, thwarting the development of increased multiculturalism in the community.

We are experiencing a nationwide increase in our multicultural society due to immigration migration within the United States because of posthurricane displacement to other areas of the country. When nursing experts are asked to predict the skills, education, and perspectives that nurses will need to prosper in the coming era, they suggest that nurses will need to demonstrate transcultural competence to employers and consumers (Alexander et al, 1998; Reeves and Fogg, 2006). However, some nurses still ask, "What's culture got to do with it?" After all, according to many Americans, healthcare is healthcare and we've got the best in the world. This ethnocentric attitude interferes with nurses' recognition and appreciation of a broad view of culture and communication. Everyone is familiar with the meaning of communication, but what is culture?

Definition of Culture, Ethnicity, and Ethnocentrism

Madeline Leininger defines *culture* as the learned and shared beliefs, values, and lifeways of a particular group that are generally transmitted intergenerationally and influence one's thinking and actions. For three decades, Leininger has emphasized the need for nurses to become informed about other cultures' healthcare beliefs and practices. Ethnicity also needs to be defined because some confuse its meaning with that of culture. According to Leininger, *ethnicity* refers to the social identity and origins of a social group due largely to language, religion, and national origin; for example, the Amish are an ethnic group. Sociologists and psychologists are more likely to use the term *ethnicity*. The term *culture* is used more frequently by anthropologists and transcultural nurses. Culture is a broader term because it refers to the holistic, patterned lifeways of a group rather than to selected ethnic features or origins (Leininger, 2002).

The term *ethnocentrism* was coined by William Graham Sumner, a social evolutionist and professor of political and social science at Yale University. He defined it as the universal tendency of people to believe that one's own race or ethnic group is the most important and/or that some or all aspects of its culture are superior to those of other groups (Salter, 2002). Furthermore, ethnocentrism perpetuates the attitude that beliefs differing greatly from one's own are strange, bizarre, or unenlightened, and therefore wrong (Purnell and Paulanka, 1998). Within this ideology, individuals will judge other groups in relation to their own particular ethnic group or culture, especially with concern to language, behavior, customs, and religion. These ethnic distinctions and subdivisions serve to define each ethnicity's unique cultural identity.

Reasons Why Nurses Need to Be Culturally Informed

There are several compelling reasons why nurses need to be informed about culture. First, shifting demographics will call for dramatic changes in the U.S. healthcare industry. The proportion of white Americans will significantly decrease by the mid–twenty-first century to approximately 51% of the total population. The literature suggests that Hispanics and nonwhites have much different patterns of healthcare than do non-Hispanic whites, with disparities in healthcare access accounting for a large portion of differences in use. It is projected, however, that demand for healthcare services by minorities is increasing as percentages within the population increase. Moreover, between 2000 and 2020, the percentage of total patient care hours that providers spend with minority clients will increase from 31% to 40% (Health Resources and Services Administration, 2006). With the increase in

nonwhite clients, it is imperative that healthcare professionals understand the importance of culture and its relationship to clients, their families, and the community (Zoucha, 2000).

Second, care is central to the concept of nursing. As technology becomes an increasingly important part of healthcare, the essence of human caring becomes the most valued aspect of nursing. The diversity of populations and the uniqueness of the caring phenomenon in these diverse practice settings provide the cultural basis of human caring (Brown, 2001).

Third, although the United States has always been a diverse society, this diversity has not always been recognized by healthcare providers, because they have long had the attitude that newcomers should adapt to "us." We as a society are beginning to recognize that this is not desirable, and it will not work in a heterogeneous society. As our patients become increasingly diverse, it is imperative that nurses be capable not only of understanding but also of working with those diverse groups in a productive (health-producing) way (Chrisman, 1993).

Furthermore, there are serious concerns that, overall, nursing education does not adequately prepare nurses to work with diverse populations. The teaching of cultural competence to nursing students commonly emphasizes cultural beliefs, values, and practices, rather than issues of race, gender, class, or sexual orientation. Although this approach has been somewhat successful in increasing practitioners' awareness of and sensitivity to cultural groups, it does not address other problems related to the nursing care of nondominant people. Culturally competent care cannot be provided unless underlying issues of discrimination are confronted (Abrums and Leppa, 2001). A study designed to uncover racial bias in nursing fundamentals textbooks found minimization of the effects of racism (Byrne, 2001). There is a concern about this educational omission because it limits students' understanding of the implications of racism to those inherent in power dynamics, namely oppression and subordination. In addition to implications for patient care such as delivery and disparity, nursing curricula typically do not include content on racism, oppression, and group dynamics within the nursing profession. When such controversial topics are omitted or minimized, students do not fully comprehend nor do they have the information necessary to detect, understand, and, therefore, change circumstances reflecting lack of cultural awareness.

Fourth, this is an age of economic imperatives. Our healthcare system is evolving toward an integrated system combining hospital and community facilities as well as physical health and mental health services, Western and traditional medicine, primary and tertiary care, technology and clinical practice, and so on. As providers and systems strive to gain market share, competition for clients increases. Regional systems, alliances, mergers, and networks have become commonplace (Chin, 2000). The increasing diversity of the overall population forces healthcare plans and organizations to ask whether their employees reflect the communities they serve. If they do, their ability to deliver culturally competent care is enhanced. If they do not, then a chance to improve the care experience for a large portion of their members is being lost, and the organization is missing an opportunity to gain a competitive edge in the marketplace.

The provision of publicly financed healthcare services is now being delegated to the private sector. Issues of concern in the current healthcare environment include the marketing of health services and the cost-effectiveness of healthcare delivery. The potential for improved services lies in state managed-care contracts that can increase retention and access to care, expand recruitment, and increase the satisfaction of individuals seeking healthcare services. To reach these outcomes, managed care plans must incorporate culturally competent policies, structures, and practices to provide services for people from diverse ethnic, racial, cultural, and linguistic backgrounds.

Finally, the issues of working with older clients and with the chronically ill are of immense importance. Chrisman (1993) suggests that there is an increasing number of cases in which healthcare personnel need to work in community settings and with whole families and in which the outcomes are not (and cannot be) the standard medical outcome of cure. Clearly, the achievement of nursing outcomes requires working with (versus working on) humans in settings in which the nurse has less control. Consequently, the client and family have more control than does the nurse, and culture has a strong effect on how people act.

In summary, nurses need to know about culture because it influences both nurses' and clients' healthcare perceptions and behaviors. Also, with healthcare moving into the community, if nurses expect to be part of this movement, they must know about the culture of diverse clients and communities. To achieve this outcome, nurses must first recognize and then overcome certain attitudes basic to the American culture.

Barriers That Interfere with Nurses' Recognition and Appreciation of Diverse Cultures

Despite notable progress in the overall health of Americans, there are continuing disparities in health status among African Americans, Hispanics, Native Americans, and Pacific Islanders, compared with the U.S. population as a whole. In addition, the healthcare system is becoming more challenged as the population becomes more ethnically diverse. Therefore, the future health of the U.S. population as a whole will be influenced substantially by improvements in the health of racial and ethnic minorities.

Cultural, ethnic, linguistic, and economic differences impact how individuals and groups access and use health, education, and social services. They can also present barriers to effective education and healthcare interventions. This is especially true when health educators or healthcare practitioners stereotype, misinterpret, make faulty assumptions, or otherwise mishandle their encounters with individuals and groups viewed as different in terms of their backgrounds and experiences. The demand for culturally competent healthcare in the United States is a direct result of the failure of the healthcare system to provide adequate care to all segments of the population.

Ethnocentrism interferes with the appreciation of diverse cultures and their accompanying beliefs and behaviors. On an international basis, the United States is considered to have the best healthcare system in the world. Western healthcare is traditionally seen as delivering topnotch high-technology care, yet being lacking because the care is reductionistic rather than holistic. Furthermore, the cost of the care is considered exorbitant relative to the outcome. Recognition of ethnocentrism is necessary to develop an appreciation of diverse cultures. One nurse put it this way:

> I always thought of myself as open, flexible, and reasonably unprejudiced; but I am not always! When caring for my friend from Saudi Arabia, I realized that, without knowing, I made value judgments. These judgments reflected my inability to accept that others handle the same data differently; and their perspectives are as important as mine.

We as nurses recognize that we need to know about delivering care to diverse clients, but how do we go about it? First, nurses need to become familiar with their own healthcare beliefs and behaviors, because without self-awareness, nurses cannot recognize that their beliefs and behaviors are not necessarily common to all. Nurses' lack of knowledge about their own culture can distort their perceptions of the beliefs and behaviors of clients from diverse cultures. It is logical that if a nurse does not understand the reasons for a client's behavior, then it is impossible for the nurse to implement appropriate interventions.

Your answers to the following questions are both interesting and important. For example, consider your answer to the question, "What did your family do to stay healthy?" If your family advocated taking a daily vitamin to stay healthy, how do you view a client who daily drinks a small amount of his own urine to promote health? How do you perceive the Cuban mother who tells you her child is very beautiful and healthy because he is fat?

"What did your family believe caused illness?" If you grew up in the United States, your family probably thought that illness was caused by germs and bacteria. This way of thinking contrasts greatly with that of a client from Thailand, who might believe that her liver cancer is a punishment for a wrongdoing, or that of a Mexican American client, who might believe his illness is a result of witchcraft.

"How were specific illnesses treated?" Americans use medication—over-the-counter or physician prescribed—to treat illnesses. Asian clients often prefer meditation rather than medication to treat illness. They believe that illness is a sign that the body is out of balance, and meditation helps restore the body's balance. How do you react when a client refuses morning care or breakfast because it is time to meditate?

"Who was responsible for deciding the appropriate treatment?" Because most Americans place a high value on individualism, the individual adult client usually decides what treatment he or she deems to be most appropriate. How do you perceive a female Hispanic client whose husband decides the preferred treatment for his wife? A nurse notes, "I had always thought the patient was the one making his decision but now I realize that many families, particularly Hispanic and Asian ones, think these are family affairs and not individual choices."

"What healthcare practitioners outside of the family were used to treat illness?" Most American families

eventually consult a medical doctor if illness persists and if home remedies do not work. How do you perceive a Mexican American client who prefers that a curandero (folk practitioner), not a physician, treat his liver disease?

It is interesting to compare the healthcare beliefs and behaviors of your family of origin with those of friends or other healthcare professionals. It often becomes apparent that your family's ideas and behaviors are not necessarily common to all. This recognition is an important step in not only identifying but also appreciating the healthcare beliefs and behaviors of diverse cultures.

Because cultures are so diverse, no one can possibly know all the unique aspects of each client's cultural healthcare beliefs and behaviors. To address this need, nurses and other healthcare professionals began to develop conceptual and theoretical frameworks for assessing, planning, and implementing culturally appropriate interventions. One of the most popular transcultural theoretical and conceptual frameworks is Leininger's sunrise model, which was designed for nursing (Leininger, 1988). Tripp-Reimer and Afifi (1989) suggest two processes that nurses may use to communicate with clients from diverse cultures: cultural assessment and cultural negotiation. Cultural assessment refers to the appraisal of a client's health beliefs and behaviors. The information is then used to determine appropriate nursing interventions. Cultural negotiation refers to the process of negotiating with the client regarding differences in the lay and professional belief systems concerning appropriate care.

Since Leininger's "first" cultural theory in nursing (1988), several transcultural frameworks or models have been proposed for nurses, including cultural assessment frameworks and models (Giger and Davidhizar, 1999; Purnell, 2002). Research suggests that culturally competent care brings positive health outcomes (Leininger, 1988; Smith, 1998; Zoucha, 1998). With the movement of healthcare to more community-based settings, nursing researchers have expanded on these models in order to predict public health outcomes of culturally competent care. Bernal (1993) suggested a framework for community-based care including the concepts of cultural self-awareness and self-efficacy. Kim-Godwin and colleagues (2001) proposed the Culturally Competent Community Care (CCCC) model built around three constructs of cultural competence, the healthcare system, and health outcomes. Four interdependent dimensions of cultural competence are caring, cultural sensitivity, cultural knowledge, and cultural skills. In the healthcare environment calling for more evidenced-based practice, the CCCC model provides specific guidelines for community-based nurses in developing and assessing cultural competence and meeting the healthcare needs of a diverse patient population.

With increasing frequency, a cultural assessment has become a standard of care in the initial client assessment in both acute and primary care settings. Consider reviewing the assessment tool that you use when you admit a client. How is the client's culture addressed in the tool? The model for cultural competence developed by Purnell and Paulanka (1998) provides you with ideas about other cultural components that may need to be addressed. The 12 domains essential for assessing the ethnocultural attributes of an individual, a family, or a group are as follows: overview, inhabited localities, and topography; communication; family roles and organization; workforce issues; biocultural ecology; high-risk health behaviors; nutrition; pregnancy and childbearing practices; death rituals; spirituality; healthcare practices; and healthcare practitioners. The domains are interconnected and have implications for health. Box 4-1 details the communication component of the model for cultural competence.

The components of communication listed in Box 4-1 provide the structure for a discussion of how culture affects communication in the context of providing healthcare to diverse clients. When cultural communication similarities and differences are identified, stereotyping should be avoided. All cultural groups share some communication practices, but broad cultural communication differences may also exist. It is dangerous to assume that all members of the same cultural group share the same communication characteristics.

Box 4-1	*Assessment of Characteristics of Clients' Communication*

DOMINANT LANGUAGE AND DIALECTS

1. Identify the dominant language of the group.
2. Identify dialects that may interfere with communications.
3. Explore contextual speech patterns of the group. What is the usual volume and tone of speech?

CULTURAL COMMUNICATION PATTERNS

1. Explore the willingness of individuals to share thoughts, feelings, and ideas.
2. Explore the practice and meaning of touch in the given society within the family, among friends, with strangers, with members of the same sex, with members of the opposite sex, and with healthcare providers.
3. Identify personal spatial and distancing characteristics during one-to-one communication. Explore how distancing changes with friends compared with strangers.
4. Explore the use of eye contact within the group. Does avoidance of eye contact have special meaning? How does eye contact vary among family, friends, and strangers? Does eye contact change among socioeconomic groups?

5. Explore the meaning of various facial expressions. Do specific facial expressions have special meanings? Do people tend to smile a lot? How are emotions displayed or not displayed in facial expressions?
6. Are there acceptable ways of standing and greeting outsiders?

TEMPORAL RELATIONSHIPS

1. Explore temporal relationships in the group. Are individuals primarily oriented to the past, present, or future? How do individuals see the context of past, present, and future?
2. Identify differences in the interpretation of social time versus clock time.
3. Explore how time factors are interpreted by the group. Are individuals expected to be punctual in arrival to jobs, appointments, and social engagements?

FORMAT FOR NAMES

1. Explore the format for personal names.
2. How does the individual expect to be greeted by strangers and healthcare practitioners?

From Purnell L, Paulanka B: *Transcultural health care: a culturally competent approach*, Philadelphia, 1998, FA Davis.

Dominant Language and Dialects

Wouldn't it be great if all of our clients spoke fluent English? It is important to realize that such thinking is grandiose and ethnocentric. Cultural diversity is the current reality. We have a growing population composed of people from a variety of cultural and ethnic groups. In the twenty-first century, nurses are confronted with the challenge of providing healthcare services to these clients. How do you care for clients when communication is significantly impaired because you do not speak the same language? One nurse describes such a situation:

> I had a Vietnamese gentleman in for hernia surgery. He had been in this country for 2 weeks, and his hernia needed to be repaired before he could start work. He spoke no English, nor did his family, and an interpreter was not available. The only tools available were body language, and hard as that was, we were able to communicate to a small degree. It was very difficult to explain anesthesia. He looked scared; he kept his eyes closed most of the time in pre-op. It was as if he was pretending he wasn't there. Surgery moves relatively fast, so there wasn't a lot of time prior to induction. I'm sure the recovery process was equally as difficult and frightening for this man.

The nurse in the preceding scenario poignantly identifies the difficulties and anxieties inherent in working with hospitalized clients who are not fluent in English. The client's anxiety is much greater than that of the staff. Hospitalization is always a crisis. Add to this crisis the anxiety in not being able to communicate your symptoms, perceptions, needs, and questions. The solution is to provide medical interpreters; they are essential to the delivery of culturally competent care. Certification of medical interpreters would help ensure a high quality of care to clients who are not fluent in English (Lester, 1998). Box 4-2 provides guidelines for communicating with non–English-speaking clients that may be useful until medical interpreters become consistently available.

Professional interpreters are better able to communicate medical terms and can be of assistance in reducing the risks of breaches in patient privacy and confidentiality. This risk occurs when medical professionals call on family members or volunteers to serve as go-betweens for the health professional and patient. Patients are often uncomfortable sharing

---

Box 4-2 | *Guidelines for Communicating with Non–English-speaking Clients*

1. IF THERE *IS* AN INTERPRETER AVAILABLE:
- Use dialect-specific interpreters, when possible.
- Give the client and interpreter time alone together.
- Avoid using children and relatives as interpreters.
- Select same-age and same-gender interpreters.
- Address your questions to the client, not the interpreter.

2. IF THERE *IS NOT* AN INTERPRETER AVAILABLE:
- Determine whether there is a third language that both you and the client speak. It is common for clients from diverse cultures to speak several languages.
- Remember that nonverbal communication is more important than verbal communication.
- Be attentive to both your own and the client's nonverbal messages.
- Pantomime simple words and actions.
- Remember: a picture is worth a thousand words. Use paper and pencil and also give them to the client.
- Talk with the administration about the importance of using trained medical interpreters when caring for the non–English-speaking client.
- Until medical interpreters are available, use both formal and informal networking to locate a suitable interpreter. If all else fails, owners of ethnic restaurants and grocery stores may be sources for locating interpreters or translators.

---

sensitive information through relatives or friends. An interpreter is focused on two-way conversation, interpreting the question from the nurse to the patient, listening to the patient's response, and then relaying the information back to the nurse. A family member who is caught up in a crisis, such as a visit to the emergency department, may relay information about their loved one but fail to direct the question from the healthcare provider directly to the patient. A trained interpreter might have avoided this problem (Greenbaum and Flores, 2004).

Because nurses care for clients from diverse cultures, they can expect that the client's first language is often a language other than English. The use of professionally trained interpreters is ideal, but such interpreters are rarely available. Clients frequently know at least a little English. Nurses often find that they need to just plunge in when communicating with a client who knows little English: "I hope I get over it, but I always feel silly when I try to communicate with someone who speaks only a little English. I feel like a little kid—I try to use a lot of gestures. It is really awkward for me; I get so embarrassed. But then I realize how awkward it is for the client to try to speak English. He's got to feel that he's in a place with a lot of foreigners who are responsible for treating him. That's got to be really scary!" Box 4-3 provides guidelines for communicating with clients who speak some English.

There is more to language than understanding the meaning of words. Tone and volume of voice are also important aspects of communication. For example,

European Americans generally talk loudly in comparison to people from Thailand. A nurse from Thailand says, "Thai people are very quiet because they believe that talking too much is a sign of stupidity and ignorance. If you talk a lot, you probably don't think a lot." Cuban Americans are frequently viewed as loud and boisterous because they speak loudly and quickly. A Cuban nurse relates: "Our language (Spanish) is everything to us. We're proud to speak it loudly—we love to socialize anywhere with family and friends." It is important that nurses not misinterpret differences in voice tone and volume; they may be cultural.

It is helpful if language interpreters are also able to function as cultural interpreters who are able to teach healthcare providers about cultural context as an adjunct to language interpretation. If the community has a large percentage of a particular cultural group, additional cultural interpreters may be recruited from the community. Community leaders might be encouraged to become involved in identifying potential volunteers and to become actively involved in their training (Green-Hernandez et al, 2004). Several years ago, one of the local health departments in the Tampa Bay area identified a migrant worker from a rural area who was well respected in the community. She was recruited as an interpreter and hired full-time by a satellite clinic of the health department to serve the Spanish-speaking migrant population who did seasonal agricultural work in the area.

Cultural Communication Patterns

Communication patterns are an important part of every culture. Box 4-4 offers general guidelines for improving cross-cultural communications.

The nurse must interact with the client to put into practice the guidelines in Box 4-3. This is very important! This is not the time to follow the old adage, "Don't talk to strangers." All too often, nurses seem to apply this saying to clients from different cultures. It is easy to avoid clients whose healthcare beliefs and behaviors are "different" (Box 4-5).

Cultural differences are seen in the willingness of individuals to share thoughts and feelings. European Americans are quite open to discussing feelings about almost any topic. This contrasts with Asian Americans, who do not value the display of strong feelings and believe that personal thoughts are to be shared only

---

Box 4-3	*Guidelines for Communicating with Clients Who Are Partially Fluent in English*

1. Assess the client's nonverbal as well as verbal communication.
2. Keep your eyes at approximately the same level as the client's. This probably means you will sit. Assess whether the client is comfortable with eye contact.
3. Speak slowly and never loudly (unless the client has a hearing impairment).
4. Use pictures when possible (remember: a picture is worth a thousand words).
5. Avoid using technical terms.
6. Ask for feedback. Provide the client with paper and pencil.
7. Remember that clients understand more than they can express—they need time to think in their own language.
8. Remember that stress interferes with the client's ability to think and speak in English.

| **Box 4-4** | *Guidelines for Improving Cross-cultural Communications (L.E.A.R.N.)* |

- **L**isten with sympathy and understanding to the client's perception of the problem.
- **E**xplain your perceptions of the problem.
- **A**cknowledge and discuss the differences and similarities.
- **R**ecommend treatment.
- **N**egotiate agreement.

From Buchwald D, Caralis P, Gany F, et al: Caring for patients in a multicultural society: five vignettes of cross-cultural care, *Patient Care* 28:105, 1994.

| **Box 4-5** | *Avoidance of Clients Who Are "Different"* |

"I've noticed nurses ignoring people who are different. I don't think they do it intentionally, but out of frustration at not being able to communicate, they stay out of the room. Recently we treated an older Cuban woman who only spoke Spanish. She wouldn't eat the hospital food and took some strange herbs. Her daughter was the only family member who spoke English. When her daughter was at her side, the interaction was easy—when her daughter wasn't, there was no interaction. She would look at us with big, wide-open eyes. It was easier to stay out of there than to go in and feel helpless."

with close friends and family. This fact is respected by the faculty of a college of nursing in California. Students are no longer required to keep journals as part of course requirements because it was not a culturally appropriate assignment for the many Asian students.

The acceptability of touch varies considerably among cultures. In Arab and Hispanic cultures, male healthcare professionals may not touch or examine certain parts of the female body (Andrews and Boyle, 1999). Visitors to France note that both French men and French women greet each other with a kiss or kisses on the cheek. Young men in India walk down the street with their arms on each others' shoulders.

Different cultures prefer different degrees of closeness in personal space. In general, the British, Canadians, and middle-class Americans feel uncomfortable when forced to stand close to people they do not know well. The United States is a vast country, and historically Americans are used to a lot of space. Latin Americans, African Americans, Indonesians, Arabs, and the French welcome physical closeness (Luckmann, 2000). In addition, maintaining direct eye contact is an important expectation in American culture. This is not a universal standard, however, as one nurse learned: "Since I am a person who values eye contact, it was interesting to me to find out that this can be cultural. Previously, I assumed a lack of eye contact correlated with a lack of self-esteem."

It is important for nurses to recognize that eye contact is often cultural. For example, some Asians and Native Americans believe that prolonged eye contact is rude and intrusive (Luckmann, 2000). Muslim Arab women may not have eye contact with males, with the exception of their husbands. Hasidic Jewish men have culturally based norms concerning eye contact with women (Andrews and Boyle, 1999).

Variation in greetings is found from one culture to another. The handshake of an East Indian woman consists of a quick touch of the palms. Most East Indians bow the head, put the palms together, and say, "Namaste," which means "I bow to you—I respect the God in you, I join my hands in prayer for you because I respect you." In American culture, a firm handshake is expected.

Cultural communication patterns take on particular significance for the nurse making home visits (Narayan, 1997). A home visit may be refused if the nurse's communication is viewed as rude or inappropriate. For example, the nurse must keep in mind the social customs that are practiced when visiting a person of a given culture. It is of the utmost importance that the nurse demonstrate respect for the client. The home is the client's turf—the client has complete control. The following points must be kept in mind: How is respect conveyed in the client's culture? Are shoes removed before entering the home? Should you bow or shake the client's hand? Is a "proper" handshake firm or just a brief, light touch of the palms? The nurse knows the name of the person he or she is visiting, but how does the client prefer to be addressed?

Temporal Relationships

Americans expect punctuality and generally attach a negative meaning to what is viewed as "lateness." We have the expression "Time is money." The value placed on punctuality plays out in a strange way with appointments in the healthcare system. Clients are expected to be on time—often to find that they must wait at least an hour to be seen by the healthcare professional. Timeliness seems to refer to clients but not to healthcare providers. This double standard of punctuality must change.

The Navajo and other Native American tribes have a present time orientation. Consequently, they often fail to understand the relationship between a person's past activities and present illness (Plawecki et al, 1994; Flowers, 2005).

Numerous other cultures are much more flexible regarding time than are Americans: "I've learned from my Filipino friend that I don't have to set a specific time when I need to talk to her. I don't have to announce myself before making a visit. I can drop by her house at any time and it will be accepted in her culture—it's not in mine."

Format for Names

It is important to call a client by the name he or she prefers. Most Americans are comfortable with calling people by their first names. This is perceived by some, however, as a failure to show respect. It is important to ask a person how he or she prefers to be addressed, because considerable cultural variation exists.

Age

In the United States, the percentage of older adults in the general population is increasing rapidly, and the percentage of ethnic older adults is increasing at an even faster rate. Although individuals providing care to older adults are aware of these trends, cultural competence training is not an integral part of a health professional's education, nor are culturally competent care standards widespread in care facilities (Swanson, 2002). Ageism refers to the devaluing of older individuals—and it exists in the American culture.

Aging is generally viewed differently in Asian cultures. Increasing age is valued and respected because it brings knowledge and experience; the opinions of elders are held in high regard. Evidence of this is seen in India and Thailand, where few nursing homes exist. Elders live with their families and are cared for by them. Furthermore, in Hindi, the national language of India, the word *Buddha* means both "wise" and "old."

Ageism is particularly problematic in American culture because our society is aging. Older adults are avid consumers of healthcare and average nearly twice as many visits to their physicians as does the general population. Older adults and healthcare professionals may experience communication problems because of ageism. Examples of ageism include the healthcare professional's use of patronizing speech or the assumption that the older person does not understand. The key to effective delivery of healthcare to the elderly is recognition and respect of intergenerational differences by healthcare professionals (Bethea and Balazs, 1997). Because nurses spend more time with clients than do any other type of healthcare professional, nurses have the perfect opportunity to practice and then role-model care that facilitates communication across generations. Box 4-6 suggests communication strategies that healthcare professionals can use to improve healthcare delivery to older adults.

That the young do patronize the old in American society is commonly accepted. Many nurses have witnessed older clients being addressed with disrespectful terms such as "honey," "sweetheart," "gramps," and "granny" and other patronizing forms of speech. Older adults often construe improper behavior and communication on the part of caregivers as mistreatment (Mouton et al, 2005). Research conducted by Giles and Williams (1994) suggests that patronization is not a one-way street. Older adults also patronize young adults by using three distinct speech patterns—nonlistening, disapproving, and parental. This finding suggests the possibility of complex communication problems between healthcare professionals and clients because of the aging of our society. Not only are clients increasingly older, but healthcare professionals are also older and are taking care of young adult clients. Clearly, nurses must be aware of the fact that in the American culture, age is often a factor that influences verbal and nonverbal communication patterns with clients. If this is true for you, consider how it affects your delivery of healthcare services.

Box 4-6	*Communication Strategies to Improve Healthcare Delivery to Older Adults*

- Develop an increased awareness of ageist stereotyping in interactions between the healthcare professional and older client.
- View each interaction as a negotiation to reduce miscommunication.
- Develop a unique relationship with each client (a relational culture unique to each relationship).
- Promote the use of repetition and sensitive interrogation to help older adult clients understand technical jargon, diagnoses, and treatment options.
- Use metaphors and examples salient to individual clients' interests to explain medical terms and procedures.
- Enhance the relational interaction on an affective level so clients will be satisfied and remain loyal.
- Develop a holistic understanding of each client by listening to client narratives and historical life reviews. Consider the use of a tape recorder to collect client information and a database management system to refer to client history before client visits.
- Understand clients in relation to their cohort membership and its effects on their expectations of the healthcare professional–client interaction.

From Bethea L, Balazs A: Improving intergenerational health care communications, *J Health Commun* 2(2):129, 1997.

Gender

Perhaps the most significant cultural communication problems are those that exist between men and women because they transcend all cultures. Males and females are socialized differently worldwide, and this is thought to account for differences in behavior.

In the United States the differences in socialization are believed to account for the fact that American women are typically credited with being more expressive and relationship oriented. Women are thought to value intimacy more than do men. Men, on the other hand, are thought to value power and social status and to be more concerned with gathering and processing information. American society provides us with many examples of the frustrations experienced because of the differences in male–female communication values and styles: country and Western music woefully describes many situations in which men and women cause each other great grief, television soap operas give day-to-day accounts of the triumphs and tragedies (mostly tragedies) that envelop male–female relationships, and a favorite topic of Broadway plays is the struggle between men and women. Comic defenses of the caveman seek to explain the differences in actions and interactions between the sexes. In the ever-popular *My Fair Lady*, Professor Henry Higgins asks, "Why can't a woman be more like a man?"

Current interest in enhancing male–female communication is evidenced by the popularity of books that focus on improving relationships between men and women. John Gray, in his bestseller *Men Are from Mars, Women Are from Venus: A Practical Guide for Improving Communication and Getting What You Want in Your Relationship* (1992), focuses on differences between men and women. He explores how gender differences can create conflicts that prevent the development of mutually fulfilling loving relationships. This best-selling book is an excellent guide for achieving deeper and more satisfying male–female relationships.

Another popular author who deals with intergender communication is Deborah Tannen. In *You Just Don't Understand: Women and Men in Conversation* (2001), she focuses on patterns of one-to-one conversational style between intimates and friends that are influenced by gender. Her book is based on the assumption that children learn styles of communication as they grow up and that they tend to play in sex-separated groups. Styles of communication that differ by gender are practiced and reinforced. She focuses on male–female communication as cross-cultural communication. Her book *Talking from 9 to 5: How Women's and Men's Conversational Styles Affect Who Gets Heard, Who Gets Credit, and What Gets Done at Work* (1994) focuses on private speaking in a public context—the talk that goes on at work. This book is particularly useful to nurses because it can be used to explore gender differences in communication within the healthcare environment. Work is a unique place because, as we talk to get our jobs done, we are evaluated in various ways, and the evaluation is often based on how we talk. This presents a special challenge to women because the ways that women are expected to talk at work frequently differ from the ways that they are expected to talk in personal relationships. Tannen suggests that no one style of speaking is best and that we need to become aware of and learn from other communication styles and develop flexibility.

Research (Michaud and Warner, 1997) validates Tannen's suggestion that consistent gender differences exist in communication styles used at work—particularly in response to "troubles talk." Men are more likely to tell a joke or change the subject—to avoid the issue. Women are more likely to offer sympathy—to be supportive.

Given that the majority of physicians are men and the majority of nurses are women, it is important to be informed about the influence that gender may have on communication. Gender issues may interfere with nurse–physician communication and the retention of nurses.

The current nursing shortage has drawn attention to the need for more effective ways to recruit and retain nurses. Rosenstein (2002) surveyed nurses, physicians, and executives in a large network of hospitals. The goal of the survey was to assess the atmosphere and significance of nurse–physician relationships and to determine the influence of disruptive physician behavior on nurse satisfaction and retention. The survey found that some of the issues of concern to nurses relate to the male-dominated physician and administrative cultures, which view nursing as a subservient role and in which disruptive physician behavior is tolerated because physicians bring revenue to the hospital. The respondents suggested the need to emphasize the connection among communication, collaboration, and teamwork, which ultimately results in improved quality of client care.

Communication between physicians and nurses in hospital settings has been found to be the single most important predictor of mortality rates. Furthermore, one of the characteristics of magnet hospitals (found to have lower mortality rates than nonmagnet hospitals) is good nurse–physician relationships (Mason, 2002).

Learning how to deal with gender issues in the current healthcare work environment may be one way of improving the delivery of comprehensive nursing care. Following are five strategies to improve communication between nurses and physicians:

1. *Level the playing field*: Nurses, who are generally women, need to understand and play by the male

rules, rather than spending time complaining about them. The rules are the following:

2. *Get to the point*: Simplicity of speech is recommended. "Just the facts" is a valuable communication strategy. Men prefer direct communication with few words. Focus on the goal, not the process. The nurse executive will find that the process skills that are helpful when working with women may be detrimental when working with men.

3. *Use powerful prose*: Fear of being viewed as aggressive has stifled many nurses from stating the obvious in client care situations. Terms and phrases such as "I'm not sure" and "maybe" are not nearly as powerful in interactions as are statements such as "I think so" and "I know." The female nursing executive must behave in competitive, aggressive ways to acquire the resources and influence that the profession of nursing requires. Men expect competition. Women are expected to be "nice." Nurses frequently equate polite behavior with professional respect, a view not necessarily shared by men.

4. *Exude expertise*: Nurses have information about clients that other members of the healthcare team need. How this information is imparted is important. A nurse who ends sentences with qualifiers and questions may come across as being unsure of what she is communicating. It is important to speak confidently and present yourself in a manner that makes it clear that you do not expect to be refuted. Women nursing executives may be faced with work environment problems that arise due to male predominance in administrative positions. They can experience short-term success by playing by male rules—be organized, get to the point, seek coaching from the boss, and maintain friendliness. Long-term success requires educating staff about gender differences (Helm, 1995).

5. *Expect respect*: Men interrupt more often than do women. A typical female response to being interrupted is to stop speaking. If nurses believe that what they have to say is important, the thing to do is change tactics and keep talking. Nurses must begin all interactions as though they expect respect.

A final way that men and women differ in communication strategies is that they often bring different rules of behavior to meetings. Men resist being influenced, particularly in public. Men are more likely to have a meeting before the meeting to get matters in order. Women often prefer to bring their ideas to the meeting for discussion with the group (Helm, 1995).

Given that men and women have been socialized differently, how do we best make use of these differences in nursing? Nurses' future success will be determined by how well they select the behaviors, either male or female, that best fit the situation. Male and female healthcare workers can learn from each other (Cummings, 1995).

Finally, a few words must be said about how Americans may view the lack of verbal communication, or silence. The meaning of silence in our culture is problematic because we tend to be verbal people. The significance may be ambiguous; does silence mean client satisfaction or suppressed dissatisfaction? Silence may also be cultural. For example, silence is highly valued in the Navajo culture. A person who hurries a conversation is thought to be rude. Lengthy periods of silence are used to think so that the spoken word will have significance (Andrews and Boyle, 1999).

Closing Thoughts

This chapter has focused on the importance of nurses' recognizing and appreciating healthcare beliefs and behaviors of diverse cultures. The QSEN initiative recommends that nurses seek out learning experiences with patients who represent all aspects of human diversity (QSEN, 2010b). Consider ways in which you may continue to build your cultural competence. Some schools of nursing have immersion courses in which you travel to another country. Participating students experienced a broader world view (Larson et al, 2010). A qualitative study of the lived experience of students who were involved in a study abroad program suggested participants gained an increase in awareness of diverse cultures as well as self-efficacy (Edmonds, 2010). As a nurse you can volunteer for a medical mission. Visit www.medicalmissions.org to see some of the current trips. A clinical experience in community health can provide service learning, where you learn about diversity while being actively involved in the community. Such courses, which include structure programs for community assessment and working with defined issues, promote the development of the delivery of culturally sensitive care (Amerson, 2010). Dealing with differences is important, but something can also be said for identifying the commonalities we

share as members of the human race. Recognition of commonalities builds bonds. For example, we all value our health and our families and we all want a better world for our children. Consideration of commonalities emphasizes the sameness of members of the human species. Recognizing and appreciating commonalities as well as differences provide a holistic or transpersonal way of viewing people. Transpersonal human caring may well be what Florence Nightingale had in mind, as reflected in her life's work and writings regarding holistic nursing (Watson, 1998).

Moments of Connection . . .
Empathy, Respect, and Genuineness

A nurse was assigned to care for an 83-year-old woman from a coastal mountain fishing village in Thailand. The client was diagnosed with liver cancer. Her two daughters served as interpreters. The client's deep religious beliefs in Buddhism were central to her life. Medications and tests were administered at times that were congruent with her schedule for religious practices (e.g., morning prayer, afternoon meditation, and evening devotion). Religious icons were allowed to be placed in close proximity to the client. It was observed that the client was drinking only the tea and juice sent on her dietary tray. Negotiations were made, with the advisement of the attending physician, to have the daughters bring traditional foods cooked at home. The nurse was made to feel welcomed when the dietary changes were made. The daughters brought in a huge basket of fruit for the unit staff. While interacting with the family, the nurse mentioned his interest in Asian cooking and in Buddhism. Soon after, the daughters brought the nurse dumplings and fragrant rice "especially for him." Within a short period of time, the unit was blessed with another huge basket of fruit and what the nurse called "the most fragrant flowers I have ever beheld." He was called into the room and was given special rare fruits that came from the Far East.

The nurse described his final interaction with the client and her family: "This would be the woman's last night at the unit, and the elderly lady reached out and touched my hand (she had never displayed something like this before). I turned to her family and noticed they were weeping. My throat thickened, and tears filled my own eyes. I bowed to my patient and walked out, knowing what it is like being in the presence of someone so much more aware of life than I will ever be."

Reflections On . . .

Understanding Each Other

Consider what you read about culture and what was new to you.

What? . . .

Write one thing you learned from this chapter.

So what? . . .

How will this affect your nursing practice?

Now what? . . .

How will you implement this new knowledge or skill?

Think about it . . .

Practicing Understanding Each Other

Exercise 1

Go to http://www.youtube.com/watch?v= o7YMuYs8VWs and listen to "Don't Laugh at Me," a song by Steve Seskin and Allen Shamblin, sung by Peter, Paul, and Mary. Or you can search for the lyrics. Write about a childhood experience of your own or one you witnessed in which being different was a source of pain.

Exercise 2

1. Write what you can remember about at least one client from another culture whom you have cared for or observed being cared for and with whom a communication problem existed.
2. Describe how application of a few of the communication techniques suggested in this chapter might have improved the outcome.

Exercise 3

Write the first words that come to mind when you contemplate being assigned to care for an "old" client. Reflect on how your expectations may influence the interaction.

Exercise 4

Identify a workplace interaction problem that may have been caused by gender differences in communication. Review the five strategies to improve communication between nurses and physicians and identify possible approaches to the workplace problem you identified.

Exercise 5

The following table depicts the minority population of Canada from the 2006 census. Assume that you have been invited to consult with a hospital serving a population with a similar breakdown in ethnic and racial population. What have you learned in this chapter that might be helpful in training the nursing staff, most of whom are probably members of the dominant white culture, to begin to develop cultural awareness? How might this have an impact on the provision of healthcare?

	POPULATION	PERCENTAGE OF POPULATION
South Asian	1,262,865	4%
Chinese	1,216,565	3.8%
Black	783,795	2.5%
Filipino	410,700	1.3%
Latin American	304,245	0.9%
Arab	265,550	0.8%
Southeast Asian	239,935	0.7%
West Asian	156,695	0.5%
Korean	141,890	0.4%
Japanese	81,300	0.2%
Multiple visible minority	133,120	0.4%
Visible minority (not included elsewhere)	71,420	0.2%
Total visible minority population	**5,068,095**	

From Statistics Canada: *2006 Census of Population*, Ottawa, 2006, Statistics Canada.

Exercise 6

Interview one person from a culture distinctly different from your own, someone who was born in another country and lived there past childhood. Discuss health practices related to that culture, selected traditional therapies used in health promotion, and maintenance and restoration, as well as any other interesting features about the culture and personal responses to the experience. Ask about remedies/treatments for a cold, pain, or other ailments. Discuss this person's view of western medicine. Write a reflective journal entry based on this experience.

WIT& *Wisdom*

Differing Gifts

There once was a class, "Diversity,"

Taught just to prevent adversity,

But we found there no rifts,

Only differing gifts,

Life being one grand university.

References

Abrums M, Leppa C: Beyond cultural competence: teaching about race, gender, class and sexual orientation, *J Nurs Educ* 40(6):270, 2001.

Alexander N, Bailey M, Curtin L: What you'll need to succeed, *Nursing* 28(5):57, 1998.

Amerson R: The impact of service learning on cultural competence, *Nurs Educ Perspect* 31(1):18, January/February 2010.

Andrews M, Boyle J: *Transcultural concepts in nursing care*, Philadelphia, 1999, JB Lippincott.

Bernal H: A model for delivering culture-relevant care in the community, *Public Health Nurs* 10(4):228, 1993.

Bethea L, Balazs A: Improving intergenerational health care communications, *J Health Commun* 2(2):129, 1997.

Brown B: Role of culture in nursing, *Nurs Admin Q* 25(3):vi, 2001.

Byrne MM: Uncovering racial bias in nursing fundamentals textbooks, *Nurs Health Care Perspect* 22(6):299, 2001.

Chin JL: Culturally competent health care, *Public Health Rep* 115:25, 2000.

Chrisman N: Personal communication, December 21, 1993.

Cummings S: Attila the Hun versus Attila the hen: gender socialization of the American nurse, *Nurs Admin Q* 19(2):19, 1995.

Edmonds ML: The lived experience of nursing students who study abroad, *Journal of Studies in International Education*, 14(5):545, November 2010.

Flowers DL: Culturally-competent nursing care for American Indian clients in a critical care setting, *Crit Care Nurse* 25(1):45, 2005.

Frohlich KL, Potvin L: The inequality paradox: The population approach and vulnerable populations, *Am J Public Health*, 98(2):216, 2008.

Giger J, Davidhizar R: *Transcultural nursing: assessment and intervention*, St. Louis, 1999, Mosby.

Giles H, Williams A: Patronizing the young: forms and evaluations, *Int J Aging Hum Dev* 39(1):33, 1994.

Gray J: *Men are from Mars, women are from Venus: a practical guide for improving communication and getting what you want in your relationships*, New York, 1992, HarperCollins.

Greenbaum M, Flores G: Lost in translation, *Mod Health* 34(18):21, 2004.

Green-Hernandez C, Quinn A, Denman-Vitale S, et al: Making nursing culturally competent, *Holist Nurs Pract* 18(4):215, 2004.

Health Resources and Services Administration (HRSA) Bureau of Health Professionals: *Changing demographics and the implications for physicians, nurses, and other health workers*, U.S. Department of Health and Human Services, 2006. http://bhpr.hrsa.gov/healthworkforce/reports/changingdemo/default.htm. Accessed April 2011.

Helm P: Getting beyond "she said, he said," *Nurs Admin Q* 19(2):6, 1995.

Humes KA, Jones NA, Ramirez RA: *Overview of race and hispanic origin: 2010*, US Census Bureau, 2011.

Kim-Godwin YS, Clarke PN, Barton L: A model for the delivery of culturally competent community care, *J Adv Nurs* 35(6):918, 2001.

Larson KL, Ott M, Miles JM : International cultural immersion: en vivo reflections of cultural competence, *J Cult Divers* 17(2):44–50, June 1, 2010.

Leininger M: Culture care theory: a major contribution to advance transcultural nursing knowledge and practices, *J Transcult Nurs* 13(3):189, 2002.

Leininger M: Leininger's theory of nursing: culture care diversity and universality, *Nurs Sci Q* 1(4):152, 1988.

Lester N: Cultural competence: a nursing dialogue, 1, *Am J Nurs* 98(8):26, 1998.

Luckmann J: *Transcultural communication in health care*, Toronto, 2000, Delmar/Thomson Learning.

Mason D: MD–RN: a tired old dance, *Am J Nurs* 102(6):7, 2002.

Michaud S, Warner R: Gender differences in self-reported response in troubles talk, *Sex Roles* 37(7/8):527, 1997.

Mouton CP, Larme AC, Alford CL, et al: Multiethnic perspective on elder mistreatment, *J Elder Abuse Negl* 17(2):21, 2005.

Narayan M: Cultural assessment in home healthcare, *Home Healthcare Nurse* 15(10 C):663, 1997.

Plawecki H, Sanchez T, Plawecki J: Cultural aspects of caring for Navajo Indian clients, *J Holist Nurs* 12(3):291, 1994.

Purnell L: The Purnell model for cultural competence, *J Transcult Nurs* 13(3):193, 2002.

Purnell L, Paulanka B: *Transcultural health care: a culturally competent approach*, Philadelphia, 1998, FA Davis.

Quality and Safety Education for Nurses (QSEN): Competency KSAs. (2010a). http://www.qsen.org/ksas_graduate.php#informatics. Accessed January 29, 2011.

Quality and Safety Education for Nurses (QSEN): Informatics Definition (2010b). http://www.qsen.org/definition.php?id=6. Accessed January 29, 2011.

RAND: *RAND Policy Brief: America becoming: the growing complexity of America's racial mosaic*. Population Matters, 2006. http://www.rand.org/pubs/research_briefs/RB5050/index1.html. Accessed January 20, 2007.

Reeves JS, Fogg C: Perceptions of graduating nursing students regarding life experiences that promote culturally competent care, *J Transcult Nurs* 17(2):171, 2006.

Rosenstein A: Nurse–physician relationships: impact on nurse satisfaction and retention, *Am J Nurs* 102(6):26, 2002.

Salter FK, editor: *Risky transactions: trust, kinship, and ethnicity*, Oxford/New York, 2002, Berghahn.

Smith LS: Cultural competence for nurses: canonical correlation of two culture scales, *J Cult Diversity* 5(4):120, 1998.

Sobralske M, Katz J: Culturally competent care of patients with acute chest pain, *J Am Acad Nurse Pract* 17(9):342, 2005.

Swanson E: Culturally competent care for older adults—we have a way to go, *J Gerontol Nurs* 28(7):3, 2002.

Tannen D: *Talking from 9 to 5: how women's and men's conversational styles affect who gets heard, who gets credit, and what gets done at work*, New York, 1994, William Morrow.

Tannen D: *You just don't understand: women and men in conversation*, New York, 2001, Quill.

Tripp-Reimer T, Afifi LA: Cross-cultural perspectives on patient teaching, *Nurs Clin North Am* 24(3):613, 1989.

Watson J: Florence Nightingale and the enduring legacy of transpersonal human caring, *J Holist Nurs* 16(2):292, 1998.

Weaver G: *Culture, communication and conflict: readings in intercultural relations*, Boston, 2000, Pearson Publishing.

Zoucha Z: The experiences of Mexican-Americans receiving professional nursing care: an ethnonursing study, *J Transcult Nurs* 9:34, 1998.

Zoucha Z: The keys to culturally sensitive care, *Am J Nurs* 100(2):24GG, 2000.

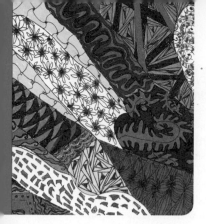

Chapter 5

Working Together in Groups

Objectives

1. Identify three essential conditions for group effectiveness
2. Identify four stages of group development
3. Examine how different mental processes affect behavior in groups
4. Identify maintenance roles of group members
5. Identify task roles of group members
6. Identify individual roles of group members that impede group progress
7. Apply the concept of emotional intelligence to groups
8. Discuss why meetings are important
9. Identify tools to promote effectiveness in meetings
10. Discuss characteristics of effective groups
11. Describe strategies to organize a committee
12. Participate in exercises to build skills in working together in groups

We have experience with groups in many arenas in our lives. A group is two or more people coming together to pursue common goals and/or interests (Varcarolis and Halter, 2010). Nurses have many opportunities to work in groups: staff meetings; patient care conferences; committees; project teams, such as quality improvement teams; multidisciplinary research teams (Weaver, 2008); and patient groups, such as support groups, either motivational or educational (Touhy and Jett, 2010). In a community setting, nurses may serve on boards or task forces as volunteers or political appointees. Psychiatric nurses may lead therapy groups. This chapter focuses on the dynamics of people working together in groups rather than on insight-oriented therapy groups, although some principles apply to all groups. Reynolds (2005) suggests that nurses need more education about group dynamics and that we cannot rely on working in groups just being common sense.

Communicating assertively in groups requires an understanding of group dynamics. This information can help you understand and modify your own behavior and help you to be a responsible group member. As you read, be thinking about your own experience in groups as a student, as a practitioner, and as a community member.

Three Conditions for Effective Group Development

Research demonstrates that three conditions must be met for effective group development: group members must trust one another; a sense of group identity must be present; and there must be a sense of group efficacy, a belief that the group can and will perform well, that the group as a whole performs better than individuals working on their own (Druskat, 2001; Gundry and LaMantia, 2001; Rosenthal, 2001). For these conditions to be met, the group must achieve high levels of participation, cooperation, and collaboration. Communication in groups is a blending of communication styles that may conflict or agree. Alessandra (2001) writes that a genuinely productive team "fully understands and savors its members' styles." Individuals must work together with a sense of belonging, yet each must still retain a sense of self, of a person with a personal history and story. Because obstacles exist to smooth communication in groups, it is important that there be a common purpose that is clear. As you learn more about the dynamics of people working together in a group, whether it be a team, a committee, or another form of group, consider that the group may be bigger in scope, intention, and power than the individuals of whom it is composed.

Four Stages of Group Development

Four stages occur in the development of a group or team, although there is no set time for these stages, and it may seem that members move back and forth among the stages. Understanding these stages promotes longevity of groups. The stages are forming, storming, norming, and performing (Tuckman, 1965; Stuart, 2009). Think about individual development and consider how these stages compare: forming is like childhood, storming is like adolescence, norming is like young adulthood, and performing is like adulthood (Box 5-1).

Effect of Personal Mental Processes on Behavior in Groups

People have preferences for and are most comfortable with certain styles of mental processing. These styles include extroversion versus introversion and intuitive versus sensing modes of perceiving. Group conflict may be a reflection of differences in the way people process data. As you read, consider how these differences can be gifts to the functioning of a group.

People characterized by extroversion talk to think. Extroverts think out loud and get their energy from fast-paced conversations with quick exchanges of partially formed ideas. They get excited about their ideas and do their best work when they have time to

| **Box 5-1** | *Stages of Group or Team Development* |

- In the *forming* stage, people are polite yet impersonal, unsure of their commitment. The team is figuring out team goals and beginning to obtain a clear idea of the work to be done. Members are testing group relationships to see how the work will get done and may want a dependent relationship with the leader or other group members.
- In the *storming* stage, overt or covert conflict may be evident. People may be hostile, engage in power struggles, be apathetic, and not be willing to work. They are resisting the process of teamwork, are resisting cohesion and collaboration, and do not have a commitment to the team. A hazard here is early termination of the group or committee when conflict surfaces and it is not understood as a healthy stage of building a cohesive group.
- In the *norming* stage, the group is getting organized, figuring out necessary rules and standards to get the work done, confronting problems and issues in a constructive way, and giving feedback. Members clarify the goals of the team, adopt new roles, define the tasks and procedures for the work to be done, and move into cohesion, collaboration, and commitment. The norms might be to turn off cell phones and beepers during the meeting, to arrive on time, to begin and end on time, to allow only one person to speak at a time, and to follow the agenda.
- In the *performing* stage, the work is getting done. People are open, can collaborate, are flexible, and are productive. They begin to do quality work, respect and support one another, motivate others by group achievement, and become flexible in their roles.

Modified from Tuckman B: Developmental sequence in small groups, *Psychol Bull* 63:384, 1965; and Stuart GW: *Principles and practice of psychiatric nursing*, ed 9, St. Louis, 2009, Mosby.

talk them through to a logical conclusion. These people are comfortable sharing an idea just to get others' reactions. This does not mean that they necessarily believe what they say.

People characterized by introversion think to talk. Introverts prefer to contemplate their ideas before sharing them. They use fewer, measured words and prefer not to share their ideas until their ideas are fully formed. They are less likely to respond quickly to questions because they wait to give their best answer.

> *Success is knowing the difference between cornering people and getting people in your corner.*
>
> **Bill Copeland**
>
> WIT&*Wisdom*

> WIT&*Wisdom*
>
> *For the Extrovert*
> It has been estimated that we have 15,000 thoughts per day. There is no need to share every one of these.

> WIT&*Wisdom*
>
> *For the Introvert*
> The giraffe can reach the tender leaves only by sticking its neck out.

Take a moment to consider whether extroversion or introversion sounds like your style. If group members are not aware of these different styles of thinking and sharing ideas, the people who talk to think, extroverts, may appear always to lead the discussion and to receive no help from those who think to talk. The extroverts resent the lack of participation of the quieter members, or perhaps they never even notice. The quieter members, the introverts, may believe their opinions are not wanted and stop trying. To honor these differences, the extroverts can practice their listening skills, understanding that silence may be needed for processing and that it does not necessarily mean consensus. They can consciously slow down and ask only one question at a time, allowing time for a response. The introverts can understand this and allow the extroverts time to process their ideas aloud. They can ask for a moment to think and take the initiative to make sure they are heard. With this knowledge, a group can avoid misunderstanding of each others' styles and confront this issue to continue to get the best of people's gifts. Some organizations provide staff with training in personality preferences, using a personality preference profile such as the Myers–Briggs Type Indicator (MBTI) and/or trained facilitators to promote richer problem solving that honors the different styles people bring to groups (Balzer Riley, 1997; Kroeger et al, 2002).

People with an intuitive style of perceiving see the big picture. Intuitive individuals look for the end product and anticipate it. They may skip steps on the way to the solution, thinking "A . . . oh, yes, D." In solving problems, they use and trust their intuition.

People with a sensing style collect data. Sensors want to know how many, how big, when, what, where, and who. They think "A . . . B . . . C . . ., and then D." They solve problems by collecting facts.

Big-picture people may present what seem like unrealistic, fantastic ideas. They may jump to conclusions without careful consideration of all the practicalities involved in implementing their ideas. These big-picture people, or intuitives, if they can laugh at themselves, will understand the one-liner, "The possibilities are endless." Data collectors, or sensors, may have trouble making a decision because they can never obtain all the data they would like. If these people can laugh at themselves, they will understand the one-liner, "Analysis paralysis."

To honor these differences, big-picture people, intuitives, can listen to the detail people, sensors, to avoid making hasty decisions. They can be more patient with the necessary process of attention to details. They can focus on the current issues to be resolved before a solution can be implemented. Data collectors, sensors, can give others time to express their ideas without rapid dismissal, so that the creativity may be harnessed. They can understand that all the little pieces fit together to make the big picture (Kroeger et al, 2002).

To apply these concepts to group decision making, consider these two kinds of thinkers as divergent thinkers and convergent thinkers. Divergent thinkers want to express their views and broaden the discussion; this approach is characterized by the generation of options, free discussion, and gathering of diverse opinions. Convergent thinkers want to move toward conclusions; this approach is characterized by the evaluation of options, summarization of key points, and sorting of ideas into categories (Kaner et al, 1996).

Task, Maintenance, and Individual Roles in Groups

In groups, people assume roles that can facilitate or impede the work of the group. Table 5-1 lists maintenance and task roles that help build group success. As you read, consider what roles you have played in groups and those you might be willing to assume. Table 5-2 describes roles that can hinder the progress of groups. Consider which of these behaviors you have observed in groups and honestly evaluate which roles you have played that you would be willing to reexamine and change.

Table 5-1 *Group Roles*

ROLE	FUNCTION
MAINTENANCE ROLES	
Encourager	To be a positive influence on the group
Harmonizer	To make/keep peace
Compromiser	To minimize conflict by seeking options
Gatekeeper	To determine the level of group acceptance of individual members
Follower	To serve as an interested audience
Rule maker	To set standards for group behaviors
Problem solver	To solve problems to allow the group to continue its work
TASK ROLES	
Leader	To set direction
Questioner	To clarify issues and information
Facilitator	To keep the group focused
Summarizer	To state the current position of the group
Evaluator	To assess the performance of the group
Initiator	To begin group discussion

Modified from Stuart GW: *Principles and practice of psychiatric nursing,* ed 9, St. Louis, 2009, Mosby.

Table 5-2 *Individual Roles That Impede Group Progress*

ROLE	DESCRIPTION
Aggressor	Annihilates other group members; destroys other members' self-esteem
Nonconformist	Finds something wrong with almost everything; very negative
Conformist	Agrees with everything
Recognition seeker	Wants to be the shining star; concerned with personal achievements
Self-confessor	Tries to use the group for therapy sessions; shares personal life
Silent one	Does not contribute
Know-it-all	Knows something about everything
Playboy/playgirl	Lacks interest and involvement; is not committed
Latecomer	Shows lack of respect for the group and wants to be seen as important

Modified from Stuart GW: *Principles and practice of psychiatric nursing,* ed 9, St. Louis, 2009, Mosby; and Balzer Riley J: *Instant tools for health care teams,* St. Louis, 1997, Mosby.

Emotional Intelligence in Groups

Emotional intelligence, a concept usually applied to individuals, is the ability to access, manage, and use one's feelings in relationships and is identified as the ingredient that distinguishes the most successful leaders in business (Goleman, 2000). In healthcare, technology may help us become more efficient but also can lead to isolation and alienation in staff as we depend on electronic forms of communication. Face-to-face meetings, led with the application of concepts of emotional intelligence, may build staff cohesion (Simpson and Keegan, 2002). Group emotional intelligence is about bringing emotions to the surface, understanding how they affect the team's work, and behaving inside and outside the group in ways that build relationships to strengthen the group's ability to face challenges. It is about small human acts in relationships that make a difference, such as saying "thank you" for extra effort from an individual (Druskat, 2001). Emotional intelligence competencies include goal commitment, empathy, confrontation, and caring

(Simpson and Keegan, 2002). See Box 5-2 for other suggestions for building group emotional intelligence for success.

> *Wise people seek solutions; the ignorant only cast blame.*
>
> **Lao Tzu (*Tao Te Ching*),**
> **as cited by Diane Dreher (1990)**
>
> **WIT&***Wisdom*

Importance of Meetings

Small groups come together frequently in our work world: to provide information, plan, problem solve, give feedback on performance, and make and evaluate decisions. If you spend 4 hours in meetings each week, that is over 9000 hours or more than 365 days in your life. Middle managers may spend as much as 35% of their work week in meetings (Doyle and Straus, 1993). This increases to 50% for those in top management. Such meetings are expensive to the organization; thus, it is important to make wise decisions about when to convene a meeting and to put in place strategies to increase the effectiveness of meetings (Doyle and Straus, 1993). Executives in one company reported that they waste 7.8 hours per week, or 2.3 months per year, in unnecessary meetings (Messmer, 2001).

To Meet or Not to Meet

A meeting is the best tool when face-to-face communication is needed. An e-mail memo and responses are no substitute for the timeliness of communicating in person and the ability to observe and respond to nonverbal behavior. The synergy of a group of people can produce creative solutions, and objections or problems can be addressed immediately. Staff meetings can create excitement and enthusiasm, more possible when people meet face-to-face (Overgaard, 2010). People who are involved in making a decision are more likely to support it. Successful meetings can increase a sense of belonging and build team spirit (Doyle and Straus, 1993). Research of nursing students working together in groups to study family health indicated higher critical thinking skills scores than those in a routine educational program (Khosravani et al, 2005). Law

---

Box 5-2	*Norms That Foster Emotional Intelligence in Groups*

- Use icebreakers to help group members get to know each other, have members share their thoughts and feelings in the group, and relieve stress with levity.
- Have a brief "check-in" from each member at the start of the meeting to see how everyone is doing and acknowledge a shift in group mood.
- Ask if each member agrees with a decision.
- Validate the contribution of members.
- Encourage members to help each other focus on the purpose or mission of the group.
- Build the expectation that the group can use humor to intervene in difficult group behaviors and encourage "inside" humor that evolves naturally from the group's history.
- Keep the group focused on problem solving, not blaming.
- Encourage team members to ask each other what they need.
- Anticipate and prepare for difficulties in the group's work.
- Periodically evaluate group effectiveness and individual member satisfaction.

Modified from Druskat VU: Building the emotional intelligence of groups, *Harv Bus Rev* 79(3):81, 2001; and Balzer Riley J: *Instant tools for health care teams*, St. Louis, 1997, Mosby.

---

students traditionally form study groups to prepare for classes.

There are instances in which a meeting is not the best use of time. Although it is not uncommon for a hospital to have large informational meetings on policy changes, there is no guarantee that people's minds are engaged when their bodies are present. Follow-up with written material may be helpful.

When one employee demonstrates a problem behavior, such as lateness to work, it is tempting for a manager to convene a staff meeting and address the "problem" of lateness. A more appropriate course, although sometimes uncomfortable, is to confront the employee with the problem to offer counseling, coaching, and eventually a reprimand if the problem is not resolved. To present this situation as a group problem creates anger and resentment.

If a decision has already been made or no option exists, it is inappropriate to call a meeting as if an employee group had the power to make the decision.

If you have only blue paint, don't ask the staff what color they would like the lounge to be painted.

Tools to Promote Effectiveness of Meetings

Provide an agenda for a meeting as an organizing framework and a template for the work to be accomplished. Distribute the agenda several days before the meeting so members can prepare their best thoughts and ideas on the issues to be discussed. Distinguish between action items, discussion items for future decisions, and informational items (Orlikoff and Totten, 2001). Include the amount of time available for discussion if appropriate.

Choose a person to function as a recorder for the meeting. The recorder takes notes on a flip chart, overhead transparency, whiteboard, or other memo board of what happens in the meeting. The recorder may abbreviate but does not paraphrase a contribution. The recorder may be someone who is not a member of the group, an appointed group member, or a volunteer member. This position might rotate among members. The record may include names of members present, members absent, and even members arriving late to draw attention to the importance of timely attendance. These notes become the basis for the minutes

or meetings notes that are kept as an ongoing record of the work of the group.

Consider the use of a facilitator, such as those in a quality improvement team. The facilitator's function is to focus on content issues; to keep the group on task; to point out process issues, or how a group works together (Schwarz, 2002); to summarize; to test for consensus; and to deal with problem behaviors that may impede the group's work if no facilitator is designated or if group members do not share the task role of facilitator. For example, to deal with the behavior of the latecomer, the facilitator might acknowledge the person: "Tom, glad you could come. You can catch up with where we are by looking at the recorder's notes." A facilitator can approach the person after the meeting and simply ask why the person was late. The facilitator can ask what would make the meeting important enough to come on time. To deal with someone who interrupts another member, the facilitator might immediately say, "Just a minute, Jane, let's let Sam finish before we hear your point." Asking the person who interrupts to assume the role of recorder may help the person to listen better and capture the energy of involvement (Doyle and Straus, 1993).

Characteristics of an Effective Group

Effective meetings accomplish the objectives of the meeting in the least amount of time possible and satisfy the participants (Haynes, 1997). Members of an effective group follow the strategies listed in Box 5-3.

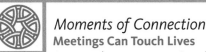

Moments of Connection
Meetings Can Touch Lives
    A nurse educator was moving after working for 13 years in training and development at a hospital. At her going-away party, one of the employees in the maintenance department sought her out to tell her that a meeting at which she spoke was the best meeting he had ever attended. She had been teaching an employee class on preventing human immunodeficiency virus infection and acquired immunodeficiency syndrome. He had listened with discomfort to the talk about the importance of using condoms but decided he needed to speak to his younger brother about it. He believed that might have saved his brother's life.

Box 5-3	*Members of an Effective Group . . .*

- Assume responsibility to share ideas and opinions and refuse to shut down. They participate willingly and communicate effectively.
- Negotiate and build consensus. They see an issue more than one way, share and value different ideas, and consider other viewpoints.
- Give and receive feedback even when it is difficult. They demonstrate a willingness to delay judgment and tolerate the confusion of a group working out its issues. They know that what seems like confusion might be a prelude to creativity.
- Commit to team goals to achieve the best outcome. They work to find a solution to which all group members are willing to commit rather than seek a quick compromise that may not receive the full support of members. They are willing to support the team's decision, knowing they have made their opinions known or chosen to support others' opinions.

Modified from Harrington-Mackin D: *The team building tool kit: tips, tactics, and rules for effective workplace teams*, New York, 1994, AMACOM; and Kaner S, Lind L, Toldi C, et al: *Facilitator's guide to participatory decision-making*, New York, 1996, New Society.

Strategies for Building Successful Committees

Understanding about working together in groups is essential for successful committee work. Pay attention to the movement of committees through the stages of group development and remember that the stage of storming is a time when committees may run into problems if group dynamics are not understood. See Box 5-4 for strategies for building a successful committee.

Box 5-4	*Strategies to Build a Successful Committee*

SELECT THE BEST MEMBERS
- Select staff who want to contribute to this particular task, such as a policy and procedures committee, and who have the energy and time.
- Select staff with appropriate work experience and education.
- Select an effective chairperson.

SELECT A WORKABLE NUMBER
- Six to eight is a good number.
- Clearly outline work.
- Communicate the tasks and responsibilities of the committee, how the committee's work is to be reported, and deadlines, if any.

SET EXPECTATIONS ABOUT ASSIGNMENTS
- To accept an assignment means to report on the work at the next meeting or on another designated date.

PROVIDE A WRITTEN AGENDA FOR EACH MEETING
- The agenda should be distributed several days before the meeting.

COMPILE WRITTEN RECORDS OF EACH MEETING
- Assign the role of recorder or obtain the commitment of a volunteer.

PROVIDE ADEQUATE MEETING SPACE
- Reserve a room with enough space and, if possible, use the same room for the duration of the committee.

WIT & *Wisdom*

The Team Pledge
We promise to:
Promote team spirit through genuine respect
for one another and consistent willingness to
cooperate, and by exhibiting a positive attitude and a sense of humor as measured by
observation and feedback.

Recognize and acknowledge each team
member's unique contribution by offering
encouragement, support, and appreciation
as measured by observation.

From Balzer Riley J: *Instant tools for health care teams,*
St. Louis, 1997, Mosby.

Reflections On . . .

Working Together in Groups

Consider what you have learned about working together
in groups and your own experience with groups and
meetings.

What? . . .
Write one thing you learned from this chapter.

So what? . . .
How will this affect your nursing practice?

Now what? . . .
How will you implement this new knowledge or skill?

Think about it . . .

Practicing Working Together in Groups

Exercise 1

Businesses are becoming innovative in finding ways
to help people work better in groups or teams. Try
the following activity from the fields of movement,
or improvisation to increase energy, understand how
team members work together, and tap kinesthetic
awareness of difference in groups.

For this you will need a bell or chime to stop, alter,
and start the movement as well as a room big enough

for all participants to walk freely through the space. If
you have only a small meeting room, divide the
groups so fewer people can move at one time, while
others observe. Explain the purpose of the activity;
invite participants to begin walking at an easy pace,
not all in the same direction or in a circle, and then
direct their walking with varied instructions such as
the following: Walk as if you are in a hurry. Walk
peacefully and contemplatively. Walk as if you are
fearful, anticipating danger. Walk with purpose and
determination. Ring the bell or sound the chime to
signal a change each time. After everyone has had a
chance to move, invite reflections about implications
for team collaboration. How are these different
courses of action similar to the action of a team?
How easy was it to navigate? (VanGundy and
Naiman, 2005).

Exercise 2

Match the following descriptions with the four
phases of group development:

_____ **1.** Forming **a.** Resistance and conflict are
expected now. There is little
or no evidence of group cohesion or team commit-
ment.

_____ **2.** Storming **b.** The work gets done. Team
members feel good about
their achievements and are
flexible in their roles to
meet team goals.

_____ **3.** Norming **c.** Team members clarify
group goals and figure out
the rules necessary to get
the work done.

_____ **4.** Performing **d.** Team members are polite,
begin to identify group
goals, and test relationships.

(Answers are at the end of the exercises in this chapter.)

Exercise 3

Review Table 5-1. Identify a group of which you are
currently a member or one in which you have been a
member. List the task and maintenance roles you
have seen in this group and the functions they ful-
filled in the group. Share your responses with another student.

Exercise 4

Review the individual roles listed in Table 5-1. Write an example of a role or roles you have played in a group and of others you have observed. Discuss this with another student.

Exercise 5

You are a nurse who is responsible for organizing the Nurse Week celebration committee. Outline the steps you will take to create an effective committee using the guidelines in this chapter and write a proposal for the creation of the committee.

Exercise 6

In a small student or staff group, plan a renewal activity, an outing together, or a potluck event. Pay attention to how your work together illustrates the content of this chapter. These skills would translate well to renewal of spirit in the workplace.

Answers to Exercise 2
1. d
2. a
3. c
4. b

References

Alessandra T: Team meetings, *Executive Excellence* 18(12):17, 2001.

Balzer Riley J: *Instant tools for health care teams*, St. Louis, 1997, Mosby.

Doyle M, Straus D: *How to make meetings work*, New York, 1993, Berkley Books.

Dreher D: *The Tao of Inner Peace*, New York, 1990, Plume/Penguin Putnam.

Druskat VU: Building the emotional intelligence of groups, *Harv Bus Rev* 79(3):80, 2001.

Goleman D: *Working with emotional intelligence*, New York, 2000, Bantam Doubleday Dell.

Gundry L, LaMantia L: Dream teams, *Executive Excellence* 18(10):13, 2001.

Haynes ME: *Effective meeting skills (50 minute series)*, Menlo Park, Calif, 1997, Crisp Publications.

Kaner S, Lind L, Toldi C, et al: *Facilitator's guide to participatory decision-making*, New York, 1996, New Society.

Khosravani S, Manoochehri H, Memarian R: Developing critical thinking skills in nursing students by group dynamics, *Internet J Adv Nurs Pract* 7(2):1, 2005.

Kroeger O, Thuesen JM, Rutledge H: *Type talk: the 16 personality types that determine how we live, love, and work*, New York, 2002, Dell.

Messmer M: Conducting effective meetings, *Strategic Finance* 82(12):8, 2001.

Orlikoff JE, Totten MK: How to run effective board meetings, *Trustee* 54(4):12, 2001.

Overgaard PM: 7 steps to highly effective staff meetings, *Nurs Manage* 41(3):54, 2010.

Reynolds F: *Communication and clinical effectiveness in rehabilitation*, Edinburgh, 2005, Elsevier.

Rosenthal MJ: High-performance teams, *Executive Excellence* 18(10):6, 2001.

Schwarz RM: *The skilled facilitator: practical wisdom for developing effective groups*, San Francisco, 2002, Jossey-Bass.

Simpson RL, Keegan AJ: How connected are you? Employing emotional intelligence in a high-tech world, *Nurs Admin Q* 26(2):80, 2002.

Stuart GW: *Principles and practice of psychiatric nursing*, ed 9, St. Louis, 2009, Mosby.

Touhy TA, Jett KF: *Ebersole and Hess' gerontological nursing & healthy aging*, ed 3, St. Louis, 2010, Mosby.

Tuckman B: Developmental sequence in small groups, *Psychol Bull* 63:384, 1965.

VanGundy AB, Naiman L: *Orchestrating collaboration at work: Using music, improvisation, storytelling, and other arts to improve teamwork*, San Francisco, 2003, 2005. [e-book], Pfeiffer, An Imprint of John Wiley & Sons, Inc.

Varcarolis EM, Halter MJ: *Foundations of psychiatric mental health nursing: a clinical approach*, ed 6, St. Louis, Mo, 2010, Saunders.

Weaver TE: Enhancing multiple disciplinary teamwork, *Nurs Outlook*, 56(3):108, 2008.

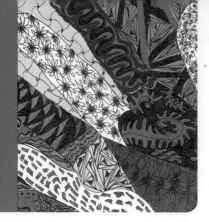

Chapter 6

The Changing World of Electronic Communication

| CONTRIBUTED BY CINDY CARTER, MSN, BSN, RN, IBCLC, RLC |

In 10 years we have seen the Internet go from a slow, stationary, information vending machine to a fast, mobile, communications appliance that fits in your pocket. Information has become portable, personalized, and participatory.

Susannah Fox (2010)

Objectives

1. Provide one reason nurses need knowledge of electronic communication
2. Discuss the role of a nursing informatician
3. Compare e-mail and texting and list one advantage for each
4. Explore the use of smartphones in healthcare
5. Discuss one aspect of social media as applicable to nursing
6. Name one healthcare application beneficial to nursing
7. Describe one type of electronic learning used in nursing
8. Name one reputable search engine for electronic nursing research
9. Examine clinical documentation in an electronic health record (EHR) system
10. Describe the dangers of electronic communication and how to avoid them
11. Participate in exercises to build skills in electronic communication

Nurses and Electronic Communication

Welcome to the world of electronic communication! You may already be deeply immersed in this world or it may be new to you. This chapter invites you to consider ways in which nursing and healthcare delivery is and will be changed by electronic communication. As you read, reflect on how you can continue to grow and stretch as the limits of our imagination are tested in this new world.

The nursing profession has changed. Nurses today are on the move. Keeping in touch requires a strategy different from that used by previous generations of nurses. Some of you may be reading this text through an electronic tool. You may be taking an online class. Nursing course delivery is changing.

If the way information is being received has changed, so has the way information is transmitted. According to a report by the Pew Internet and American Life Project (Rainie, 2009), communication in the United States is changing among people at all income levels and ages, with 73% of the American population now using the Internet or e-mail. Further research by the same organization has shown that 59% of those adults are accessing the Internet wirelessly (Smith, 2010).

With this rapid increase in mobile communication access, it is important for nurses to add an electronic communication skills set to their repertoire. The ability to type and computer literacy are necessary skills for busy nurses today (Cronenwett et al, 2007). Delaney (as cited by J. Karnas; Delaney, 2007) also agrees: "Informatics competencies are required for all nurses, whether generalists or specialists, to function in the 21st century."

In fact, socialization into nursing has a new context, with the focus today being on "building nursing intellectual capital" (Simpson, 2007). Simpson states that the changing healthcare environment "will demand nurses for whom technology use is as inherent as critical thinking." The National League of Nurses (NLN) agrees. One of their position statements recommends "preparing . . . nurses to practice in a technology-rich environment" (NLN, 2008).

According to the Quality and Safety Education for Nurses (QSEN) Initiative, informatics skills are vital for future nurses (QSEN, 2010a). As such, QSEN calls nursing informatics one of the six pillars of safe and effective nursing care, recognizing this competency as one of the required Knowledge, Skills, and Attitudes (KSAs) needed to promote patient safety. According to their definition, nurses should be able to "Use information and technology to communicate, manage knowledge, mitigate error, and support decision making" (QSEN, 2010b). It is recommended that these KSAs be part of simulations during nursing school to allow the student to begin to practice these core competencies needed by the nursing profession; as a result, they have found their way into the core curriculums of many universities and colleges. According to QSEN, registered nurses (RNs) are now required to be knowledge workers, system thinkers, and complex adaptive system managers, all of which require excellent communication skills in the midst of such a dynamic, interactive, and ever-changing practice.

Referring to the TIGER initiative recommendations (Technology Informatics Guiding Education Reform, 2007): "All nurses in every role must be prepared to make HIT [healthcare information technology] the stethoscope of the 21st century" (Westra and Delaney, 2008). Westra and Delaney also emphasized computer skills, informatics knowledge, and informatics as a skills triad needed by every nurse, from the bedside nurse to the chief executive nurse. Also recognizing this need, the Agency for Healthcare Research and Quality (AHRQ) has created several toolkits for healthcare IT, to facilitate the process of assisting all healthcare providers to become competent in healthcare IT (AHRQ, 2010).

Because of the challenges within the electronic side of healthcare in the past few decades, a new professional role has arisen: the nurse informatician. According to the American Nurses Association *Nursing Informatics: Scope & Standards of Practice*, nursing informatics is defined as "a specialty that integrates nursing science, computer science, and information science to manage and communicate data, knowledge, and wisdom in nursing practice" (American Nurses Association, 2008). As a nurse with education and experience on both the clinical side of nursing and IT, the nursing informatician focuses on the nurse workflow from the end-user point of view. Rather than having the nurse adjust his or her workflow to meet the electronic guidelines, this role works to have technology meet the nurse's current workflow. According to Simpson, a pioneer among nursing informaticians, "information technology can transform nursing tasks into nursing knowledge" (Simpson, 2007). The world of electronic communication within healthcare has changed forever.

Electronic Communication Defined

Telephones, radio, and television were some of the original electronic communication tools. Today technological capabilities involve so much more. The NASA space program's innovations have contributed many of the electronic advances used in the present healthcare environment (NASA, 2010). e-Mail is a fast and inexpensive way to communicate, yet has the permanence of a written letter. It is an asynchronous type of communication because the sender and receiver do not have to be online at the same time. Even without at-home computer access, nurses can use free services at most public libraries. Many hospitals additionally offer company e-mail and computer access for their employees' use at work. Often busy nurse managers communicate unit updates with e-mail blasts to staff members.

Capabilities of Electronic Communication

Depending on your Internet connection, you can share ideas, pictures, videos, audio, or more in a matter of seconds. You can design your e-mails with stationery backgrounds and request recipient receipts when opened. You can send files as attachments and collaboratively work on a presentation project with classmates or co-workers. These are just a few examples of electronic sharing. Internet connections can include dial-up, DSL, 3G, 4G, or more, depending on the connections offered by your Internet service provider (ISP). The type of connection will be the deciding factor on how quickly information sharing is handled.

Databases, Spreadsheets, Word Processing, Presentations, Desktop Publishing

All of the above are common communication tools for the student or professional nurse. Whatever type of document, spreadsheet, or presentation you create, one of the most important steps is how you save your work. Saving should begin when you open a document by creating a unique title and placing it on the hard drive of your computer. You should also save frequently throughout the creation process. Some people even create their detailed e-mails in a word-processing program, and then cut and paste the information into the e-mail to send. This is especially helpful if you are submitting assignments. Also, always have a back-up plan for document storage, whether CDs, DVDs, or memory sticks (also called *flash* or *jump drives*) in addition to the computer hard drive. Nothing is worse than working on a project for work or school, only to have it disappear because of a computer crash. Another suggestion is to mail yourself the finished project as an attached document. In this way, it is saved within the e-mail provider's files as well and can be easily retrieved. Software, even professional software, is constantly changing, so investing in brand-name applications will serve you well during your educational endeavor. Professional visual presentation software is also changing, with emphasis today more on visually interactive sessions in which participants use cell phones or iClickers to vote in audience polls and thus contribute to the communication during the session.

Computer Technology and Learning

According to an Australian study, being computer savvy with social networking and communication, however, does not necessarily translate into a desire to learn electronically (Curran, 2008). Even members of the Net Generation, who have been called *Digital Natives* by some, were found to prefer less electronic communication when it applied to learning and more hands-on and traditional face-to-face sessions (Gregor et al, 2008). Bennett and colleagues (2008) also reported on the same phenomenon. From the preliminary research, even the most computer literate students appreciate variety in the teaching methods of online classes, a hybrid blend of online and face-time, for learning electronically is not the same as socializing electronically.

e-Learning

The availability of online higher education courses has been the largest change in education in the past decade. Online college courses may be either synchronous (real-time) or asynchronous, but they usually have components of both. Podcasts or webinars represent one way to communicate electronically and can be a part of higher education course delivery or a way to provide professional continuing education credits. In a *podcast*, the lecturer (instructor or professor) is in a particular physical location, and typically is using some type of multimedia presentation. The presentation may have in-class participants, but it is also being recorded and broadcast to one or more locations simultaneously. For this reason it is often referred to as a *simulcast*. The recorded podcast is then placed in the organization's internal intranet for access by those participants as needed. Current personal digital assistants (PDAs), iPods, smartphones, iPads, MP3 players, and computers can be programmed to accept such podcasts for watching at a later time. Instant messaging and chat rooms also allow synchronous interactions that mimic real conversations in which participants exchange dialogue. When a user signs on to an instant messaging server, the user's designated "friends" can see if that user is online and available for conversation. The same is true in the educational environment in a chat room. In a classroom setting, these friends included in the chat room are normally certain peers all working on a group project. Another innovation in electronic communication is the ability to take review courses and examinations totally online. From college classes to certification examinations to the National Council Licensure Examination (NCLEX), this type of convenience has never been easier. Whether used for friends or as a part of a class, this type of electronic communication allows for connections that are instantaneous or synchronous.

Asynchronous learning opportunities, such as discussion boards, also enrich the online course delivery. Normally, the instructor posts assignments and each student answers online over the course of several days, and then responds to other posted comments. Thoughtful reflection and critical thinking skills are often unveiled as the students explore various topics in this manner. Another type of asynchronous activity in a learning community is web journal writing or blogging (Cohen, 2005). Originally a web-log (hence the word *blog*), blog spots have now become popular on a variety of subjects. Many professional nursing organizations offer a blog or link to their social networking site, as well as a listserv, a type of automatic feed from the organization to a participant's e-mail on certain topics. Students are encouraged to participate in such organizations to explore their intended nursing field further.

RSS (Really Simple Syndication) Feeds

How do you currently get your news? Do you watch the nightly news? Do you start your morning with the news? Or are you one of the people who now gets an RSS feed to their electronic device almost when it happens? RSS feeds are a quick and easy way to access news. Whether it be from the national media or the most current nursing journal, since we have so much information at our fingertips, it becomes part of the job of the nurse to assess the quality of whatever information is received (see Box 6-2).

Electronic Journals/Books

Principles, platforms, and technologies are changing the world of nursing education. Electronic textbooks combine the ease of cyberspace access with tactile study tools such as electronic highlighting and organizing. Most publishers offer these tools as a part of their e-books, where a student's personal changes are saved into an account. This type of cloud computing, in which your changes within the textbook are stored not on your home computer but in cyberspace, is becoming more prevalent each year. In addition, with all of the new e-books, the industry created an electronic reader a few years ago to address the concern of eye strain, which several manufacturers now offer.

Traditional nursing care plans created on paper may soon become a thing of the past, as more instructors are sending students to electronic nursing care plan constructors. There are also websites that host genealogy projects, pedigree trees, and other common traditional written nursing assignments or projects.

Researching journals has never been easier for students today. Instead of wading through stacks of hard copy journals, students can use a few search engines for articles and immediately have access to the specifics. Another added benefit of electronically searching for articles is the ability to limit your searches to specific authors, publications, or dates. Google Scholar is probably one of the quickest ways to look for journal articles, even without access to any other database. CINAHL (Cumulative Index to Nursing and Allied Health Literature) is an excellent resource available through public libraries, for it focuses specifically on nursing and healthcare journals. PubMed is also a favorite with healthcare providers (HCPs), for it houses the majority of interdisciplinary professional journals from all types of medicine, nursing, pharmacology, and so on.

Another important part of electronic communication is knowing how to reference the information that you gather. The professional world of nursing recommends using the American Psychological Association (APA) form of citation. Another new way is to use a digital content identifier (DOI), which is a way to directly link to an electronic document (Science Direct, 2010).

One cautionary note on searching the Internet for reliable references for scholarly and professional papers: Although Wikipedia is a quick way to find a definition or description of a multitude of items, it is not a peer-reviewed source. Wikipedia is simply a collection of thoughts of thousands of people who chose to share their personal definitions on one site. Peer-reviewed journals publish articles that have been evaluated by scholars within the same profession who have confirmed that the information presented is valid and appropriate.

Not only has the way information is now sought changed, but electronic communication has also changed the way educational information is shared. No longer does a great idea have to be shared individually for years before it can catch on. More than one group of nursing students has found a unique way to memorize the steps of a certain procedure and then shared the method with the world on YouTube. The phenomenon of YouTube has been yet another distinctive contribution of the Internet. Through this medium, people have shared what they found meaningful with others, and creative nursing students find ways to use its capabilities as an educational source.

Skype is also becoming a favorite among students. Skype is a personal video conferencing application run through an Internet connection between two or more computers that are equipped with a camera, a *webcam*, so the participants can see as well as hear each other. It is basically a free Internet video conferencing service. Many students have found this a wonderful way to participate in study groups, with the capability to show the textbook diagram or picture as needed. It also eliminates the distance barrier, since students can partner with those hundreds or even thousands of miles away. Students away from home can connect with families for support.

Professional video conferencing, online meetings such as GoToMeeting, take the Skype concept one step further, providing live cyberspace applications such as audio, visual, and software applications at the same time. In this way, participants at different locations not only can see and hear one another, they can also view an electronic presentation such as a PowerPoint at the same time. Organizations and hospitals often use GoToMeeting for intradepartmental meetings. Even many of the required continuing education courses for nurses are now conveniently available in online modules.

Web 2.0-Social Media

Living in an interconnected world, the fastest mode of communication is often the preferred method. As fast as e-mail is compared with postal mail, the new social networking environment has created even faster ways to communicate. Texting outperforms e-mail as a fast way to send quick, time-sensitive material. With text messages, the participants often type in shortened versions of normal words. In fact, text messages have developed a language all their own called the SMS language, with abbreviations and representations of particular words with certain patterns. (Most often, texting language omits the vowels from most words to shorten them.) However, as efficient as text messages can be in communicating, they are not always the most effective means in a professional or educational setting. (For example, during clinical rotations a student wanting assistance with a procedure may relate this to their faculty via a text. However, because texts normally do not include the sender's name, the faculty still would not know either the student's identity or location.)

Another social phenomenon, *tweeting* (done at the Twitter website), has arisen that is even faster than texting when communicating with multiple people at the same time. When tweeting, the participant can electronically share even the smallest of details of their daily life with their friends in seconds. In fact, one speaker at an informatics conference referred to this new type of experience as living on "Twitter Time" (Novak, 2010). In the professional world, many companies and innovative hospitals have instituted an internal professional social network called *Yammer*. Similar to tweeting, yamming is an online program that allows participants to share specific details of current work projects, and so on. Yammer, unlike Twitter, is a closed social networking site; participants who work at that particular company with a company work e-mail address can join in the conversations. In-hospital social networking sites such as Yammer have just crossed the million participant marker (Yammer, 2010). Employees post about projects in which they are involved, offer advice and shortcuts, or discuss the latest equipment relevant to their profession. This form of intranet communication is very applicable to the healthcare environment as a place to share lessons learned. Whether texting, tweeting, or yamming, all of these can be delivered and used through a smartphone.

Another effective company-based electronic communication tool is Microsoft SharePoint. In many ways, it is similar to a discussion board for an online college course, only with increased capabilities. At SharePoint sites, employees can post documents, pictures, and so on, for their department. Others in the department can access the documents, make changes, and then repost. It is a wonderful way to communicate and share projects among several people in a department as well as to keep one project calendar for the department. Because nurses often work in a shared-governance type of atmosphere, such sites are very useful for their profession.

Trending Now

Developing out of the generation of PDAs, the new smartphones have texting, media, e-mail, and social networking features as basic components to the phone. According to the Pew Research Center, 9 of 10 young adults now own a phone with these types of capabilities and use these enhancements on a regular basis (Smith, 2010). Cell phones have become so prevalent in America that according to one study, many would find it "very hard to give up" (Rainie, 2009). One employee asked to go home shortly after arriving at work and explained that she had inadvertently left her cell phone at home and did not think she could make it through her shift without that access. So what is the proper use of cell phones in the workplace, especially in nursing? Many employers have begun to create specific policies about cell phone use during work hours and whether employees may keep phones with them during their shift. There is good reason for this. One recent study correlated the number of interruptions a nurse has during the process of medication administration with an increase in medication errors (Westbrook et al, 2010). Surely our patients depend on a focused nurse who is able to provide safe and effective care.

With a sense of community being at the heart of the social media explosion, electronic communication capabilities are constantly expanding. Cell phones or smartphones with the ability to take digital pictures, audio, and share the clips quickly have now presented a unique problem in healthcare settings. Any phone carried by the nurse during a shift can add an additional layer of possible interruptions. Because one purpose of such phones is to be instantly connected to friends and family, what if a boyfriend or girlfriend decides to break up via a text message in the middle of a nurse's shift? What happens to the focus and mental clarity of the nurse whose very role requires single-minded diligence to care for the patients? What about a staff nurse who sees an interesting trauma or wound and decides to take a digital picture or video clip of it to show to some friends. Would you be offended to find your or your family's private information shared in such a way on YouTube? Contemplating the long-term effects such actions could set in motion, you can understand why some hospitals are so concerned that they have written policies requiring that all cell phones be left in the locker room, to be used only during breaks or at the end of the shift.

Social networking has far surpassed all expectations and moved into the mainstream as a form of electronic communication. Facebook is the most used form of social networking in the United States, comprising at least 500 million active users in 2010 (Facebook, 2011). One of the business formats for social networking, LinkedIn, had more than 50 million participants in 2009 (LinkedIn, 2009). As with any of the forms of electronic communication, it is important to remember that everything said in a social media format becomes a part of the permanent record somewhere in cyberspace. For healthcare, the social media explosion has left major questions still to be answered about what is appropriate to share and what is not. Is it a violation of the Health Insurance Portability and Accountability Act (HIPAA) to discuss a patient's condition at a social networking site? If so, should a nurse be held to the same standards according to HIPAA as if he or she had discussed the patient in the elevator at work? Should nurses lose their license over such an indiscretion? Such questions are being discussed by several state boards of nursing as they consider how to handle the social phenomenon of nurses freely posting descriptions related to patients on social networking sites (Spector, 2010). The question is, how will the additional capabilities of Internet-based electronic communication affect you and your ethical, safe nursing practice?

Social Media Capabilities

Social networking also has applicability beyond the social media sites such as Facebook and MySpace. Similar techniques are being used within the healthcare environment as more health-related sites arise for patients, families, and professionals. For example, there are sites dedicated to patient support such as DailyStrength (2011) and CaringBridge (2011). Such sites offer a positive way to disseminate information quickly among a large number of peers, which can save time for patients or family members trying to provide updates to others in the midst of their treatments. Friends can post notes of encouragement back to the site. There are online support group discussion boards for patients, based on their particular illness or injury. A new site has appeared as a part of the Pew Research Center dedicated simply to patients interacting with other patients (Fox, 2010).

LinkedIn can be used to promote your career, having a place for résumés to be uploaded and a posting board to highlight your education and other accomplishments. You may join a professional listserv or distribution list to stay current in nursing. Another web-based service allows you to create an electronic portfolio, holding word processing–type data and scanned copies of your college diplomas, awards, certificates, professional presentations, and so on, all in one concise format. Once it is all stored, you, as the owner, can update it regularly and provide access to other interested parties, such as a potential employer.

Healthcare Apps

Another form of electronic communication is called *apps*. Instead of being found on the hardware of a computer, apps are a cyberspace-based software (or application) that can be accessed through some type of network device such as a smartphone or tablet, another example of cloud computing. Some network devices offer touch screens whereas others use miniature keyboards. Consider that more than 3 billion apps were downloaded in the first 18 months after the launch of the Apple App Store alone (Apple Corporation, 2010). A quick investigation using one of the Internet search engines for medical and nursing apps will reveal hundreds of healthcare applications for smartphones and tablets. From radiology to laboratories, medical terminology to an eye chart, clinicians can now have almost unlimited references at their hands instantly. As a patient advocate, a nurse can lead patients who are technologically savvy to use such apps to help keep up with data concerning their particular health issues.

Electronic Health Records/ Electronic Medical Record

The new form of patient documentation, the electronic health record (EHR) system, is usually a software application loaded into multiple computers through a hospital's intranet system. According to Robles and Karnas (as cited by B. Beaty; Robles and Karnas, 2007, p. 7), "the electronic medical record shifts the paradigm of nursing." The EHR "crosses the continuum of care" with the ability to add to the patient's story with each entry, not rewrite it (as cited by B. Beaty; Robles and Karnas, 2007, p. 7). Timely charting is even more important because an HCP could be at the office viewing the patient's chart, making decisions, and entering orders according to such information. Current intake and output data could affect the order for a diuretic.

The vital essence of this transition from paper to electronic charts has led a U.S. government task force to define the meaningful use of EHRs. The government has further established guidelines that require all healthcare providers to implement EHRs by a certain deadline, with incentives paid according to a provider's current stage of implementation. The Health Information Technology for Economic and Clinical Health Act (HITECH) "authorized incentive payments through Medicare and Medicaid to clinicians and hospitals when they use EHRs privately and securely to achieve specified improvements in care delivery" (Blumenthal and Tavenner, 2010, p. 3).

Electronic communications are also being used in rather unexpected ways within the EHRs. In days past, a nurse would document a pressure ulcer or possible abuse case by hand-drawing the approximate size and area of a wound onto a paper-based figure of a human body and placing it in the chart. Today, nurses often use digital cameras to document pressure ulcers or abuse and upload the visible evidence into the patient's EHR. Quality reviews and risk management are also being taken to a new level with the new form of electronic communication in the hospital setting.

The new electronic communication devices are not limited to just the documentation portion of a patient's hospital stay, for even the tests, procedures, and interventions have changed. Think of the electronic medication administration record (e-MAR BMV, where "BMV" stands for bedside medication verification, an additional level of verification added to ensure that no mistakes are made). This type of delivery of medication changes the workflow of the nurse from traditional medication administration. It is basically a safety device created to prevent medication errors. The drug interaction software alone found within the EHRs is a giant step toward promoting increased patient safety, for it alerts the staff to possible negative reactions between certain medications.

According to Delaney (as cited by J. Karnas; Delaney, 2007), "Nanotechnologies are fundamentally changing every aspect of health care delivery." Again, these new technological advancements from surgery to laboratory can inhibit or enhance our communication and patient relationships and, ultimately, our ability to deliver safe and effective care as nurses. As a part of the incentives in the HITECH legislation, certain financial incentives can be received only when such clinical decision support tools are used (Blumenthal and Tavenner, 2010, p. 4).

The Institute of Medicine reports that "about 20% of the United States population lives in rural areas, but only 9% of physicians practice there" (as cited in Effken and Abbott, 2009, p. 442). Effken and Abbott have cast a vision for a new type of healthcare, "health IT–enabled care," whereby nurses can play a greater role as the HCP through telehealth and tele–home care for underserved populations.

The EHRs make this increasingly possible. How will electronic communication affect the future ability of nurses to actually provide primary care for patients?

According to Demiris and colleagues (2008, p. 8), healthcare information technology can also empower patients to move from a passive to active role in their healthcare. When a patient begins to use patient-centered healthcare apps (as discussed previously) or when a patient reviews the literature and illness-specific information on the Internet, the patient becomes involved in the decision-making process, opening communication channels between the HCP and patient. Demiris and colleagues describe portable monitoring tools and mobile devices that further allow electronic communication data to be fed back to the HCP for evaluation.

Not all of the literature on EHRs has been positive. One review found the attitudes of HCPs to be a significant factor in whether the EHRs were accepted in practice (Ward et al, 2008). Another study looked at the old adage of nursing documentation or the lack of it, that is, "if it isn't written down, it wasn't done" (Carroll-Johnson, 2008), and how the lack of timely charting in the EHRs world can be a pitfall. Sassen describes how nurses feel about the EHRs. The inability of the EHRs to actually "capture the invisible work of nurses" is one of the major barriers (Sassen, 2009, p. 282). There is a learning curve when a healthcare environment changes over to an EHR. According to Courtney and colleagues (2008), nurses have to move from novice to expert in the area of information technology. Overcoming this knowledge gap can be challenging. Because of the informatics competency issue, some companies start by evaluating the basic computer skills of their employees before they ever start EHR training. The nurse must learn to prioritize in a manner different from that used with paper documentation. Without a doubt, EHRs change a nurse's workflow, so it is important for nurses to be involved when information technology decisions are made for the end-user. Without adequate input into the design, nurses will just create work-arounds (in which a nurse figures out a way to by-pass the EHRs just to get the job done). In the end, these work-arounds are costly to the staff, hospitals, and patients. This is another reason for the rise in the role of the nursing informatician: to provide the end-user's viewpoint and to create EHRs that accommodate nurse workflows.

Electronic Feedback

Some innovative hospitals have also begun to offer additional electronic communication services in which family members or friends can send e-mail messages, called *e-Cards*, to inpatients. Some hospitals encourage staff members to use a web-based accolade system to recognize co-workers for outstanding performance. Some rehabilitation facilities are being changed as computer interaction consoles and exercisers talk the patients through their workouts. With positive reinforcement being inherent in the game itself through electronic communication, Nintendo's Wii is being used in many rehabilitation facilities as a way to provide interactive games appropriate for patients. Residents in assisted living facilities are being bussed to other facilities for Wii bowling tournaments. All of these use electronic communication as a means of feedback to the patients or staff in order to facilitate their growth and empowerment in the midst of healthcare.

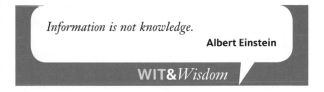

Information is not knowledge.

Albert Einstein

WIT&*Wisdom*

Dangers of Electronic Communication

Without the benefit of nonverbal clues and body language, the written word can be more easily misunderstood. Be sure your professional electronic communications, whatever form they may take, come across as professional (Box 6-1). Rarely use the option to "Reply All," for too many e-mails bog down others' e-mail and the option increases your risk of sending something inadvertently. Another hint is, don't trust every website. If you are sending information that needs to be secure (such as a credit card number for an online order), look at the hyperlink address. Instead of an "http://" address, it should be an "https://" address. The extra letter "s" in this case stands for data-secured site.

Viruses, worms, and hackers are real dangers in the world of electronic communications. It is wise to invest in a good antivirus program. Do not open e-mails with

---

Box 6-1 *Best Practices for e-Mail*

- Use the subject line to identify the content.
- Make the message and format appropriate for the person to whom you are writing.
- Do not type in all caps (unless you want to be perceived as shouting).
- Recognize that messages may not be read or answered immediately.
- Do not indiscriminately forward jokes and warnings to everyone you know.
- Use a virus protection program and keep it up to date.
- Do not send confidential messages via e-mail (unless both parties agree).
- If you need a faster form of communication, call or text the person.

---

attachments that look suspicious. Perform a system check on your home computer on a regular basis.

Passwords can be a hassle, especially the type within a school or work account that requires a change every 3 months. However, passwords are for your safety. Not only are they important in the healthcare environment, your protected password guarantees that you and you alone will be documenting under your name. Because your name in an EHR is your legal acceptance of what was documented, this becomes even more important. Never, never share your password with anyone or allow others to document, even vital signs, under your password.

Stranger danger is as real in the electronic communication environment as ever. Be careful with whom you share information. Common interests do not guarantee common goals or the same belief system. Be careful what you share on the Internet. Safety rules for within social media include not listing your home address or phone number, to prevent someone from tracing your web presence to your physical address. Also, be aware that once a picture is posted on a social media site, access to it is free to anyone who wants it by simply right-clicking it and saving it to their computer.

Another danger with the Internet occurs when clients (and professionals) are defrauded by faulty or misleading information. Because more and more

people are turning to the Internet for health information, it is important for nurses not only to be advocates, teaching patients how to seek credible Internet information, but also to become healthcare leaders in the realm of electronic communication. See Box 6-2 for specific information on evaluating websites.

Electronic communications is a new world indeed. When combined with nursing, it has the potential to increase our time for actual patient care in a safer environment. However, as with any new skill, electronic communication also has quite a learning curve. For those who are willing to give it their all, the benefits in the long run far outweigh climbing the steep mountain to learn.

Man is still the most extraordinary computer of all.

John Fitzgerald Kennedy, 35th President of the United States

WIT&*Wisdom*

Box 6-2 *Evaluation of Health Information Web Pages*

- Who wrote this web page? What are the credentials of this person?
- Who is the page written for—healthcare providers? patients? prospective customers?
- What is the intent of the page—to provide objective information? persuade? sell?
- When was the page written, and when was it last updated?
- What sources were used for the information?
- Who is paying for the web page to be on a web server?
- Who is advertising on the page? Is the difference between information and ads clear?
- What information does the page collect about visitors? How does it use this information?

Data from the Health on the Net Foundation (http://www.hon. ch/HONcode/Conduct.html) and the Sheridan Libraries of the Johns Hopkins University (http://guides.library.jhu.edu/ evaluatinginformation).

The ability to send photographs by e-mail or post them on web pages has given parents an easy and economical way to send pictures to grandparents. Many hospitals provide a service that allows parents of new babies to have a picture of the baby placed on a website so that family members can see the baby even before the parents have time to send a picture.

Moments of Connection . . .
Electronic Communication

I was visiting a hospice client in her home. She was anxiously awaiting a telephone call to announce the birth of her first grandchild. On my next visit, she proudly showed me a picture of her granddaughter that her son-in-law had e-mailed her. She was going to make a screensaver for her computer from the file.

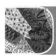

Reflections On . . .

Electronic Communication

Consider what you read about electronic communication to answer these questions.

What? . . .
Write one thing you learned from this chapter.

So what? . . .
How will this affect your nursing practice?

Now what? . . .
How will you implement this new knowledge or skill?

Think about it . . .

Practicing Electronic Communication

Exercise 1
Visit http://www.senate.gov/ and find the web pages for the two U.S. senators from your state or use www.google.com to find an official website of the government of your country. Write one paragraph about what you learned.

Exercise 2
Search online using the search engine www.askjeeves.com, where you type a question. For example, because obesity is such a major health concern, search, "How can I lose weight?" Create a list of resources.

Exercise 3 — QSEN
Competency in informatics crosses all other quality and safety competencies. The knowledge, skills, and attitudes that comprise competency in informatics help nurses with database searches to locate and evaluate evidence-based information, use decision support tools in making care decisions, record information and communicate among the many disciplines involved in a patient's care via the electronic health record, and manage information confidentially. Use the questions below to assess how informatics is integrated throughout the unit. At the end of a clinical learning experience discuss the questions below in small groups to identify ways that informatics are a part of nursing practice on a daily basis and can be used to improve quality and safety.

1. *Patient-centered Care*: Patients and families often search for information about their illness using the World Wide Web. How can you help guide them in using appropriate sites and evaluating the information found?
2. *Teamwork and Collaboration*: When handing off a patient from one provider to another, there is an increased opportunity for errors and missed information that can be critical for making care decisions. Describe how automated checklists can ensure that accurate and complete information is shared in the hand-off between providers.
3. *Evidence-based Practice*: Can you cite the evidence for the care you deliver? Demonstrate use of a database search to investigate a question you encountered in delivering care to your patient.
4. *Quality Improvement*: Demonstrate how you would access sites that share quality care standards. What electronic quality improvement tools are used to measure the outcomes of care on your unit and compare these with the industry standard?
5. *Safety*: Ask if there are automated safety alerts embedded in the electronic health records on your unit to notify staff of a possible error. What
Continued

are the benefits and challenges of having auto-mated safety alerts?

6. *Informatics*: Define decision support tools used to help staff make informed decisions. What decision support is available to the staff on your unit?

QSEN competency: Informatics

Exercise 4

Select a chronic illness to research on the Internet. Review Table 6-1 and search appropriate sites for useful information. Try using the search engine www.google.com to search for information about the illness. Then, for the same chronic illness, search for support groups or chat rooms that might be useful to clients with this illness. With another student or in a group, discuss the benefits and liabilities of such support via the Internet.

Exercise 5

Search www.google.com to find creative sites to teach your patients. For example, play some of the games at http://www.kidshealth.org/kid/closet/, a children's website to help children explore their health and the human body. Write a paragraph discussing the application of this content to your clinical practice.

Table 6-1 *Websites with Information Relevant to Healthcare and Nursing*

WEBSITE	ADDRESS
GOVERNMENT SITES FOR HEALTHCARE PROFESSIONALS	
Agency for Healthcare Research and Quality	http://www.ahrq.gov
Centers for Disease Control and Prevention	http://www.cdc.gov/
CINAHL	http://www.ebscohost.com/cinahl/
PubMed Central/NCBI/NLM/NIH	http://www.ncbi.nlm.nih.gov/sites/entrez?db+pmc
Medline Plus	www.nlm.nih.gov/medlineplus
National Guideline Clearinghouse	http://www.guideline.gov
National Library of Medicine	http://www.nlm.nih.gov/
Office of the Surgeon General	http://www.surgeongeneral.gov/
Healthy People 2010	http://www.health.gov/healthypeople/
GOVERNMENT SITES FOR HEALTHCARE CONSUMERS	
Healthfinder	http://www.healthfinder.gov
National Institutes of Health (NIH)	http://health.nih.gov/
NIH information for consumers	http://medlineplus.gov/
President's Council on Physical Fitness	http://www.fitness.gov/
Closing the Health Gap—health information especially for communities of color	http://www.healthgap.omhrc.gov/
Information about clinical research studies	http://clinicaltrials.gov/
National Women's Health Information Center	http://www.4woman.gov/

Table 6-1 *Websites with Information Relevant to Healthcare and Nursing—cont'd*

WEBSITE	ADDRESS
U.S. Department of Agriculture nutrition information	http://www.nutrition.gov/
Consumer Product Safety Commission	http://www.cpsc.gov/
GOVERNMENT SITES FOR OLDER ADULTS	
Seniors' health topics	http://www.nlm.nih.gov/medlineplus/seniorshealth.html
NIH senior health	http://nihseniorhealth.gov/
National Institute on Aging	http://www.nia.nih.gov/
FirstGov for Seniors	http://www.nia.nih.gov/
PRIVATE SITES FOR HEALTHCARE CONSUMERS	
Mayo Clinic health information site	http://www.mayoclinic.com/
Harvard University Medical School health information site	http://www.intelihealth.com/
American Heart Association	http://www.americanheart.org/
American Diabetes Association	http://www.diabetes.org
American Cancer Society	http://www.cancer.org/
SITES ABOUT GOVERNMENT AGENCIES AND RESOURCES	
U.S. gateway to all government information	http://www.usa.gov/
Library of Congress	http://loc.gov
NURSING ORGANIZATION SITES	
American Nurses Association	http://www.nursingworld.org/
National Council of State Boards of Nursing	http://www.ncsbn.org/

References

Agency for Healthcare and Research Quality (AHRQ) (website). http://healthit.ahrq.gov. Accessed 11/23/2010.

American Nurses Association: *Nursing informatics: scope & standards of practice*, Washington, DC, 2008, American Nurses Association Publishing.

Apple Corporation: *Apple's App Store Downloads Top Three Billion*. http://www.apple.com/pr/library/2010/01/05appstore.html. Accessed 11/23/2010.

Bennett S, Maqton K, Kervin L: The 'digital natives' debate: a critical review of evidence, *Br J Educ Technol* 39(5):775, 2008.

Blumenthal D, Tavenner M: The "meaningful use" regulation for electronic health records, *N Engl J Med* 363(6):501, 2010.

CaringBridge: *Connecting family and friends when health matters most.* http://www.caringbridge.org. Accessed 3/18/11.

Carroll-Johnson RM: If it isn't written down, it wasn't done, *Oncol Nurs Forum* 35(3):331, 2008.

Cohen JA: The mirror as metaphor for reflective practice, *Annu Rev Nurs Educ* 3:313, 2005.

Courtney KL, Alexander GL, Demiris G: Information technology from novice to expert: implementation implications, *J Nurs Manag* 16(6):692, 2008.

Cronenwett L, Sherwood G, Barnsteiner J, et al: Quality and safety education for nurses, *Nurs Outlook* 55(3):122, 2007.

Curran CR: Faculty development initiatives for the integration of informatics competencies and point-of-care technologies in undergraduate nursing education, *Nurs Clin North Am* 43(4):523, 2008.

DailyStrength: *Find your online support group*. http://www.dailystrength.org/support-groups. Accessed 3/18/11.

Delaney C: Nursing and informatics for the 21st century: a conversation with Connie Delaney [interview by Joan Karnas]. *Creat Nurs* 13(2):4, 2007.

Demiris G, Afrin L, Speedie S, et al: Patient-centered applications: use of information technology to promote disease management and wellness. A White Paper by the AMIA Knowledge in Motion Working Group, *J Am Med Inform Assoc* 15(1):8, 2008.

Effken JA, Abbott P: Health IT-enabled care for underserved rural populations: the role of nursing, *J Am Med Inform Assoc* 16(4):439, 2009.

Facebook: *Pressroom: Statistics*. http://www.facebook.com/press/info.php?statistics. Accessed 3/18/11.

Fox S: *The power of mobile*. Prepared for e-patients.net, a project of the Society for Participatory Medicine. http://e-patients.net/archives/2010/09/the-power-of-mobile.html#more-7226. Accessed 11/23/2010.

Gregor E, Kennedy TS, Judd A, et al: First year students' experiences with technology: are they really digital natives? *Australian J Educ Technol* 24(1):108, 2008.

LinkedIn: *LinkedIn: 50 million professionals worldwide*. http://blog.linkedin.com/2009/10/14/linkedin-50-million-professionals-worldwide. Accessed 10/14/2009.

National Aeronautics and Space Administration (NASA): *Innovative Partnerships Program: NASA Spinoff*. http://www.sti.nasa.gov/tto/. Accessed 11/23/2010.

National League of Nurses (NLN): *Preparing the next generation of nurses to practice in a technology-rich environment: an informatics agenda [position paper]*. http://www.nln.org/aboutnln/positionstatements/informatics_052808.pdf. Accessed 07/02/08.

Novak, D: *Patient–organization interaction via social media*. Presented at Texas Regional Conference, May 13–14, Addison, Tex, 2010. HIMSS Chapters Southern Regional Conference Agenda. http://www.himssregional.com/agenda_materials.html. Accessed 11/23/2010.

Quality and Safety Education for Nurses (QSEN): *Competency KSAs*. http://www.qsen.org/ksas_graduate.php#informatics. Accessed 11/23/2010.

Quality and Safety Education for Nurses (QSEN): *Informatics* [definition]. http://www.qsen.org/definition.php?id=6. Accessed 11/23/2010.

Rainie L: *Baby boomers in the digital age*. http://www.slideshare.net/pewinternet/baby-boomers-in-the-digital-age?type=powerpoint. Accessed 01/11/09.

Robles J, Karnas J: The Electronic Medical Record: shifting the paradigm. A conversation with Jane Robles and Joan Karnas [interview by Beth Beaty], *Creat Nurs* 13(2):7, 2007.

Sassen EJ: Love, hate, or indifference: how nurses really feel about the electronic health record system, *CIN: Computers, Informatics, Nursing* 27(5):281, 2009.

Science Direct: *SciVerse: Creating a DOI link*. http://help.sciencedirect.com/flare/sdhelp_Left.htm#CSHID=doi.htm. Accessed 11/23/2010.

Simpson RL: Information technology: building nursing intellectual capital for the information age, *Nurs Adm Q* 31(1): 84, 2007.

Smith A: *Mobile access 2010. [an overview of mobile access]*. http://www.pewinternet.org/Reports/2010/Mobile-Access-2010.aspx. Accessed 11/23/2010.

Society for Participatory Medicine: *E-patients.net: Because health professional can't do it alone. The power of mobile*. http://e-patients.net/archives/2010/09/the-power-of-mobile.html#more-7226. Accessed 11/23/2010.

Spector N: Boundary violations via the internet, *Texas Board of Nursing Quarterly Newsletter* 41(3):6, 2010.

Technology Informatics Guiding Education Reform (TIGER): *The TIGER Initiative: Evidence and informatics. Transforming nursing: 3-year action steps towards a 10-year vision*, 2007. http://www.tigersummit.com/uploads/TIGERInitiative_Report2007_Color.pdf.

Ward R, Stevens C, Brentnall P, et al: The attitudes of healthcare staff to IT: a comprehensive review of the research literature, *Health Info Libr J* 25(2):81, 2008. Available from doi: 10.1111/j.1471-1842.2008.00777.x

Westbrook JI, Woods A, Rob MI, et al: Association of interruptions with an increased risk and severity of medication administration errors, *Arch Intern Med* 170(8):683, 2010.

Westra BL, Delaney CW: Informatics competencies for nursing and healthcare leaders. In *American Medical Informatics Association Symposium Proceedings*, 2008, 804. Available from PubMed: PMCID: PMC2655955.

Yammer: *Yammer continues strong growth in record-breaking Q2*. http://www.marketwire.com/press-release/Yammer-Continues-Strong-Growth-in-Record-Breaking-Q2-1293292.htm. Accessed 11/23/2010.

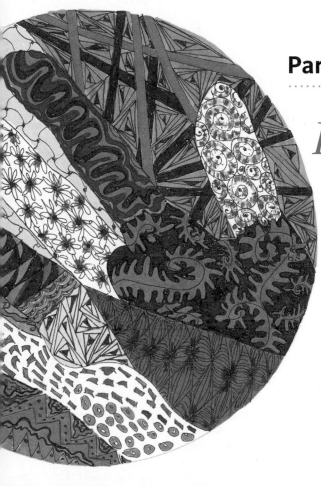

Part 2

*Building
Relationships*

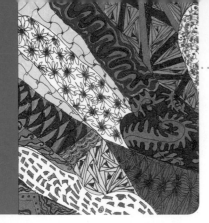

Chapter 7

Warmth

| PORTIONS OF THIS CHAPTER CONTRIBUTED
BY MARGARET E. ERICKSON, PhD |

> *All the statistics in the world can't measure the warmth of a smile.*
>
> **Chris Hart**

Objectives

1. Discuss the benefits of warmth in communication with clients and colleagues
2. Identify behaviors that demonstrate warmth
3. Review a tool to analyze warmth in interpersonal communications
4. Describe a variety of ways in which warmth is displayed and articulate the importance of warmth in human interactions
5. Become aware of opportunities to embellish your life with warmth in day-to-day encounters with clients and colleagues
6. Participate in exercises to build skills in demonstrating warmth

Close your eyes for a moment and imagine someone for whom you feel warmth. Experience this sense of warmth. Now ask yourself, "If I feel warm toward someone, how do I show it?" Consider what you experienced in this brief exercise and reflect upon how you can demonstrate warmth in your nursing practice.

"Speak with me in a warm and caring voice" (Lee-Hsieh et al, 2004, p. 26). Let your voice inflection say, I care about you as we share this moment (Pullen and Mathias, 2010). Warmth is the glue in the bonding between people and the magnetism that draws us to a closer intimacy with others. It is a special ingredient, even a catalyst, in our human relationships. It is comfort, as in the lines of a prayer, "May comfort be yours, warm and soft like a sigh" (Tabron, 2001). The expression of warmth makes us feel welcomed, relaxed, and joyful. Although clients may not be able to judge our intelligence, certifications, or degrees, they can judge our hearts by the care we give and the warmth we demonstrate at their sides (Carver, 1998). A student nurse struggling with injection skills and the potential effect of her lack of confidence on her clients reflected that "a dose of genuine warmth is as essential as skill with a syringe" (O'Connor, 2005, p. 28).

Warmth has been identified as an essential attribute in psychotherapists. The therapist's warmth, along with empathy and genuineness, contributes to client improvement and leads to more open, full relationships for clients in and out of therapy. Warmth sets the tone for clients, families, and colleagues to share their own stories. Baker and Diekelmann (1994) called these "connecting conversations." Most of you will not be psychotherapists. Your expression of warmth to your clients, however, will make them feel welcomed and not judged. These positive emotions will foster feelings of well-being and likely promote healing. The warmth communicated in family support has a direct effect on the well-being of clients because family members can often offer better support than staff (Cooper and Powell, 1998). Caring acts that show warmth and genuineness have been associated with increased hope in clients with cancer (Koopmeiners et al, 1997). In a study to identify and validate the dimensions for caregiver reciprocity in intergenerational exchanges, warmth and regard were found to be important factors (Carruth, 1996). Clients who sense your warmth are more likely to engage in dialogue and provide information about their health conditions. This communication helps the nurse to make a nursing diagnosis, determine expected outcomes, work out a nursing care plan, and evaluate the progress of nursing care with the client.

> *Warmth, kindness, and friendship are the most yearned-for commodities in the world. The person who can provide them will never be lonely.*
>
> **Ann Landers**
>
> **WIT&***Wisdom*

Exchanging warmth with colleagues makes the workplace a more pleasant environment. Warmth enhances closeness, which has social and work-related benefits. A study by the American Management Association (Ekeren, 1994) identified eight traits that often lead to failure for executives. The first two were "insensitivity to co-workers" and "aloofness and arrogance." Extending our warmth to our colleagues makes us more approachable. Increased communication among colleagues ensures that important messages about clients or unit policies and procedures are transmitted.

Although we often refer to others as warm, as a human quality warmth is difficult to describe and one of the most difficult interpersonal communication behaviors to learn. Warmth involves not only attitudinal and psychomotor behavior but also a total way of offering oneself to another person. Showing warmth to others means conveying that you like to be with them and that you accept them as they are. In this sense warmth is a way of showing respect to clients and colleagues.

Warmth is not communicated in isolation. It enhances and is enhanced by other facilitative communication behaviors that you will learn about in later chapters (such as respect, genuineness, and empathy). By itself, warmth is not sufficient for building an effective helping relationship, developing mutual respect, or solving problems, but warmth enhances these processes.

According to Levine and Adelman (1982), a study conducted in the United States found that 93% of a message is transmitted by tone of voice and facial expression and only 7% by words. We may possibly tune into the nonverbal expression of emotions and attitudes more than the verbal. Because expression of warmth is predominantly nonverbal, it is wise to heed these findings.

Ways to Display Warmth to Your Clients and Colleagues

Warmth is displayed primarily in a nonverbal manner. Subtle facial and body signs, as well as gestures (small movements of a hand, brow, or eye), convey our inner relaxation and attentiveness to another person (Table 7-1).

Table 7-1 *Facial Signals of Warmth*

FACIAL FEATURE	HOW WARMTH IS DISPLAYED
Forehead	Muscles are relaxed, and forehead is smooth; there is no furrowing of the brow
Eyes	Comfortable eye contact is maintained; pupils are dilated; gaze is neither fixed nor shifting and darting
Mouth	Lips are loose and relaxed, not tight or pursed; gestures such as biting a lip or forcing a smile are absent; jaw is relaxed and mobile, not clenched; smile is appropriate
Expression	Features of the face move in a relaxed, fluid way; worried, distracted, or fretful looks are absent; the face shows interest and attentiveness

There is a lot that you do with your face to convey warmth. When you are talking to another person, attention is largely focused on the face, so it is important to know how to make facial expressions that maximize your warmth.

During interaction, your face can communicate information regarding your personality, interests, and responsiveness, as well as your emotional state. Your facial expression can open or close a conversation. The context, including the relationship, determines the meaning of facial expressions. Also, the degree of facial expressiveness varies among individuals and cultures. In relationships with clients and colleagues, it is wise to remember that although people from other cultures may not express emotions (such as warmth) openly, this does not mean that they do not experience these emotions.

Americans express themselves to varying degrees. People from certain ethnic backgrounds in the United States may use their hands, bodies, and faces more than others. Warmth can be expressed in a variety of ways, but to have a poker face or deadpan expression is usually considered suspicious.

We may interpret insufficient or excessive eye contact as communication barriers. No specific rules govern eye behavior, except that to stare, especially at strangers, is considered rude. Eye contact can have different meanings in different cultures.

Your posture can communicate warmth. Movements or ways of holding yourself that encourage communication and indicate interest and pleasure in being with the other person constitute warmth (Table 7-2). The list in Table 7-2 may sound like your mother telling you to sit up straight at dinner, yet the details provide solid guidelines for communicating the warmth you feel even if you are anxious.

Warmth indicators include a shift of posture toward the other person, a smile, direct eye contact, and motionless hands. In a study by Knapp (1980), gestures such as looking around the room, slumping, drumming fingers, and looking glum detract from warmth. In a dialogue situation, positive warmth cues, coupled with verbal reinforcers such as "mm-hmm," are effective in increasing verbal output from the interviewee (whereas verbal cues alone are insufficient). These findings from an early study have implications for nursing, in which so much client information is gathered through interviewing.

Purtilo and Haddad (2002) pointed out that in addition to whole-body posturing and positioning, gestures

Table 7-2 *Postural Signals of Warmth*

POSTURAL FEATURE	HOW WARMTH IS DISPLAYED
Body position	Client is faced squarely, with shoulders parallel to the client's shoulders
Head position	Head is kept at the same level as the client's; periodic nodding shows interest and attentiveness
Shoulders	Shoulders are kept level and mobile, not hunched and tense
Arms	Arms are kept loose and able to move smoothly, rather than held stiffly
Hands	Gestures are natural, with no clenching or grasping of a clipboard or chart; distracting mannerisms such as tapping a pen or playing with an object are avoided
Chest	Breathing is at an even pace; the chest is kept open, neither slouched nor extended too far forward in feigned attentiveness; a slight forward leaning shows interest
Legs	Whether crossed or uncrossed, legs are kept in a comfortable and natural position; during standing, knees should be flexed and not locked
Feet	Fidgeting, tapping, and kicking are avoided

involving the extremities—even one finger—can suggest the meaning of a message. Think about how the following gestures would affect your message of warmth: shrugging your shoulders, folding your arms over your chest, rolling your thumb, shuffling your foot, or silently clenching your fist. Even if other parts of your body are focused on conveying warmth, these partial gestures might minimize or erase the message of warmth you are trying to send.

Remember not all gestures have universal meaning. A wink or a hand gesture may not be received in the same mood of warmth in which it is delivered. For example, the American "OK" sign (circle made with thumb and forefinger) is a symbol for money in Japan and is considered obscene in some Latin American countries.

The spatial distance or closeness we create between us and our clients and colleagues can affect the perception of warmth. For Americans, distance in social conversation is about an arm's length to 4 feet. In our exuberance to display warmth, we may invade this unseen but well-defined circumference. Not all clients or colleagues feel comforted by this gesture; some may feel intruded upon, and others may feel threatened and act defensively.

Touching is another way to affectionately transmit warmth. From the briefest pat on the shoulder to an embracing hug or extended hand, you can convey warmth to others. Your comfort or lack of comfort with touch is communicated. The gentle, sincere touch of your hand can express warmth, caring, and comfort (Reynolds, 2002; Gleeson, 2004).

Warmth can be conveyed verbally as well as nonverbally. The volume of the voice is related to warmth. Softer, modulated tones convey warmth more than loud, aggressive tones that are harsh to the ears. A pitch that seems comfortable for the speaker transmits warmth more than an unnatural pitch that seems to be out of the speaker's range. The pacing of words is also important. Pressured, stilted, or stoic speech detracts from the warmth that can be conveyed through rhythmic speech, whose pacing is in keeping with the speaker's natural breathing. The actual words also have the power to extend warmth to others. Loving, soft words are warmer than harsh, thoughtless words: "So, you've never exercised before and now you think you'll become a 'super-jock' and take up jogging?" is cold and judgmental compared with "You'd like to improve your fitness level so you're taking a new lease on life and learning to jog."

As you may have noticed, many of the features of warmth are those of a relaxed person. Not only must you be relaxed, but you can communicate warmth only when you have a genuine interest in the other person and a wish to convey that welcome and pleasure to him or her. A desire to be warm is based on the belief that each person you encounter is worthy of receiving the acceptance and comfort that your warmth generates. The ability to be warm was so valued by a psychiatric facility in Surrey, England, that it was included in an online recruitment ad. When you display high-level warmth, you are completely and intensely attentive to the interaction between yourself and your clients or colleagues, making them feel accepted and important. The opposite—cold behavior—conveys disapproval or disinterest.

Stories of Warmth in the Actions of Nurses

A collection of Moments of Connection stories demonstrates the tapestry woven from lessons learned in our professional and personal journey and illustrates the warmth that is so central to the caring art of nursing.

Extension and Withdrawal of Warmth

Any time you wish to become closer to one of your clients or colleagues, or to provide the message that you really care, an expression of warmth is appropriate. There are degrees of warmth. An attitude of "I like that client (colleague); I feel warmly toward him with all his strengths and weaknesses" is warmer than "I don't feel dislike for my client (colleague)." The warmth you express should reflect your genuine feelings. Your expression of warmth to a colleague whom you would like to date will likely be more open and intense than the warmth you might express to a client in your care.

 Moments of Connection . . .
**For Our Loved Ones
and Yours in Their Final Hours**
"My father died suddenly in 1992, alone in a hospital far from family. I can only hope and pray that a kind nurse was with him or, hopefully, held his hand or said a prayer with him as he passed away. I tend to want to hold my patients' hands or pray—or be kind—so their family members can rest assured that a kind person was with their loved one."

 Moments of Connection . . .
Pain Management: More Than Analgesia
"I was caring for a pain management patient who was reluctant to take medication. After talking with him, I learned he had lost his only child 3 months before in an automobile accident. He needed to talk. He was frightened and wanted a hand to hold. Despite my busy schedule, I knew this was where I belonged. I left when he was more comfortable. As I walked down the hall, I thanked God for giving me the talent and knowledge to help another person."

Moments of Connection . . .
A Pillow, a Washcloth, and Myself

"As an operating room nurse I had a patient with muscular dystrophy. Her surgery was delayed, and I spent about 30 minutes with her. She was in her twenties and we laughed and joked. I repositioned her arms and legs for her (she was already quite crippled) and gave her pillows and wet washcloths. Our time meant a lot to her, and she asked me if I would see her after surgery. When I did, she was thrilled and asked me to take my hat off so she could see me better. She visited me each time she came to the hospital. Later I learned she and her mother lived alone. She did not have any friends until we met. These comfort measures were just part of my work, but they meant a lot to her."

Factors that make it possible to convey warmth are the physical ability to control the facial, postural, tactile, and verbal indicators of warmth, and the ability to overcome any of the cognitive or affective influences mediating against warmth. What are some of the factors working against the expression of warmth? Any thoughts or feelings that distract your attention from other people block the expression of warmth. Being rushed, overcome with strong emotions, shocked, and judgmental about others' behaviors are distractions that divert your attention. When you feel hurried, you are focused on yourself and are unable to enjoy the people around you. Remember to take a deep breath and bring your attention back to the person.

It is only natural to withdraw your warmth when you are angry with another person. When you feel hurt, bitter, irritated, or enraged with a client or colleague, trying to convey warmth would be insincere. At times you may feel insecure about whether you will be accepted or rejected by another person. Then, you might hide behind a crisp façade until you feel safe enough to allow your warmth to surface.

Moments of Connection . . .
Off the Clock

"My story is about my own unplanned C-section. I have been a pain management nurse for 5 years and know many people in the hospital. We all know it can be tough to care for another nurse. A special nurse from the postanesthesia care unit inserted my Foley catheter for my male RN friend who was the circulating RN that day. Then she clocked out after seeing my nervousness and anxiety in the holding area. She comforted me and followed me through surgery. She did everything for me to provide warmth and comfort, including holding my hand during the epidural. I could just picture that 3-inch spinal needle! She took the video for my husband so he could enjoy the first moments of our daughter's life. She provided comfort not only physically but emotionally as well. I will never forget her caring."

Moments of Connection . . .
When the Client Is Scared

"I had just begun to work with cancer patients when I met a young woman dying with sarcoma. She required many boluses of medication to relieve her pain, which was worst at night when she was most fearful. I held her hand and patted her shoulder gently to soothe her until the medication took effect."

Moments of Connection . . .
Showing Our Sympathy

"Working in the chronic pain setting, we do not have many deaths. When someone does die, as Pain Clinic Coordinator, I call the family to offer condolences. We also send a sympathy card. This time a daughter of a patient was killed in an accident and we chose to send flowers. The patient and family expressed their appreciation for this connection to them at a difficult time."

On the other hand, there may be occasions when you withhold your feelings for fear of being too warm. Perhaps you have romantic thoughts about a client or an unavailable colleague that are inappropriate to express. Sometimes you may have very strong negative feelings toward someone. It is likely that we all have encountered someone who has treated us coldly, with disdain, or even with rudeness or contempt. It would be difficult for most of us to be warm with those who have treated us in this way. When we want to protect ourselves from perceived or actual uncaring or disinterest, we may withdraw our warmth or refrain from offering it.

It is assertive to express your warmth to clients and colleagues when you wish. It is nonassertive to withhold the warmth you feel. In contrast, it is aggressive to exude a warmth beyond the measure of your feelings. When you sincerely convey the warmth you feel, you bring to life the assertive position: "I like myself; I like you." This warmth is nonpossessive and allows others room to be themselves.

The following exercises can make you aware of your warmth and provide you with pointers on how to convey your warmth when you choose.

> *Professionals are those who do their best even when they do not feel like it.*
>
> **Author unknown**
>
> **WIT&***Wisdom*

> *Kind hearts are the garden, kind thoughts are the roots, kind words are the flowers, and kind deeds are the fruits.*
>
> **Hungarian proverb**
>
> **WIT&***Wisdom*

Reflections On . . .

Warmth

Consider what you read about how to demonstrate warmth and its importance in making real connections with clients. It is easy to become focused on the technical skills you are learning in order to work with clients. Often the small acts of warmth are what embellish our work with an indication of who we are, and become our signature.

What? . . .
Write one thing you learned from this chapter.

So what? . . .
How will this affect your nursing practice?

Now what? . . .
How will you implement this new knowledge or skill?

Think about it . . .

Practicing Warmth

Exercise 1
Before you start observing or changing your own behavior, take a few days to observe the warmth displayed by colleagues and friends. Keep notes of what you see and your reactions. What did you notice about the following:

- Facial expressions
- Posturing
- Verbal expression
- Touching

What felt good? What warmth behaviors would you like to emulate? Compare your observations with those of your classmates. What did you learn from each other about the communication of warmth?

Exercise 2
For a few days, focus on your delivery of warmth. What is it you do to show your loved ones that you care? How is this expression different from your display of warmth to co-workers and to clients? How is it the same? Would you like to display more affection for others than you do? Make note of what you could change to be warmer. Find a partner in the class and exchange notes on the self-observations you have made.

Exercise 3
Find a full-length mirror and take a good look at yourself. Make a statement about the warmth your image projects. Does the set of your face convey warmth? Why? Why not? Note how you are holding your facial muscles. Do your eyes twinkle, or are they cold? Are your lips softly mobile, or are they tightened? Now, change your expression to make it warmer. Note what you do. How does it feel to soften your facial expression? Recall that feeling—you need that memory to call upon when you want to convey warmth to another person (when you don't have your mirror handy).

Next, turn away from the mirror and attempt to recapture that same warm facial expression. Then turn to check in the mirror. Have you got it? Or does your head need tilting, your smile broadening, or your eyes crinkling?

If you want to convey warmth, you need to practice these nonverbal gestures so that you feel confident
Continued

that you are sending out the message of warmth you want your clients and colleagues to receive.

Exercise 4

Identify a situation in which you felt warm toward someone, perhaps one who makes you smile. You might have seen a parent and child playing together or have been playing with your own child. Write a haiku poem describing the scene. This is a Japanese form of poetry, a three-line, 17-syllable poem, that captures a moment in time, from the perception of the poet and usually involves nature.

Use five syllables in the first line, seven in the second line, and five in the third line. An example is:

> *Head on my shoulder*
> *Baby-sleep warmth spreads throughout*
> *New mother delight.*

Exercise 5

This is an assessment of warmth skills. This exercise helps you develop skills in assessing warmth and provides you with feedback on your own warmth skills.

Work in groups of four for this exercise. During the week, all group members make 10-minute videotapes of themselves individually interviewing clients. (If clients are not available, group members can interview each other about a topic of personal significance to the interviewee.)

The members of each small group meet to view the videotapes. As one member shows his or her individual videotape to the rest of the group, the other members use the Warmth Content Analysis Sheet (Figure 7-1) to check off the warmth behaviors they see demonstrated by the interviewer.

Instructions for the Warmth Content Analysis Sheet: Each time you observe the interviewer demonstrate one of the warmth behaviors listed during a 1-minute interval, place a check mark in the appropriate column. For example, if during the first minute the interviewer smiles, has a warm vocal tone, and leans slightly forward, place checks in the 1-minute column beside the appropriate rows. Even if the interviewer engages in a behavior more than once during a 1-minute interval, put only one check mark. During each interval check off only whether a behavior occurs—how often it occurs doesn't matter. When a minute is up, move to the next minute column and check off any behaviors that occur during that minute interval. During each

1-minute interval you will be making a separate set of ratings. When the interview is over (or when 10 minutes has passed), add up your check marks in each row and write the total in the last column.

At the end of the 10-minute interview, after all group members have totaled their scores on the Warmth Content Analysis Sheet, all members use the Warmth Rating Scale (see Figure 7-1) to rate how warm they felt the interviewer's behavior was overall.

Note that these two tools measure different aspects of warmth. The content analysis sheet provides information on specific behaviors that occurred during the interview. The rating scale provides an overall assessment of the quality of warmth provided by the interviewer.

When the ratings are complete, group members give each other feedback on their warmth scores. This feedback includes the overall warmth rating and the specific behaviors used to communicate warmth. As the group members complete their feedback, they should finish by telling the interviewer the one thing the interviewer did best to show warmth.

Repeat these steps with each group member until everyone has had a turn at receiving feedback.

Exercise 6

Make your warmth assessment and care plan. At this point you have considerable information about your ability to express warmth. List those areas in which your communication of warmth is strong and in keeping with how you wish it to be. You might write something like this:

> Facial and body expression of warmth to others adequate when feeling inwardly calm, respected by the other person, and caught up in my work.

There may be situations in which the expression of your warmth is less than you would like. You might write something like this:

> Diminished expression of facial warmth in situations in which I'm expecting criticism. Absence of facial warmth (to the point of coldness) and absence of postural warmth (to the point of rigidity) when encountering an angry client because of fear of disapproval or dislike.

Pinpointing areas of concern helps you realize how specific and isolated the occasions for improvement are and directs you in developing a plan for improvement.

Name of person rated:_____   Name of rater:_____

Interviewer's behavior	1-Minute intervals										Total
	1	2	3	4	5	6	7	8	9	10	
1. Maintains eye contact											
2. Faces interviewee "squarely"											
3. Leans forward slightly											
4. Uses open posture: arms											
5. Uses open posture: legs											
6. Maintains relaxed posture											
7. Nods head to show interest											
8. Smiles											
9. Jokes											
10. Uses warm voice tone											
11. Face shows interest, attentiveness											
12. Speech content shows interest											

Warmth rating scale

Instructions: Place a check mark (✔) in the box beside the rating that indicates how warm you felt the interviewer's behavior was.

4.0 ☐ Very good response: very warm
3.5 ☐
3.0 ☐ Good response: warm
2.5 ☐
2.0 ☐ Poor response: cool
1.5 ☐
1.0 ☐ Very poor response: cold

FIGURE 7-1 Warmth Content Analysis Sheet. From Gerrard B, Boniface W, Love B: *Interpersonal skills for health professionals*, Reston, Va, 1980, Reston Publishing.

Exercise 7

Look for ways to evaluate improvements in your expression of warmth. One of the most important barometers of your warmth is your inner feelings. Are you feeling more relaxed and caring with clients and colleagues? Do you feel like you are expressing more affection and engaging more fully with others?

Are your expressions of affection flowing more freely?

For an external evaluation, you can monitor the verbal and nonverbal feedback you obtain from your clients. Do your clients talk more, look at you more, ask questions of you, shift to a relaxing position

Continued

in the chair, and indicate that they feel cared for by you?

You might wish to receive even more specific feedback about your warmth ability. One way to obtain this feedback is to ask a colleague to watch your interactions with clients and colleagues and to let you know the ways in which your warmth is conveyed and the areas in which you might improve.

Exercise 8

Customer service inventories report the value of kindness and warmth in health caring relationships. Discuss the value of warmth rather than defensiveness when a client or family member makes a complaint. Consider these phrases to demonstrate warmth. "Tell me about your concerns." "What can we do to make this better for you?"

Flowers leave fragrance in the hand that bestows them.

Filipino proverb

WIT&*Wisdom*

References

Baker C, Diekelmann N: Connecting conversations of caring: recalling the narrative to clinical practice, *Nurs Outlook* 42(2):65, 1994.

Carruth AK: Development and testing of the Caregiver Reciprocity Scale, *Nurs Res* 45(2):92, 1996.

Carver I: Healthcare with a human touch, *Nurs Spectr* 8(18):7, 1998.

Cooper MC, Powell E: Technology and care in a bone marrow transplant unit: creating and assuaging vulnerability, *Holist Nurs Pract* 12(4):57, 1998.

Ekeren GV: *Speaker's sourcebook, II: quotes, stories, and anecdotes for every occasion*, Englewood Cliffs, N.J., 1994, Prentice Hall.

Gleeson M: The use of touch to enhance nursing care of older persons in long-term mental health care facilities, *J Psychiatric Ment Health Nurs* 11(5):541, 2004.

Knapp ML: *Essentials of nonverbal communication*, New York, 1980, Holt, Rinehart & Winston.

Koopmeiners L, Post-White J, Gutknecht S, et al: How healthcare professionals contribute to hope in patients with cancer, *Oncol Nurs Forum* 24(9):1507, 1997.

Lee-Hsieh J, Fang Y, Kuy C, et al: Patient experiences in the development of a caring code for clinical nursing practice, *Int J Hum Caring* 8(3):21, 2004.

Levine DR, Adelman MB: *Beyond language: intercultural communication for English as a second language*, Englewood Cliffs, N.J., 1982, Prentice-Hall Regents.

O'Connor K: A dose of genuine warmth is as essential as skill with a syringe, *Nurs Stand* 19(32):28, 2005.

Purtilo R, Haddad AM: *Health professionals and patient interaction*, Philadelphia, 2002, WB Saunders.

Pullen RL, Mathias T: Fostering therapeutic nurse–patient relationships, *Nursing Made Incredibly Easy* 8(3):4, 2010. www.NursingMadeincrediblyeasy.com.

Reynolds M: Reflecting on paediatric oncology nursing practice using Benner's Helping Rose as a framework to examine aspects of caring, *Eur J Oncol Nurs* 6(1):30, 2002.

Tabron S: A prayer. In Knight B, editor: *Blessed are the caregivers: a daily book of comfort and cheer*, Albuquerque, 2001, Hartman Publishers.

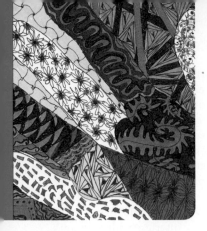

Chapter 8

Respect

| PORTIONS OF THIS CHAPTER CONTRIBUTED
BY MARGARET E. ERICKSON, PhD |

> *Respect is like air. If you take it away, it's all people can think about.*
>
> **Patterson and colleagues (2002), as cited by Kaplan and colleagues (2010)**

Objectives

1. Discuss the benefits of respect in the relationships in healthcare
2. Identify behaviors that demonstrate respect in relationships
3. Participate in exercises to build skills in demonstrating respect

Recognizing the Benefits of Respect

Respect, the foundation of helping interventions (Egan, 2006), is the communication of acceptance of the client's ideas, feelings, and experiences (Haber et al, 1997). When we show respect to our clients and colleagues, we are sending them the message, "I value you. You are important to me." Together, warmth and respect form what is called unconditional positive regard (Stuart, 2009). When helpers demonstrate that they care in a nonpossessive way, they transmit unconditional positive regard. This means accepting others for what they are, not on the condition that they behave in a certain way or possess special characteristics. Respect for the client is part of maintaining the person's dignity (Milika and Trorey, 2004; Griffin-Heslin, 2005).

Receiving respect makes people feel important, cared for, and worthwhile. These examples illustrate such reactions. Your co-worker tells you: "I love going to my new physician. Besides being a good clinician, she makes me feel so important. She's on time for my appointments, her receptionist remembers my name, and she follows up on all my requests." Your neighbor tells you about her recent experience with the nursing staff on the unit in which her husband is hospitalized: "The nurses are busy, of course, but they seem to have time to say 'hello' and pause for a few minutes to tell me something new about Jack. They never seem too busy for the little touches that make you feel so special. Not like the unit he was on before, where they scowled if you asked for something and gave you the impression that they didn't have time for you."

In contrast, when people do not receive respect, they feel hurt and ignored. For example, a middle-aged woman complains about the health unit coordinator on a busy hospital unit: "She didn't even have the courtesy to raise her head to speak to me when I asked her where Dad's room was. I might as well not have been there." A nurse reports her frustration at the disrespect she encountered: "Boy, I'm glad I don't work there! When I came down to borrow some syringes, the two nurses ignored me and kept on talking! It didn't even register that I was in a hurry and needed the stuff quickly." When people sense that they are not being treated with respect, they feel angry and rejected.

Experience shows that a positive correlation exists among respect, warmth, empathy, and successful treatment outcomes in psychotherapy clients. Indirect evidence supports the notion that respect, in terms of access to the desired physician, provision of convenient clinics, and reduced waiting times for appointments, has a beneficial influence on client compliance with the therapeutic regimen.

Moments of Connection . . .
Respect for the Sacred Relationships in Marriage

"I was the home health nurse for an elderly woman who was dying. Her husband was her primary caregiver. They had been married for more than 50 years and had always slept together. Now, however, the patient was sleeping in a hospital bed. One day the husband seemed more upset than usual. I asked him what was wrong and whether he needed more help. He began to cry and talked about missing her. I suggested he get into her bed with her and snuggle. He was afraid he would hurt her. I convinced him it would probably mean as much to her as it did to him. At the next visit she was comatose. He confided that he had gotten into bed with her the night before and slept all night with her. She had slept through the night without pain medication. He was so grateful I had made the suggestion."

Showing Respect to Your Clients

Respect is communicated principally by the ways nurses orient themselves toward and work with clients. The following ideas about respect reflect the philosophy of holistic nursing. To respect a client is also to have the humility to appreciate that the client is more than a set of symptoms classified as a disease. A person is body, mind, and spirit. These parts of the person are interrelated in such a way that the sum of them is greater than the parts, a whole with inseparable parts. "The whole is in dynamic interaction within itself, between and among other humans and with the universe. When all parts are balanced and in harmony, maximum well-being exists. Well being can exist in the presence or absence of physical ailment. Although health can be discussed in several ways—physical, social, emotional, cognitive, or spiritual health—to be truly healthy, one must experience a sense of well-being. An imbalance and disharmony within the human, human to human, and human to universe interfere with a person's well-being" (Erickson, 2007, p. 140).

Thus, the effect of treatments, medicines, and nursing interventions is influenced by all parts of the person. A person who is sad may be pessimistic and not open to getting better. A person who has a positive attitude about life, believing that every moment is precious, may not consider a physical symptom or a diagnosis of a disease as the most important thing, the focus of life. This is the person who looks for meaning in illness, a way to reflect upon what is most important in a life limited in time but not in the quality of embracing joy in life even in small moments.

To respect a client we try to "develop an image and understanding of the client's world, as the client perceives it" (Erickson et al, 1983, p. 254). "Through this process of 'Modeling' the nurse respectfully gains greater understanding of the client's model or world view. Based on the client's model of their world the nurse is then able to facilitate and nurture the individual in attaining, maintaining, or promoting health through purposeful interventions" (Erickson et al, 1983, p. 254). To respect a client is to appreciate that a person has an inherent ability to grow and become the most he or she can be, an inner voice or inner wisdom, self-care knowledge. To respect a client is to listen to what the person identifies as a need and to work to incorporate meeting that need into nursing care. To respect a client is to recognize the power of caring in the nurse–client relationship in which a "caring field" (Watson, 1979) is established . . . when the nurse and client connect on an energetic level . . . in caring moments . . . in a relationship that can "create new possibilities for the well-being" (Erickson, 2007, p. 150) of the nurse and client.

Although respect starts as an attitude, this mental outlook needs to be translated into behavior to demonstrate respect. A behavior that demonstrates respect is acknowledgment.

Acknowledging Clients

Feeling respect for your clients is not enough. They will receive the message that you think they are important and worthwhile only if you deliver the message clearly and directly. The following list provides concrete actions you can take to show respect to your clients.

- Look at your client.
- Offer your undivided attention.
- Maintain eye contact.
- Smile if appropriate.
- Move toward the other person.
- Determine how the other person likes to be addressed.
- Call the client by name and introduce yourself.
- Make contact with a handshake or by gently touching the individual.

Acknowledgment means demonstrating your awareness of your clients as individuals. One nurse wrote about a touching experience with a man sitting in an intensive care unit waiting room across the hall from where she was struggling with paperwork. Seeing his sadness, she walked over to him, sat down, and asked if she could help. Receiving no response, she simply placed her hand on his and sat in silence with him. After a time of silence, he revealed that both his wife and his son had recently died and that now he had been asked to donate his son's organs. The nurse told him she knew this was a difficult time for him and that she was there for him. After more silence, he told her he had made a decision, looked at her sadly, and left.

Moments of Connection . . .
Respect in Quiet Moments

"I work in an out-patient chronic pain center. We needed a piece of equipment that was unavailable, so I went to the intensive care unit to borrow the machine. The nurse told me I could take it from a room in which a patient had just died. I went into the room, which was very quiet, with no sounds of talking family or life-sustaining equipment. I stood in the quiet and honored that person who had died, saying a silent prayer. We face sadness, horror, and death, but in this quiet moment I felt peace, respect, and honor for that person—I felt a connection."

Simple gestures may communicate feelings when words miss the mark (Taylor, 1994). Copp (1993) identified the waiting room as a place of "lost lessons" and comments that students of nursing could learn about the demonstration of caring by being sensitive to the "weary travelers" who have come long distances, the waiting relatives who feel unsure of how to care for the loved one at home, or the waiting friends or relatives who have put their own lives on hold to be there.

Showing respect involves using verbal and nonverbal skills. Looking at our clients or colleagues as they speak shows attention, but it is the quality of our facial expressions that reveals whether we are interested in what our clients or co-workers are saying.

In the United States, introductions are accompanied by a firm, brief handshake. This custom may not be the same in all countries from which clients or colleagues come. In some cultures handshaking is prolonged, and taking our hands away too quickly could be misinterpreted as rejection. Within reason, it is best to allow the client to end the handshake.

In addition, after opening acknowledgments are made, a period of small talk usually follows, during which impersonal and trivial subjects (such as the weather) are discussed to break the ice. Some cultures prolong this period of discussion.

Establishing the Nature of the Contact

After you have acknowledged your client, several actions can convey respect at the outset of a new or ongoing client–nurse encounter.

For a first-time contact:

- Make it clear who you are and what your role is in the agency.
- Wear your name pin or identification badge.
- Ask what the other person needs or wants.
- Be clear about how you can be of help.
- Indicate how you will protect your client's confidentiality.

For an ongoing relationship:

- Ensure that the client recalls who you are and your role in the agency.
- Determine the client's needs at this point.
- Indicate that you recall details about the individual.
- Review the issue of confidentiality.
- Refrain from gossiping about other clients.
- If appropriate, suggest a referral so that the client will receive the required assistance.

As nurses we must remember that the most intensely private and personal aspects of clients' lives are revealed in times of crisis and illness, whether in a hospital setting, an outpatient clinic, or the home. At the outset of a client–nurse relationship, we have a duty to tell clients of others with whom we are likely to share the information they give us, so that they understand the parameters of confidentiality in the agency. Some private information may need to be shared with other members of the healthcare team in developing a treatment plan. We are obliged to diligently protect the confidences of our clients unless required to reveal them by law, or unless our clients give us permission to share these details. Releasing the status of a client's condition to the news media or general public does not create liability exposure, but disclosing more detailed information or a photograph without the client's consent should be avoided. In healthcare facilities in which there is public stigma, such as a psychiatric or drug abuse treatment center, even releasing a client's name would be an automatic invasion of privacy. Clients expect that the information they give will be kept strictly confidential. The need for disclosure should be carefully evaluated before information is shared. Maintaining confidentiality demonstrates respect for the rights of the individual (Erlen, 1998).

Moments of Connection . . .
Respect for the Dying Client
"I had a 19-year-old client dying of cancer. His dad had died in Vietnam and his mom could no longer cope. They had no other family and I would go sit with him, hold his hand, and talk. Finally, the mother said good-bye to him and left. He died 4 hours later. I couldn't leave. I stayed and held him and prayed with him. It was the greatest lesson of my nursing career."

Although the following ethical guidelines for confidentiality were written for psychiatric nurse specialists, these principles are applicable guides in any situation in which nurses are striving to respect clients by protecting their confidentiality (Colorado Society of Clinical Specialists in Psychiatric Nursing, 1990):

- Keep all client records secure.

- Consider carefully the content to be entered into the record.
  - Release information only with written consent and full discussion of the information to be shared, except when release is required by law.
  - Use professional judgment regarding confidentiality when the client is a danger to himself or herself or to others. Do not promise the client that you will keep secrets and acknowledge that you will use your judgment about shared information that might indicate potential harm to the client or someone else.
  - Use professional judgment deliberately when deciding how to maintain the confidentiality of a minor. The rights of the parent or guardian must also be considered.
- Disguise clinical material when used professionally for teaching and writing.
- Maintain confidentiality in consultation and in peer-reviewed situations.
- Maintain the anonymity of research subjects.
- Safeguard the confidentiality of the student in teaching and learning situations.

Establishing a Comfortable Climate

The following list describes the steps necessary to establish a comfortable environment for the client:

- Indicate at the beginning how much time you have so that your client can gauge the length of the discussion and prepare for your leaving.
- Arrange to meet at another time if the allotted period is too brief for the content to be discussed.
- Ensure privacy before engaging in a discussion of confidential matters.
- Ensure that telephones or other people do not interfere with your giving undivided attention to your client.
- Arrange the room so that no barrier, such as a desk, separates you and your client, and avoid standing over a person in a wheelchair.
- Ensure that the environment is comfortable by making space for your client, having a place for a coat and other personal belongings, and adjusting the room temperature and lighting.
- Take care to be on time for appointments and try to avoid inconveniencing a client by switching appointments.

- If you are late or have to change an appointment time, explain the reason to your client so that it is clear that the delay was unavoidable.

Promptness for appointments is important to Americans, and we consider it irresponsible to miss scheduled appointments. For Americans time is tangible, as is reflected by the phrases "find time," "spend time," "waste time," "save time," and "kill time." Because clients from other cultures may proceed at a pace different from Americans and have different ways of perceiving, regulating, and dividing time, we may have to be creative about considering time customs when making appointments. Clients from cultures with different values about time might have to learn about canceling and rescheduling appointments.

An aspect of mutuality is a sense of equality in the partnership. One nonverbal way to achieve an egalitarian relationship with clients is to arrange the seating so that you are both at the same height.

> Authority can be communicated by the height from which one person interacts with another. If one stands while the other sits, the former has subconsciously placed himself or herself in a position of authority. . . . Height is unwittingly used to project a submissive role onto a patient when he or she is confined to a bed, a treatment table, or a wheelchair (Purtilo and Haddad, 2002).

Discussing Sensitive Subjects

Some health issues have an associated stigma or evoke judgment, such as the epidemic problem of obesity in America. Overweight and obesity are grouped as a leading health indicator in *Healthy People 2010*, which details the nation's health objectives for the first decade of the twenty-first century (U.S. Department of Health and Human Services, 2001). Although it is easier to avoid addressing such health concerns with a client and family, there are respectful ways to accept this responsibility. A nurse practitioner wrote about her sensitive intervention with an 11-year-old boy weighing 265 pounds. She wanted to preserve his dignity but responsibly address this major health issue. She established rapport, addressed other presenting health issues, then respectfully discussed the challenge of obesity, offering referral to a dietitian for a customized weight-management plan and introducing the child to the activity pyramid (Bollinger, 2001).

Terminating Contact

How nurses end their discussions with clients is just as important as other phases of the interaction. Following are guidelines for terminating the contact:

- If you have to leave early, prepare your client in advance.
- Summarize what you have discussed.
- Follow through with what you said you would do.
- Make notes of any points you want to remember for future contact.

For ongoing relationships, do the following:

- Prepare your client for discharge several visits before termination.
- Allow time and space for the client to talk about the feelings that termination may bring up.
- Express your thoughts and feelings about termination as a way of showing that you care.
- If you are going to be away for a limited period of time, make arrangements for client coverage and be sure to check with your client to make sure that these arrangements are suitable.

To maintain cost effectiveness in American hospitals, the length of stay of patients is decreasing; clients are being discharged earlier. This limits the time for discharge planning, and the transition period from hospital to home is briefer and possibly not as smooth as it once was. Nurses in some hospitals follow a callback system to check on clients at home after discharge for early problem solving. This kind of follow-up demonstrates respect through a willingness to work with clients by being available and interested in their healthcare problems. Adopting the mutual problem-solving approach is also respectful because it shows good faith in our clients' ability to use their self-care knowledge and self-care resources to facilitate their own healing, health, and well-being (Erickson et al, 1983). Self-care resources refer to the individual's "internal, as well as additional resources . . . that will help them gain, maintain, and promote an optimum level of holistic health" (Erickson et al, 1983, p. 254). By facilitating and respectfully recognizing the client's self-care knowledge and resources, the nurse affirms that the client has the means, control, and knowledge necessary to heal and achieve their greatest state of well-being (Erickson et al, 1983). Attempts to overcome a language barrier with clients and families is another way of demonstrating respect. Check with the hospital's patient advocate or human resources department to identify employees who could serve as interpreters. Language Line Services can be purchased for over-the-phone interpretation of 170 languages, 24 hours a day, 7 days a week (call 1-800-752-6096 for information).

Showing Respect to Your Colleagues

You can apply many of the suggestions given earlier to show respect to your colleagues as well as to your clients. Being courteous, attentive, and mindful of the unique contribution each colleague makes to the total healthcare team are all ways of conveying respect to colleagues.

The Joint Commission (http://www.jointcommission. org/), a hospital-accrediting organization, requires a process to create a definition of and policy for addressing disruptive, disrespectful behavior among colleagues. Maimonides Medical Center (Brooklyn, N.Y.) created a code of mutual respect. This code has been implemented in the operating room, where disrespect can be common. In an operating room "measures of productivity, efficiency, and safe patient care" are higher when healthcare providers respect one another (Kaplan et al, 2010).

A lack of respect of colleagues has contributed to morale and productivity problems in the American workplace and may contribute to high levels of stress associated with emotional outbursts and violence. Electronic communication may serve as a buffer so that people do not have to face each other. A study of the manufacturing industry was described, in which employees reported they believed they had been treated rudely, disrespectfully, or insensitively by a co-worker, and 78% of respondents reported that civility had decreased in the previous 10 years (Verespej, 2001). Civility is an ethical principle of respect for people. Incivility is "morally destructive patterns of self-absorption, callousness, manipulation, and materialism so ingrained in our routine behavior that we do not even recognize them" (Peck, 1994). Consider your reaction to the extreme effects of a lack of respect for others in the workplace as you reflect on the importance of respect.

Schools of nursing are addressing student incivility. Behaviors that are disrespectful to faculty and other students reflect a lack of value for human dignity and altruism, qualities essential for professional nursing. Incivility is rudeness and breaches of common courtesy.

Examples of incivility in the classroom are lateness, leaving the class early, inattentiveness, threatening language, or physical violence (Luparell, 2005). Some schools of nursing have instituted disruptive student behavior policies.

Being respectful embodies assertiveness. When we show respect, we are upholding the other person's right to be treated with dignity (Carson and Koenig, 2008) and consideration, while at the same time not ignoring our own needs to manage our time effectively and carry out the role for which we are qualified. Being respectful means acknowledging others' needs to be attended to, understood, and helped within the limits of nurses' abilities and time.

We, as nurses, must understand the effect we can have on people in every single encounter. Being respectful means showing our finely tuned sensitivity to others with the full realization that we can affect their well-being. As nurses, we need to be aware of the power we have to make our clients and colleagues feel cared for, and, more important, to use that power consistently and with good intent. Respect for a client is part of nursing excellence. A study was conducted to examine how the coping behaviors of nurses whose own family of origin was dysfunctional helped build competent caring behaviors. It was concluded that the very behaviors that helped these nurses adapt to their own circumstances were valuable behaviors in fine-tuning their sensitivity to clients and their families. One nurse indicated that her own drive to show clients and families respect arose because that was what she longed for as a child (Biering, 1998).

One factor that facilitates nurses' demonstration of respect is the strong conviction that others have the right to be treated with respect for their feelings of worth. Nurses with less well-integrated values of human dignity might be less consistent in demonstrating their respect. If you find you are inconsistent in conveying respect, examine which of your values conflicts with being respectful in some situations. What is more powerful in influencing your behavior than your desire to be respectful?

Moments of Connection . . .
Respect for the Fearful, Grieving Client
"Suzanne was a 36-year-old woman who had experienced a ruptured ectopic pregnancy the day before. She had abdominal pain and was taken back to the operating

room. In the postanesthesia care unit she had difficulty breathing and required admission after a computed axial tomographic scan. I accompanied her for the scan. I introduced myself, held her hand, and told her that I didn't know what she was going to go through but that I would be with her. She was obviously scared and held onto my hand and closed her eyes. I took care of her the whole next week. After she was discharged, her husband brought me a teddy bear she wanted me to have and told me how grateful she was that I had stayed with her. I felt like I had made a difference."

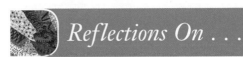

Reflections On . . .

Respect

Consider what you read about respect in relationships. How do you demonstrate respect in your relationships with clients, families, and staff?

What? . . .
Write one thing you learned from this chapter.

So what? . . .
How will this affect your nursing practice?

Now what? . . .
How will you implement this new knowledge or skill?

Think about it . . .

Practicing Respect

Exercise 1

Take a moment to identify a time when you were disrespectful to someone else. Write a brief journal entry about the situation. What happened? In what way were you disrespectful? What were the consequences? How did you feel? Putting yourself in the other person's position, how might that person have felt about the situation? What would you do differently if this happened again? What did you learn from the incident?

Exercise 2   QSEN

Patient-centered care is a fundamental concept in creating cultures of safety and in facilitating continuous improvements in quality. Mindfully engaging with each client and family as you interact and guide their care can help reduce the potential for error and improve care outcomes. Mindful engagement in a caregiving encounter helps to individualize care and to include the client and family as equal partners in their care. As you plan care for your client, consider this method for patient-centered care based on respect for the client's preferences:

- Clear your mind of distractions and focus on clients as unique people with hopes, with values, with health beliefs, and who are members of their own community.
- What is the essential information you need to know to plan effective care for these patients?
- To demonstrate respect for what patients know and believe, what choices can you offer the patients and family?

Applying evidence-based standards helps improve the quality of care, but at what point is it appropriate to respect clients' preferences and make exceptions to the standard in order to accommodate their wishes?

QSEN Competencies: Patient-centered Care; Evidence-based Care

Exercise 3

Find a partner with whom to work. For the first part of this exercise one of you talks and the other listens, and then you switch roles. When the speaker is talking, the task of the listener is to be blatantly disrespectful. For example, when you first come together, do not acknowledge the other person. Give limited attention to the other person's concerns and demonstrate rude behavior such as reading, looking at your mail, forgetting the other's name, or terminating the conversation abruptly. After 4 minutes, stop talking and discuss the interaction.

As the speaker: How did it feel to receive disrespectful communication?
As the listener: How did it feel to be disrespectful?

Share these feelings with each other as a way of learning about the negative effects of disrespect. Now switch roles so that each of you feels what it is like to be caught in a disrespectful encounter.

Exercise 4

For this exercise work in pairs. One person is the speaker and the other the listener. This time the listener shows as much respect as possible throughout the interview by exhibiting the respectful behaviors discussed earlier in the chapter.

After talking for several minutes, pause and have the speaker provide feedback to the listener on how it felt to receive respectful communication. Switch roles and repeat this.

In the class as a whole, discuss what participating in these exercises has taught you about the importance of respect in interpersonal relationships.

Exercise 5

Situation: Susan Weeks, a registered nurse, has been working for several days with Mrs. Green, an inpatient. Mrs. Green has elected to refuse chemotherapy for the treatment of cancer, leave the hospital, and be transferred to hospice care. The nurse does not agree with the client's decision although she believes it to be an informed decision. Discuss how the nurse can demonstrate her respect for Mrs. Green's right to make her own end-of-life decisions.

Exercise 6

We speak of the indignities of aging when we speak of the changes in the body as a result of aging and the losses incurred. Discuss how you can demonstrate respect to an elder client.

> *When people bring us their problems, they are often asking not for solutions but for understanding.*
>
> **Author unknown**

WIT&Wisdom

References

Biering P: "Codependency": a disease or the root of nursing excellence? *J Holist Nurs* 16(3):320, 1998.

Bollinger E: Applied concepts of holistic nursing, *J Holist Nurs* 19(2):212, 2001.

Carson VB, Koenig HG, editors: *Spiritual dimensions of nursing practice*, West Conshohocken, Pa, 2008, Templeton Foundation Press.

Colorado Society of Clinical Specialists in Psychiatric Nursing: Ethical guidelines for confidentiality, *J Psychosoc Nurs* 28(3):43, 1990.

Copp LA: Teaching site: the waiting room, *J Prof Nurs* 9(1):1, 1993.

Egan G: *The skilled helper: a problem-management and opportunity-development approach to helping*, ed 7, New York, 2006, Brooks/Cole.

Erickson H, Tomlin E, Swain MA: *Modeling and role-modeling: a theory and paradigm for nursing.* Englewood Cliffs, N.J., 1983–2010. Prentice-Hall; second–ninth printing, Cedar Park, Tex: 1988–2009; EST Co; tenth printing, Cedar Park, Tex, 2010, Unicorns Unlimited.

Erickson HL: Philosophy and theory of holism, *Nurs Clin North Am* 42:139, 2007.

Erlen JA: The inadvertent breach of confidentiality, *Orthop Nurs* 17(2):7, 1998.

Griffin-Heslin VL: An analysis of the concept of dignity, *Accid Emerg Nurs* 13(4):251, 2005.

Haber J, Krainovich-Miller B, McMahon AL: *Comprehensive psychiatric nursing*, St. Louis, 1997, Mosby.

Kaplan K, Mestel P, Feldman DL: Creating a culture of mutual respect, *AORN J* 91(4): 495, 2010.

Luparell S: Why and how we should address student incivility in nursing programs, *Annu Rev Nurs Educ* 3:23, 2005.

Milika RM, Trorey G: Perceptual adjustment levels: patients' perception of their dignity in the hospital setting, *Int J Nurs Stud* 41(7):735, 2004.

Patterson K, Grenny J, McMillan R, et al: *Crucial conversations: tools for talking when stakes are high*, New York, 2002, McGraw-Hill, p 71.

Peck S: *A world waiting to be born: civility rediscovered*, New York, 1994, Bantam Books.

Purtilo R, Haddad AM: *Health professional and patient interaction*, ed 6, Philadelphia, 2002, WB Saunders.

Stuart GW: *Principles and practice of psychiatric nursing*, ed 9, St. Louis, 2009, Mosby.

Taylor C: Communicating without words: what's left unsaid can make a difference, *Nursing* 94(24):30, 1994.

U.S. Department of Health and Human Services, Office of the Surgeon General: *The surgeon general's call to action to prevent and decrease overweight and obesity 2001*, Washington, D.C., 2001, U.S. Government Printing Office. http://www.surgeongeneral.gov/topics/obesity/. Accessed August 12, 2010.

Verespej M: Human resources: a call for civility, *Industry Week*, February 12, 2001. http://www.industryweek.com/articles/human_resources_—_a_call_for_civility_2087.aspx

Watson J: *Nursing: the philosophy and science of caring.* Boston, 1979, Little Brown.

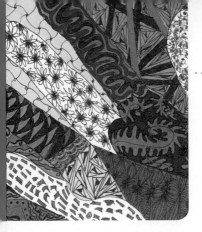

Chapter 9

Genuineness

| PORTIONS OF THIS CHAPTER CONTRIBUTED
BY MARGARET E. ERICKSON, PHD |

> *Rather a heart without words than words
> without heart.*
>
> **Sudanese proverb**

Objectives

1. Differentiate between genuine and nongenuine behavior
2. Discuss the importance of being genuine with clients and colleagues
3. Participate in exercises to build skills in demonstrating genuineness

Benefits of Genuineness in Interpersonal Relationships

If we say a person is genuine, what does it mean? Why is it important to be "your natural self" in human relationships? According to the Gallup Organization's 2010 annual poll, nurses ranked number one on professional honesty and ethical standards. Our clients care and notice that we are honest and genuine in interpersonal relationships. A woman diagnosed with cancer shared one thing she thinks nurses need to know that is a demonstration of genuine concern. She asked that when you enter a client's room, you stop and see the person first. "Here's what would be so healing that won't take but a moment" (Guilmartin, 2010, p. 18). "Could you soften your gaze as you look at me? As you approach my bed could you consider whether I need a gentle touch or a positive thought to remind me that I am more than one additional task in a tough day?" Guilmartin (2010) relates this story when she discusses the power of a pause. Here a pause is a few moments, perhaps, one deep breath, that can reframe how you see your work and its meaning and communicate your genuineness. Carl Rogers (1980), a pioneer in the study of communication, used the two synonyms *realness* and *congruence* for genuineness, which he claims is the basis for the best communication. A fundamental feature of genuineness, in Rogers's view, is the presentation of our true thoughts and feelings, both verbally and nonverbally, to another person. It is not only the words you say or how you say them, but also your facial expression and body posture that signify genuineness. Being genuine means that you send the other person the real picture of you, not a distorted one that differs from how you really think or feel. Genuineness is a spontaneous expression conveying an individual's experience (Haber et al, 1997). It is the opposite of self-alienation, in which a person suppresses spontaneous reactions to life (Stuart, 2009). You can be open to new possibilities in meeting clients' needs when you are truly present and trust the authenticity of your intention to care for and serve (Bruce and Davies, 2005).

In the classic children's story *The Velveteen Rabbit* (Bianco, 1922/1996), toys talk about what it means to be real.

> When a child loves you for a long, long time, not just to play with, but REALLY loves you, then you become real . . . by the time you are Real, most of your hair has been loved off, and your eyes drop out and you get loose in the joints and very shabby. But these things don't matter at all, because once you are Real you can't be ugly, except to people who don't understand.

To Be Real Is to Be Yourself

In the helping relationship with clients and in mutually supportive relationships with colleagues in the workplace, being genuine does not mean impulsively dumping your reactions on others. To "hit" clients and colleagues with feelings and then "run" is aggressive. In a therapeutic relationship, genuinely presenting your thoughts and feelings to others can be done assertively and constructively.

As nurses, we make an important judgment call in deciding to genuinely share our inner thoughts and feelings with others. The literature advises nurses to be genuine "when it is appropriate to do so." Appropriateness is linked to whether our revelations will benefit our clients (or colleagues) and/or our relationships. Read carefully the counsel of Peck (1997) on dedication to the truth:

> So the expression of opinions, feelings, ideas and even knowledge must be suppressed from time to time in . . . the course of human affairs. What rules, then, can one follow if one is dedicated to the truth? First, never speak a falsehood. Second, bear in mind that the act of withholding the truth is always potentially a lie, and that in each instance in which the truth is withheld a significant moral decision is required. Third, the decision to withhold the truth should never be based on personal needs, such as a need for power, a need to be liked, or a need to protect one's map from challenge. Fourth, and

conversely, the decision to withhold the truth must always be based entirely upon the needs of the person or people from whom the truth is being withheld. Fifth, the assessment of another's needs is an act of responsibility which is so complex that it can only be executed wisely when one operates with genuine love for the other. Sixth, the primary factor in the assessment of another's needs is the assessment of that person's capacity to utilize the truth for his or her own spiritual growth. Finally, in assessing the capacity of another to utilize the truth for personal spiritual growth, it should be borne in mind that our tendency is generally to underestimate rather than overestimate this capacity.

We take a risk when we are genuine because sometimes genuineness involves expressing negative thoughts and confronting others with our reactions. When we are genuine, whether expressing negative or positive reactions, the message we give to our clients and colleagues is "You are strong and worthy of my engaging fully with you." When we are genuine, we give careful attention to listening to the other person. We extend ourselves and take the extra step to do the hard work of listening, and oppose the "inertia of laziness or the resistance of fear" (Peck, 1997). We enter into a relationship with a client with a fresh perspective, aware that information we have read or heard about a client could influence our ability to be genuine and see him or her as unique. Focusing on making your own observations of the client's behavior will help you avoid stereotyping or stigmatizing a client (Sundeen et al, 1998).

Nurses who are genuine seem to their clients to mean exactly what the words they are saying connote, and their accompanying affective behavior matches their words (Arnold and Boggs, 2011). When our verbal message does not correspond to our facial expression, posture, tone of voice, and body language, clients and colleagues decode the disparate information as two distinct and dissimilar messages. It is not hard to imagine that this incongruence of conflicting or mixed messages puts our credibility in question. Furthermore, a meaningful relationship is unlikely to ensue when our clients or colleagues doubt our trustworthiness.

As nurses we have expectations about the behaviors that accompany our assumed roles. Some of the behaviors expected of nurse-advocates are providing competent nursing care based on current standards, serving on committees to ensure quality care, and coordinating all services used by clients in an attempt to restore, maintain, or promote health. The roles we assume have cultural, gender, and situational performance expectations. These roles are comforting because they provide guidelines for performance. Being genuine means remembering that roles are filled by individuals with unique personalities, styles, and ideas (Nuwayhid, 1984). Realness means being free from the bonds of the role and not hiding behind the façade of the role. Being a person and a nurse at the same time involves spontaneity; we cannot weigh every word we say or talk in scripts that seem planned or rigid. Congruence includes an openness to sharing without always waiting to be asked, to express directly what is going on inside us without distorting our messages.

Genuineness is a "what you see is what you get" phenomenon. People experiencing your genuineness can trust you because they know you are not sending false signals or hiding something from them. This building of trust is the most important reason for being genuine (Box 9-1). When we believe that we can count on others, we can start to relax in the relationship. We stop worrying about what others might really be thinking and feeling. The energy freed from worrying can be put into the relationship, both deepening it and moving it in the direction for which it was established. Being genuine as a nurse is one major step in gaining credibility with clients and colleagues.

Box 9-1 | *Benefits of Nurse Genuineness for Clients and Colleagues*

NURSE GENUINENESS
- Speaks deep from within without apology
- Expresses thoughts, feelings, and experiences in the here and now
- Shows spontaneity
- Conveys openness

BENEFITS FOR CLIENTS AND COLLEAGUES
- Feel free to express their true thoughts and emotions
- Develop a feeling of trust for the nurse
- Are provided with information they can use in the relationship here and now
- Can unwind in a relaxed atmosphere
- Enjoy a climate of realness

Incongruence

When a mismatch exists between nurses' experiences of their thoughts and feelings and their awareness, this incongruence is called *denial of awareness* or *defensiveness* (Rogers, 1995). You may notice, for example, that your colleague looks angry. She is stamping her foot, pointing her finger, becoming red in the face, and raising her voice in an accusatory way. When you suggest that she is angry, however, she brushes it off and denies her obvious feelings.

When a mismatch exists between nurses' thoughts and feelings and their communication of this internal experience, it is usually considered falseness or deceit (Rogers, 1995). For example, if you disapprove of the new policy to merge your unit with another unit in the hospital but you hide your anger and tell your boss you think the merger is a good idea because you want to make a good impression on her, this is deceit.

If we pretend that our thoughts and feelings are different from what they really are, then we will say things that we do not believe. If we act on thoughts and feelings that we do not have, we give people the wrong impression about us, leading them astray. In contrast, expressing our genuine thoughts and feelings about issues makes what we stand for absolutely clear to our clients and colleagues. The research findings of Rogers (1957) and Shapiro and colleagues (1969) establish that genuineness on the part of the therapist has positive therapeutic outcomes.

Even if we can control our verbal communication when we are trying to deceive another about our true thoughts and feelings, our nonverbal cues can give us away (Knapp, 1995). Nonverbal behavior can reveal the information we are hiding or indicate that we are attempting to deceive without indicating specific information about the nature of the deception (Knapp, 1995). We are skilled at manipulating our facial expressions and our postures to coincide with our verbal message, but the way we move our feet, legs, or hands can betray incongruence with our verbal messages—showing that we are not genuine. Some of the foot and leg movements that might alert others to our incongruence are aggressive foot kicks, flirtatious leg displays, autoerotic or soothing leg squeezing, abortive restless flight movements, tense leg positions, frequent shifts of leg posture, and restless or repetitive leg and foot motions. Revealing hand movements might include digging our hands into our cheeks, tearing at our fingernails, or protectively holding our knees while smiling and looking pleasant. Knapp reports studies revealing that one of the reasons we may not expend much effort inhibiting or dissimulating feet and hand behavior is that, over the years, we have learned to disregard internal feedback, and we do not learn to control areas of our bodies from which we receive little external feedback (Knapp, 1995). Another way we might reveal our incongruence is by neglecting to include the nonverbal action that customarily would accompany the verbal message. Our omission is a signal to clients and colleagues that something is wrong (Box 9-2).

You may ask yourself how anyone could act in any way but genuinely. Occasionally it feels risky to reveal what we think and feel to others. What if they do not agree? What if they think we are ignorant? Sometimes we fear that clients or colleagues might reject us if they do not like what we say. We worry that others might laugh at us, argue with us, put us down, or gossip about us. We may be threatened by fears that if we are honest, a colleague might refuse to work with us or a client may request the services of another nurse.

When feeling vulnerable to rejection, we might modify what we think and feel to make ourselves more acceptable to others. We change in an attempt to give others what we think they wish to hear. In so doing, we begin the entanglement of presenting a false impression of ourselves. If others are fooled, they expect the behavior to be repeated, and then we are trapped. We can continue to try to act falsely or we can confess. If our lack of authenticity is spotted, then others will stop trusting us, question our word, or ask for a second opinion. It is ironic that when we behave insincerely to avoid rejection, our worst fears of rejection can come true.

When we are genuine, we have no guarantee that our clients or colleagues will accept us or agree with us, but they will usually be touched by our willingness to present ourselves as we are and our courage to risk rejection. Our honesty is reassuring and refreshing. If others choose to withdraw from a relationship with the genuine us, then they leave us with the satisfaction of knowing we have been honest with ourselves. Being genuine is being assertive; it is an action of standing up for our legitimate rights to express our point of view. When we are authentic, our concept of ourselves as assertive nurses is strengthened.

Demonstration of Genuineness with Clients and Colleagues

The following examples illustrate how to be genuine with clients and colleagues.

For several days Joyce, a nurse, has been assigned to care for a client who has been flirtatious. He has asked for her telephone number, looked at her seductively, and touched her, as if by accident, as frequently as possible.

Joyce's thoughts: She knows it is her responsibility to behave as a professional. Because the behavior has persisted, she knows she must deal with it. This young man is in a vulnerable position as a patient and needs to have access to a professional who can care for him. A social relationship might alter his ability to make his needs known.

Box 9-2	*Negative Effects of Nurse Incongruence for Clients and Colleagues*

NURSE INCONGRUENCE

- Puts up a façade or pretense
- Withholds thoughts or experiences
- Shows a mismatch between verbal and nonverbal messages
- Communicates in a rigid and contrived way that sounds as if it is scripted

NEGATIVE EFFECTS ON CLIENTS AND COLLEAGUES

- Distrust the nurse
- Are suspicious of the nurse
- Relate to the nurse in a strained, tense way
- Omit valuable information from the interchange
- Decode the message as two distinct and dissimilar ones
- Feel confusion
- Believe only the nonverbal message
- Question the nurse's credibility
- Have difficulty maintaining a meaningful dialogue in the presence of mixed messages
- Do not believe that they are talking to a real person
- Feel that the nurse is trying to impress them rather than connect with them

Joyce's feelings: She is attracted to this client but sees his behavior as inappropriate and as a barrier to her providing him with the care he needs. She is worried about embarrassing herself and him by behaving inappropriately.

The genuine communication is to explain to the client that her relationship with him is professional, not social.

Genuine response: "Our relationship here is that of client and nurse. I would ask you to think of it that way so I can provide you with the professional care you deserve."

This statement assertively communicates Joyce's thoughts and feelings in a way that is in keeping with her personal and professional values, making her trustworthy. If she had refrained from expressing her point of view, she would have communicated in a nonassertive and nongenuine way.

Nongenuine nonassertive response: "Well, I might go out with you . . . we'll see."

This message does not clarify the professional nature of the relationship. It might invite more of the flirtatious behavior Joyce wants to avoid.

Nongenuine aggressive response: "You guys are all the same. You're a chauvinist . . . you treat nurses like playthings. Cool it, mister! I have a job to do here."

This approach creates bad feelings and may interfere with Joyce's ability to provide nursing care.

Consider this situation between colleagues in the workplace. A fellow nurse tells you that she has promised a client that her husband could bring in their cat when he comes to visit her. She explains to you, "I thought it might cheer up Mrs. Kent; she misses her cat so much. You don't mind, do you?"

The truth is, you do mind. The hospital has strict rules about not having pets on the unit and you agree with them. You are in charge on this shift, and you do not want any negative repercussions from breaking the rules.

Your thoughts: It is unfair to show favoritism by breaking the rules for one client. Good reasons exist for excluding animals from the unit.

Your feelings: You are annoyed that your colleague has made this decision without consulting you, since you will bear the brunt of any consequences. You wish to correct your colleague without putting her down.

The genuine way to communicate would be to state your disagreement and disappointment and ask your colleague to reverse her decision.

Genuine response: "It's unfortunate that you didn't discuss this issue with me first. I believe strongly that we shouldn't show favoritism, and I agree with the health unit's rationale for restricting pets from the unit. Will you tell Mrs. Kent that she won't be able to have a visit with her cat while she's in the hospital?"

This assertion makes it clear to your colleague what you think and feel, and does so in a way that respects her feelings.

Nongenuine nonassertive response: "Gee, I don't think we should be allowing a cat on the unit, do you? I guess there's nothing we can do about it now."

By passively allowing the rule to be broken and not expressing your annoyance and opinions in a clear, direct way, you are denying the expression of your genuine reaction.

Nongenuine aggressive response: "You what? Well, forget it. Go and tell Mrs. Kent that you've made a mistake. Don't ever make that kind of decision without consulting me."

This angry outburst is incongruent with your desire to communicate respectfully with your colleagues.

Being genuine is an assertive act. In expressing our thoughts and feelings, we need to take care that they are clear, direct, and respectful of the positions of others.

Factors Influencing Genuineness

Our genuineness springs from three main sources: our self-confidence, our perception of others, and our environmental influences.

When our self-confidence is blossoming, we feel strong enough to risk revealing our true selves. When our self-confidence is withering, it is easier to try to impress others with what we think they want to hear to feel accepted and important. Self-confidence is not something with which we are born, but is something that we must nourish. When we risk being authentic, we feel good about being true to our thoughts and feelings. This good feeling is translated into self-confidence.

When we perceive that others have power and influence over us, we might refrain from being authentically ourselves. If we decide that other people are smarter, more deserving, or more worthy, then we are more likely to show off for these people than relate to them in a way congruent with our thoughts and feelings. Learning to take charge and empowering ourselves to trust our own reactions help us to perceive others as equals with whom we can dare to reveal our true thoughts and feelings.

Environmental variables also influence our ability to be genuine. In front of a large group, many of us might shy away from revealing our true thoughts and feelings. Limited time may prevent us from being genuine. If we know that expression of our thoughts and feelings could cause a reaction in others that would require more than the available time to work out, then we might wait for a better time to express ourselves genuinely.

In one study of patients' perceptions of nurses' knowledge and presence, nurses identified shortened hospital stays, paperwork, and time pressures as barriers to the development of relationships with patients. Both patients and nurses valued the "little things," such as using each other's names or remembering nicknames (Cohen et al, 1994).

To be congruent we need to be aware of our thoughts and feelings (Rogers, 1995). As we get to know ourselves better, expanded self-awareness builds and deepens our self-concept. This greater self-awareness is something we need to relate more genuinely to others (Rogers, 1980).

Palliative Care: A Call to Authenticity

Palliative care nursing is the active, total care of clients who are not responsive to curative treatments, in which control of pain, other symptoms causing distress, and spiritual stress are paramount (Ferrell and Coyle, 2001). Post–World War II babies, known as *baby boomers*, are in their 60s now, and both clients and nurses are turning their thoughts to their own mortality and quality of life. The approaches used in palliative care nursing, in which the nurse's relationship with client and family has a major impact, are applicable to all nursing and offer intimate opportunities for the nurse to respond genuinely as an authentic caregiver. Healing of the body, mind, and spirit

(the word *heal* means "to make whole") can occur as the client is dying. It has been said that to "facilitate the process of healing in others, it is necessary to awaken the healer within the self" (Wells-Federman, 1996). The vulnerability of clients and their families becomes a vehicle for the expression of the nurse's authenticity as a real person with genuine empathy and compassion. If we seek to protect our vulnerability, our expression of genuine emotion, we may dehumanize clients. Our own suffering and grief help us to remain compassionate and participate in the healing, in which pain and suffering are transformed into wisdom in shared moments (Mulder, 2000).

Evaluation of Your Genuineness

You are the most important judge of your genuineness. If you are behaving in ways that are true to your thoughts and feelings, then you will feel more relaxed and self-assured. The comfort that you feel derives in part from the freedom that comes from living in harmony with yourself. Being genuine protects your right to be integrated. In other words, being genuine is being respectful of yourself.

When you are authentic, it is likely that others will react positively by communicating with you, seeking out your trustworthy companionship, and, in turn, revealing their true feelings and thoughts.

Moments of Connection . . .
Genuine Grief for Real People
    "Some of my sweetest experiences have been going to viewings and funerals of patients who have died. The family members share their grief and hug the nurses who cared for their loved ones. They know that we cared with our hearts as well as with our hands and that they don't have to hide their emotions or act 'brave' with us. Although nurses don't go to every funeral of a patient who dies, there are some that give us closure and help us to remember that not all success is measured by patient outcomes. Sometimes success is the ability to connect at a level that is meaningful to the nurse and the patient and family."

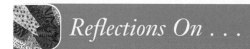 *Reflections On . . .*

Genuineness

Consider what you read about the meaning of being genuine and relating to the client as a unique individual. It takes courage and focus to be genuine and not to seal yourself off emotionally in the face of the demands of nursing.

What? . . .

Write one thing you learned from this chapter.

So what? . . .

How will this affect your nursing practice?

Now what? . . .

How will you implement this new knowledge or skill?

Think about it . . .

Practicing Genuineness

Exercise 1

Read Virginia Satir's poem, "My Declaration of Self-Esteem," available at http://www.kalimunro.com/declaration-of-self-esteem.html, or search by title at www.google.com. It is said that Virginia Satir, a family therapist, wrote this in 1975, as a letter to an angry 15-year-old patient. It begins: "I am me. In all the world, there is no one else exactly like me. Everything that comes out of me is authentically me, because I alone chose it—I own everything about me. My body, my feelings, my mouth, my voice, all my actions, whether they be to others or to myself . . . ." Reflect upon this poem about being genuine and write a journal entry about what you think and feel about its message.

Exercise 2

For the next several days, observe the genuineness in those you encounter daily. When you believe that others are genuine, stop and ask yourself what it is about their communication that makes you arrive at that conclusion. Conversely, when you assess that other peoples' communications are insincere, determine what makes them untrustworthy. Was it what they said or the style in which it was delivered? Making these observations will help you discover more about genuineness and will expand your ability to examine your own authenticity.

After you have done this exercise on your own, get together with your classmates and compare your findings about genuineness.

Exercise 3

Assess your reactions to being on the receiving end of genuine and nongenuine behavior. What are the differences in how you feel? Which feels better and why? What do your reactions tell you about how you would like to communicate with others?

In the classroom, collate your various observations about your reactions to genuine and nongenuine behavior with those of your classmates.

Exercise 4

In your day-to-day activities, notice when you are naturally and easily genuine and when you are untrue to yourself. After several days, note the factors that make it easier for you to be genuine and those that make it more difficult. Assessing your genuineness in this way will make clear where you are congruent and where you need to work harder at being integrated.

Exercise 5

This exercise is the same as Exercise 4 except that you observe your behavior at work. Note when you use your courage to be real and avoid hiding behind a professional façade. Observe when it is more difficult for you to be authentic about what you are thinking, feeling, or experiencing. What can you learn about your genuineness in relation to these situations? What information do you obtain about your genuineness or incongruence from the people in the situation?

After you have completed Exercises 4 and 5, ask yourself if there are any differences in your genuineness when you are on duty and when you are off. What does your answer tell you?

References

Arnold E, Boggs K: *Interpersonal relationships: professional communication skills for nurses*, ed 6, Philadelphia, 2011, WB Saunders.

Bianco MW: *The velveteen rabbit*, New York, 1996, Avon/Camelot. (Reprinted from Williams M: *The velveteen rabbit, or how toys become real*, London, 1922, Heinemann.)

Bruce A, Davies B: Mindfulness in hospice care: practicing meditation-in-action, *Qual Health Res* 15(10):1329, 2005.

Cohen MZ, Hausner J, Johnson M: Knowledge and presence: accountability as described by nurses and surgical patients, *J Prof Nurs* 10(3):177, 1994.

Ferrell BR, Coyle N, editors: *Textbook of palliative nursing*, New York, 2001, Oxford Press.

Gallup: *Nurses top honesty and ethics list for 11th year*, 2010. http://www.gallup.com/poll/145043/nurses-top-honesty-ethics-list-11-year.aspx. Retrieved July 6, 2011.

Guilmartin N: *The power of pause: how to be more effective in a demanding, 24/7 world*, San Francisco, 2010, Jossey-Bass.

Haber J, Krainovich-Miller B, McMahon AL: *Comprehensive psychiatric nursing*, St. Louis, 1997, Mosby.

Knapp ML: *Essentials of nonverbal communication*, New York, 1995, International Thomson Publishing.

Mulder J: Transforming experience into wisdom: healing amidst suffering, *J Palliat Care* 16(2):25, 2000.

Nuwayhid KA: Role function: theory and development. In Roy SC, editor: *Introduction to nursing: an adaptation model*, ed 2, Englewood Cliffs, NJ, 1984, Prentice-Hall.

Peck MS: *The road less traveled and beyond: spiritual growth in an age of anxiety*, New York, 1997, Simon & Schuster.

Rogers CR: *A way of being*, Boston, 1980, Houghton Mifflin.

Rogers CR: *On becoming a person: a therapist's view of psychotherapy*, New York, 1995, Mariner Books.

Rogers CR: The necessary and sufficient conditions of therapeutic personality change, *J Consult Psychol* 21(2):95, 1957.

Shapiro JG, Krauss HH, Truax CB: Therapeutic conditions and disclosure beyond the therapeutic encounter, *J Couns Psychol* 16(4):290, 1969.

Stuart GW: *Principles and practice of psychiatric nursing*, ed 9, St. Louis, 2009, Mosby.

Sundeen SJ, DeSalvo Rankin EA, Stuart GW, et al: *Nurse–client interaction: implementing the nursing process*, St. Louis, 1998, Mosby.

Wells-Federman C: Awakening the nurse healer within, *Holist Nurs Pract* 10(2):13, 1996.

Suggestion for Further Reading

Raiten-D'Antonio T: *The velveteen principles: a guide to becoming real, hidden wisdom from a children's classic*, Deerfield Beach, Fla, 2004, Health Communications, Inc.

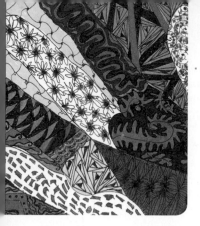

Chapter 10

Empathy

Objectives

1. Define empathy
2. Identify the preverbal, verbal, and nonverbal aspects of empathy
3. Discuss the benefits of empathy with clients and colleagues
4. Identify six steps to empathic communication
5. Examine steps in breaking bad news
6. Practice a centering exercise
7. Participate in exercises to build skills in demonstrating empathy

What Empathy Is

Empathy is the act of communicating to our fellow human beings that we understand something about their world (Dunne, 2005). As a nurse, your practice reflects your understanding of human behavior. How you listen, how you talk, and how you demonstrate empathy and concern are powerful ways to connect with another person (Gallagher, 2009). You are always being observed as a role model, as a communicator . . . you are "on" all the time (Keefe, 2006). In your education and experience you grow in self-awareness, build self-confidence, sharpen listening skills, and work on developing nonjudgmental attitudes (Davis, 1990). It is important to note that nurses may become more task oriented than client centered and patients experience this as a lack of empathy (McCabe, 2004). Taking time to inquire about how the patient is doing, appearing relaxed, and not constantly looking at your watch may demonstrate empathy (McCabe, 2004). You may have the experience of learning and working alongside role models of compassion and empathic communication and negotiate to work with nurses and in settings to foster such ideals. It has been theorized that the ability to experience empathy is the result of a developmental and maturational process (Davis, 1990; Alligood and May, 2000; Olsen, 2001). As a student and novice, you assume the responsibility to work on any problem behaviors such as "prejudice, self-preoccupation, excessive nervous talking, poor listening and poor assertiveness skills, and low self-esteem . . . that block empathy and interfere with healing" (Davis, 1990). As your own sense of self-identity, personal values, and boundaries develops, it is easier to retain your own identity in interactions with clients and thus to feel at one with others without judgment. You move to the highest level of empathy, in which you recognize the other's humanity and personhood regardless of the illness, its circumstance, or stigma. Empathy is more complex than the other interpersonal communication behaviors you have mastered so far. By the end of this chapter you will understand what empathy is and be able to explain its importance in interpersonal communication. A number of exercises provide you with the opportunity to practice demonstrating empathy with supervised feedback. Such rehearsal begins the journey to the empathic maturity that benefits clients and colleagues.

Think of empathy as occurring in three overlapping stages. The first, self-transposition, occurs when we listen carefully and seek to put ourselves in the client's place. The second, a crossing over, is an emotional shift from thinking to feeling, a deepening of our understanding, and an awareness of the client's experience. This has been called the I–Thou relationship (Buber, 1955), dialogue, or a "shared moment of meaning" (Davis, 1990). The Moments of Connection in this textbook are examples of interventions that occurred at this level of connection with clients, family, or colleagues. The third stage, getting our "self" back, is when we stand side by side with the other in heartfelt understanding about the experience just shared (Davis, 1990).

American psychologist Carl Rogers contributed immensely to defining the meaning and significance of empathy for helping professionals. He died in 1987, and in honor of his gifts to us, his direct words are quoted to expand your understanding of the meaning of empathy. This passage is from his book *A Way of Being* (1980):

An empathic way of being with another person has several facets. It means entering the private perceptual world of the other, and becoming thoroughly at home in it. It involves being sensitive, moment by moment, to the changing felt meanings which flow in this other person, to the fear or rage or tenderness or confusion or whatever that he or she is experiencing. It means temporarily living in the other's life, moving about in it delicately without making judgments; it means sensing meanings of which he or she is scarcely aware, but not trying to uncover totally unconscious feelings, since this would be too threatening. It includes communicating your sensings of the person's world as you look with fresh and unfrightened eyes at elements of which he or she is fearful. It means frequently checking with the person as to the accuracy of your

sensings, and being guided by the responses you receive. You are a confident companion to the person in his or her inner world. By pointing to the possible meanings in the flow of another person's experiencing, you help the other to focus on this useful type of referent, to experience the meanings more fully, and to move forward in the experiencing.

A synonym for *empathy* is *communicated understanding*. When we are convinced that others fully understand us, without judging us for how we are feeling, questioning why we are reacting that way, or advising us to feel differently, we experience a wonderful sense of acceptance. The process of empathy involves the unconditional acceptance of the individual in need of help; judgments and evaluation of feelings are never offered (Pike, 1990).

This nonjudgmental reception by our fellow human beings is accompanied by feelings of relief and freedom. Once we know we have been understood and accepted, we do not have to struggle to get our point across, nor do we have to justify our reactions to others. When we receive empathic responses, we can relax because we no longer fear being misunderstood or rejected. Acknowledgment of our feelings reassures us that we have a right to be who we are. We may wish to change, and we might change our feelings and reactions in the future, but there is nothing so accepting as having others verbally acknowledge that they understand our feelings.

Another skill associated with empathy is active listening. We can listen passively or actively. Listening passively includes attending nonverbally to our clients or colleagues with eye contact, head nodding, and verbally encouraging phrases such as "uh huh," "mm-hmm," "I see," "yeah," or "I hear you." It is easy to delude ourselves into thinking that when we listen passively, we truly communicate that we understand. Passive listening, however, does not include an actual articulation of others' feelings, so it lacks the conviction and reassurance of active listening. The receivers of passive listening have to assume, hope, or pretend that they are being understood. Active listening removes this guesswork. It specifically provides speakers with the knowledge that we know how they are feeling—and understand why. Receivers of active listening know that they have been understood.

Natural empathy has been described as a natural and instinctive trait, an intrinsic ability to understand the feelings of others. It contrasts with clinical empathy, a tool or skill that is consciously and deliberately employed to achieve a therapeutic intervention (LaRocco, 2010; Pike, 1990). The goal of empathy is to aid in the establishment of a helping relationship. It is not empathy by itself that is beneficial, but the intention of the giver and the perception of the receiver. An empathetic nurse helps meet the client's basic need to be understood, an important part of establishing a healthy nurse–client relationship (Davis, 2009).

If empathy is truly a curative factor, it must somehow be both communicated to and received by our clients. It is more than a state of mind or attitude. As a concept, empathy is a value-neutral tool that can be used for destructive or manipulative purposes. To be used in a therapeutic or curative way, it must be used to accept, confirm, and validate the total experiences of others. It must be used with the intention of helping.

As nurses in the changing healthcare climate come to accept that the business and caring aspects of patient care must be linked, patients' satisfaction with their caregivers becomes essential. Customer service has become another way to look at delivery of excellent patient care. Patten (1994), in an article about therapeutic hospitality, concludes that "staff interaction skills correlate more highly with patient satisfaction than technical skills." She discusses the ancient practice of hospitality, which has evolved into three levels: public, private, and therapeutic. Therapeutic hospitality involves a high degree of intimacy with a deep personal connection that is the therapeutic use of self. Empathy is an important part of this therapeutic use of self in service recovery when customers' expectations are not met.

> *Don't confuse empathy with pity. Our work is to support others, respecting their own dignity and choices, without fixing, rescuing, or judging.*
>
> **Guilmartin (2010)**
>
> **WIT&** *Wisdom*

How to Communicate Empathically

Empathy includes the ability to reflect, accurately and specifically, in words what our clients or colleagues are experiencing, drawing on the nonverbal behaviors of warmth and genuineness.

Preverbal Aspects of Empathy

In her review article on empathy, Pike (1990) summarizes the literature on the mental processes of empathy before the response becomes verbal. Empathy is not total transport into the world of another, in which the self is lost in the process. "While there is momentary abandonment, the empathizer never loses sight of her own separateness; she is always aware that the feelings of the other are not her own." Clinical, therapeutic empathy is not subjective. After experiencing the private world of their clients, nurses achieve objectivity by tuning into their situations. Although they understand what the clients' situations feel like, nurses feel tension and discomfort, which prompts them to action. The empathy is transformed into a verbal connection with the client for the purpose of being helpful (Pike, 1990). This mental shifting requires flexible ego boundaries. Nurses shift from their world into that of their clients, and then back to a processing part of the mind in which they confirm knowledge of their clients' feelings and develop a plan of what to say or do that will be in the clients' best interests.

Verbal Aspects of Empathy

The verbal part of the skill of empathy is reflecting to your clients or colleagues your understanding of their feelings and the reasons for their emotional reactions. The goal is to offer a verbal reflection that is accurate, without exaggerating or minimizing what you are being told. Ideally, the feeling words you use match what the speaker intended; the nuance and strength of the feeling need to be expressed. Your reflection of the rationale for the speaker's feelings specifically needs to be what the speaker intended. The two qualities of verbal empathy that have just been described are accuracy and specificity. It is unrealistic, however, to think that after knowing a client a short time you can always meet these goals. Later you will read about a technique to check the accuracy of your reflection.

Being empathic does not mean repeating verbatim what others have told you. Parroting only irritates speakers and implies that you have not really processed or understood their situation and subsequent reaction. When you respond empathically, you should choose your own words and respond in your own style, yet still be accurate and specific. The following example illustrates how you can accomplish this.

A young patient who has been married for only 6 months has just been told that she has cervical polyps. As she talks, you notice her brow is furrowed, her eyes are glistening, and she hesitantly says, "Can you tell me . . . what I mean is . . . I really love my husband . . . and will these polyps . . . I mean, I hope I can still make love with my husband."

You pick up several reactions from this young woman. Her stammering and tremulous speech suggest that she is embarrassed about discussing sex. You can most therapeutically deal with her embarrassment by responding in a forthright manner. Her main concern, however, is being able to continue a normal sexual relationship with her husband. You reply empathically as follows:

> I can see that you are worried that these polyps you have on your cervix will interfere with your sex life with your husband. Let me explain about cervical polyps. I think I can reassure you.

This response meets the criteria for accuracy and specificity. Your use of the word *worry* accurately reflects the verbal and nonverbal clues you noticed. Reflecting the word *fear* would have been too strong, and using the words *wonder about* or *curious about* (the sexual relationship) would have been too neutral for the level of emotion she expressed. The feeling words the listener reflects must mirror the nuance the speaker is conveying (Box 10-1). The phrase "that these polyps you have on your cervix will interfere with your sex life with your husband" specifically captures the reason for her worries.

By using your own words and phrasing things in your own style, you avoid parroting and clearly demonstrate that you have understood her worries. Because she felt your understanding before you begin the lesson on polyps, your client is more receptive to the teaching. Hearing a sense of understanding from another person provides a sense of relief and leads us to believe that what the listener says is trustworthy.

Nonverbal Aspects of Empathy

The nonverbal features of empathy are just as important as the verbal aspects. A singer might correctly enunciate each word of a song yet fail to express the mood of the piece; thus the song lacks vitality. Just as an audience would feel unconnected on hearing an emotionless song, so disengagement can occur when empathy is delivered without warmth

Box 10-1	*Choosing the "Right" Empathic Word*

Following is a list of adjectives describing feelings of being afraid, tense, or worried, which gives you an idea of the range from which you can select the feeling word or phrase.

Afraid	Hesitant	Scared
Agonizing	Ill at ease	Shaken
Alarmed	In a cold sweat	Tense
Anxious	Jittery	Terrified
Apprehensive	Jumpy	Trembling
Cautious	Nervous	Troubled
Concerned	On edge	Uncomfortable
Disturbed	Panicky	Uneasy
Dreading	Petrified	Wary
Fearful	Quaking	Worried
Fidgety	Quivering	
Frightened	Restless	

From Hills M, Coffey M: *On delivering care: an interpersonal skills training manual for nurses*, unpublished manual, 1982.

and genuineness. It is possible to articulate a technically perfect empathic response that meets the criteria for accuracy and specificity but does not positively affect the other person.

Only when your empathy is accompanied by warmth and genuineness do the true caring and concern for what your clients and colleagues are experiencing come across. It is important, however, not to overplay your warmth to the point that your intended empathy seems gushy or too sympathetic. Being empathic is not equivalent to feeling sorry for another person. Empathy is free of the judgment of condolence. It is a value-free message showing that you understand the other person's point of view. The warmth you express with empathy should convey genuine caring, not honeyed insincerity. An example might clarify the necessity for an appropriate level of warmth.

Your colleague has just told you that she is pregnant and is therefore upset because she will not be able to continue her full-time nursing career. If you were to smother her with a hug or become overly solicitous, your attentive warmth would come across as sympathy. Sympathy focuses on your own feelings rather than the other person's feelings. Being too warm in this situation might suggest that you think her predicament is hopeless. Empathy with the appropriate warmth, such as a concerned facial expression and a gentle touch on the shoulder, tells your colleague that you understand. Now she can approach her problem unburdened by your overprotectiveness.

Feeling genuine empathy for others is essential. If you decidedly do not care about how your clients or colleagues are feeling, then using an empathic response would be incongruent. Even if the verbal part of your empathy is correct, your nonverbal behavior can give away your lack of caring. Usually our expression of warmth is diminished when we do not genuinely care about the feelings of others. This diminished warmth may speak louder than the words of our empathic response, so that the message received is one of not caring. The mixed message of caring words and uncaring gestures can only be confusing for clients and colleagues.

In summary, empathic communication requires a specific and accurate verbal response accompanied by genuine caring and a receivable level of warmth. These attributes of empathy must be packaged in your own natural style of speaking. In an essay on the lived experience of cancer, a woman writes: "The capacity to recognize and respond to others' distress may be a deep and permeating element of a person's characterological build. For those endowed with the capacity for empathy, its absence is perhaps as unimaginable as color blindness or tone deafness are to those endowed with color perception and perfect pitch" (Charon, 1995).

> *Through wisdom a house is built and by understanding it prospers.*
> **Finnish proverb**
>
> **WIT&***Wisdom*

Moments of Connection . . .
In the Right Place at the Right Time
"When I was a student nurse, I was in my pediatric rotation and had the opportunity to work with a 17-year-old single mom of a child with a cleft palate and lip. The child was 3 months old, and her mom wasn't visiting or holding the child. I asked to speak with her

and asked some questions about the baby. I have faint but visible scars from cleft lip surgery, and the mother felt able to talk to me. She told me her parents said the baby was born that way because of the mother's sin of being a single mother. When I asked what she wanted for her child, she replied, to grow up and be able to sing. I was filled with a warm feeling and told her that her little girl could do anything, that I sing, and then I sang a little song for her. I told her that God doesn't punish. Sometimes you have to search for the blessing. After our talk, the mother began to visit the baby and take part in feeding and caring for the baby. The baby underwent corrective surgery 3 months later."

When to Communicate Empathically

Rogers (1980) asserts that in some situations empathy has the highest priority of the attitudinal elements and makes for growth-promoting human relationships. When clients or colleagues are hurting, confused, troubled, anxious, alienated, terrified, doubtful of self-worth, or uncertain as to identity, then understanding is called for.

Every day nurses encounter clients who are in this kind of pain. Nurses have many opportunities to know their clients' most intimate thoughts and feelings. Dicers (1990) warns that empathy is intrusive and cautions nurses to ask themselves, "How far should I go?" She reminds us that there is a tremendous amount of freedom related to empathy. "Empathy is a concept by intellection, like 'justice' or 'love,' as opposed to a concept by observation like 'chair' or 'bottle.' Such concepts are seductive because there is so much room to play around." It is the clinical and ethical judgment of nurses that guides them in deciding when to verbalize empathy. Follow this advice: "Whenever we enter another's mind, we must remember to be respectful and take off our shoes."

We nurses know that we have as much responsibility for clients' needs to express their feelings on intimate matters as we do for their privacy. We might ask ourselves: "How much should I encourage my clients to tell me? Am I at risk of crossing the line between facilitating communication (with my empathy) and aggressively pursuing their private reactions?" Being empathic can be helpful or invading, and as nurses we must strive to use our empathic skills with the intent of being helpful.

Dicers (1990) argues: "Empathy is a dangerous notion if it is thought to be mindless, experiential, existential connectedness. Surely every patient encounter requires an openness to the other's experience, for only when one is open to another can one perceive needs. But surely, not every encounter will benefit from empathy; some will require theory, or applied experience, or even translation or consultation."

It is helpful to be empathic any time people share their thoughts and feelings with you. An empathic reply can be used on its own or with another message or communication strategy. For example, empathy can be used with the following:

- *Statements*: "You feel frustrated because the clinic is not open in the evenings, when it would be more convenient for you to come and have your blood pressure checked. There have been several other requests for extended hours, so I will raise this issue with our office manager." In addition to knowing your plan to follow up on such a complaint, it is reassuring for a client to have you acknowledge the situation and the feelings related to it.
- *Questions*: "Yes, I can see that you are pretty excited about being discharged from the hospital earlier than you had expected. Have you had time to arrange for your babysitter to start earlier and give you a hand with your toddler and your new baby?" Your empathic beginning potentiates the effect of your concern for your client's discharge plans.
- *Alternate points of view*: "You feel pretty adamant that your pack-a-day smoking habit won't harm your health, since your grandfather smoked and lived to be 95. I have a different way of looking at smoking, since I've recently known several clients who have died of lung cancer. The statistics do indicate a high positive correlation between smoking and lung cancer." Most clients and colleagues hear our side of an argument if we give equal recognition to their point of view.
- *Explanations*: "Being moved to a semiprivate room has really upset you, and you feel that your privacy has been invaded. Switching rooms truly was our last alternative. We need a single room to carry out isolation techniques for an infectious client to protect everyone on the unit." By first acknowledging your client's feelings, you can help pave the way for acceptance of your decision.
- *Invitations for more information*:
  With a client: "You're worried about the sharp pains in your kidney area. Have you had any other unusual signs and symptoms lately?"

With a colleague: "From your point of view our new charting system is cumbersome and pretty frustrating. Do you have any suggestions for streamlining the recording of our nurses' notes?"

Most people engage more fully in our request for additional information when they hear that we understand what they have already told us.

Missing opportunities to convey empathy can create a gulf between speakers and listeners, and make speakers feel ignored. When we do not hear others, a new struggle is created for them. They are disappointed at not being understood and in turn either withdraw with wounded feelings or fight to convince us of their feelings. When empathy is not offered, our clients and colleagues feel cheated, frustrated, and ignored. Including empathy with other communication strategies lets our clients and colleagues know beyond a doubt that they have been heard and understood.

In any therapeutic relationship it is important that our partners feel cared for. Client–nurse relationships are ones in which we have established ourselves as helpers. That label means that we acknowledge and make public our desire to support others. Empathy is one concrete way to show our caring.

Sometimes when stress levels are high we get lost in our own concerns and forget that our colleagues have concerns of their own. Simple acts help get us back on track.

How Empathy Benefits Clients and Colleagues

Clients and colleagues share their thoughts and feelings in order to be understood, but often it is uncomfortable for them to reveal themselves. As listeners, it is not good enough for us to understand how our clients or colleagues feel without verbally sharing that empathic understanding explicitly and accurately. Communicating our understanding has many payoffs for clients and colleagues, and for our relationships with them. In a survey of more than 1 million clients, "staff sensitivity to the inconvenience that health problems and hospitalization cause" was found to be the top consideration in a person's decision to recommend a healthcare facility (Press Ganey Associates, 1996).

Empathy increases the feeling of being connected with another person. This positive feeling of belonging helps reduce negative feelings of loneliness and isolation. Although it has often been said that we are ultimately alone in our journey through life, empathy is a bridge that connects us with others, providing confidence and hope. A healthcare administrator compared the changes and stress created by downsizing in healthcare organizations to climbing a mountain. He commented that he felt the desire to say, "Let's stay close" (Clark, 1996). For colleagues to know they are not alone, to respond to each other with empathy provides comfort in times of challenging transitions. The knowledge that you understand your clients and colleagues helps them continue on their way, secure that their feelings have been acknowledged as normal human reactions. The companionship you extend through empathy, however brief the engagement, creates a human bond that adds to your clients' or colleagues' personal strength. Rogers (1980) puts it simply: empathy dissolves alienation. Consider, too, the family caregivers with whom you come in contact, those giving full-time care in the home or keeping long vigils at the client's bedside in the hospital. These have been called the hidden patients. Look for signs of exhaustion due to a lack of personal time, problems with the behavior of the care recipient, and the demands of their own employment (Ostwald, 1997).

Curry (1994) offers this description of the empathic experience:

> When I look at patients, I see friends and loved ones on a battlefield of illness and pain. I see my father in the face of a man who can no longer speak because of a brain tumor, but whose eyes still shine when his grandchildren visit. I feel my mother's hands in those of an elderly woman whose memories have been claimed by Alzheimer's disease. I see my brother in the gaunt young man with AIDS whose family and friends have deserted him.

Empathy can contribute to feelings of increased self-esteem on the part of those to whom you extend it. The fact that you take the time to listen, hear, process, and reflect what your clients or colleagues say makes them feel important. Caring enough to show that you understand makes others feel significant and worthwhile.

It is impossible to accurately sense the perceptual world of another person unless you value that person and his or her world, unless you, in some sense,

care. Hence, the message comes through to the recipient that "this other person trusts me, thinks I'm worthwhile. Perhaps I am worth something. Perhaps I could value myself. Perhaps I could care for myself." (Rogers, 1980)

Your empathy demonstrates that you accept how your clients and colleagues feel and helps them to trust that you genuinely accept them as they are.

Your withholding of judgment or advice enhances this trust. Empathy is a skill you can use to deepen your relationships with clients and colleagues. When you unconditionally accept others as they present themselves, they can relax and feel free to be who they really are. Your acceptance helps your clients and colleagues to accept themselves.

A consequence of empathic understanding is that others feel valued, cared for, and accepted as the people that they are (Rogers, 1980): "True empathy is always free of any evaluative or diagnostic quality. The recipient perceives this with some surprise: 'If I am not being judged, perhaps I am not so evil or abnormal as I have thought. Perhaps I don't have to judge myself so harshly.' Thus, the possibility of self-acceptance is gradually increased." Finely tuned understanding by others gives us all a sense of personhood and identity. Rogers shows us that empathy gives that needed confirmation.

Your empathy can help your clients and colleagues move on to new feelings and change their behavior.

The acceptance your empathy offers frees your clients and colleagues from having to defend or rationalize their feelings; as a result, they are able to experience alternative reactions, freed of any clinging to defensive feelings. When you do not give empathy, then your clients and colleagues believe they have to justify their feelings.

Receiving empathy helps them to be open and move on to different ways of experiencing. It is perfectly natural for people to change their reactions as new information is processed or old data are reexamined in a new light. The acceptance you provide through empathy helps your clients and colleagues remain flexible enough to move to a new awareness. Just as being stuck in one place retards self-growth, so having the option to move on or change fosters self-growth.

In our personal and professional lives we are often in relationships with individuals who must make difficult decisions about their lives. More often than not, that person does not need more information, certainly does not need a judgmental presence, and probably does not want the answer or the decision taken from them. What they require from us is real presence that will support them, empower them, and give them the courage to decide. (Marsden, 1990)

Presence means more than just showing up. It is the ability to "empathize, listen, reflect and observe." (Potter and Frisch, 2007, p. 218)

In some instances your empathic reflection can help your clients or colleagues comprehend more fully how they are reacting.

Hearing your reflection of their feelings may increase their self-awareness. Not only is this enlightenment satisfying, but it can widen their perspective of the whole situation. Consider this example:

You have just empathically reflected to Douglas, one of your clients in the diabetic clinic, that it just doesn't seem fair that he has diabetes while his roommate's good health allows him the freedom to eat and drink what he wants and to party until all hours of the night.

> *Douglas:* "Yes, you're right! That's exactly how I'm feeling. I hadn't realized how it gripes me that he isn't restricted like I am. I guess I think about the medical expenses that I have, not to mention the time-consuming treatments I have to put up with. No wonder I'm so short with him when I see him having a good time. In fact, sometimes I'm quite miserable to him . . . I'd better not let this situation get out of hand."

Your empathic response increased Douglas's understanding of his behavior and himself. The literature on empathy reports that psychotherapists high in empathy, genuineness, and warmth elicit greater self-exploration in their clients (Shapiro et al, 1969).

The insight and expanded self-awareness sometimes triggered by your empathic responses can help your clients and colleagues decide how to handle a situation.

Knowing how you feel about a situation and how those feelings are affecting your way of coping with the situation are important factors in deciding on a course of action. Good problem solvers take their own feelings into account when confronted with any situation, problem, or issue. Having knowledge of our feelings helps us determine whether the situation should be changed so that we will feel better or whether it is more appropriate to change our feelings and outlook on the situation so that we will feel better adjusted.

In the previous example, now that Douglas is aware of his feelings about his roommate's health and freedom, he can use this self-awareness to help him handle his situation. Douglas could consider all kinds of possibilities. In terms of changing his situation, he could get a roommate with a chronic illness so that he would not have to deal with these feelings, or he could brainstorm ways to minimize the restrictions in his diabetic regimen so that he could live his life more naturally. In terms of changing his feelings, he could stop comparing himself to others and increase his gratefulness for the lifestyle he can lead, or he could be hostile toward his roommate until the roommate can no longer tolerate it and decides either to leave or to fight back.

The knowledge of their feelings and awareness of the impact these emotions have on their situations as provided by your empathic response can give clients and colleagues more information with which to generate effective solutions. Your empathy can inspire clients to listen to themselves more empathically.

The nonevaluative and accepting quality of the empathic climate enables clients to take a prizing, caring attitude toward themselves (Rogers, 1980). Being understood makes it possible for clients to listen with greater empathy for their own reactions to what they are experiencing. This greater understanding and prizing of themselves can open new facets of experience, which bring into their awareness a more accurate picture of themselves and a clearer self-concept.

Research has demonstrated that empathy accounts for improvement in psychotherapy clients (Cartwright-Dymond and Lerner, 1963; Truax et al, 1966; Shapiro et al, 1969). Rogers (1980) cites research from the late 1960s and early 1970s on therapist–client relationships indicating that clients who eventually show more therapeutic change (in comparison with those who show less) receive more expressions of the therapist's empathic understanding, acceptance, and genuineness. Therapist empathy was the most significant factor distinguishing more and less effective therapists (Lafferty et al, 1989). The research findings of Lafferty and colleagues support the significance of the therapist's empathy in effective psychotherapy. Patients of more effective therapists felt more understood than patients of less effective therapists.

The argument can be made that empathic responses from nurses can enhance healing and well-being in all clients. Illness and hospitalization cause fear, dependency, and upheaval in clients' daily lifestyles and relationships, whether the health problem is surgical, medical, obstetric, or psychiatric. Empathic nurses can tune into their clients' feelings in a helpful way. Empathy on the part of health professionals can improve the success of the complete clinical problem-solving process and enhance client compliance because of increased client involvement.

Practicing nurses confirm the benefits of empathy in the workplace. Results of a survey of 67 nurses at an ambulatory surgery conference indicate that empathic communication can add joy to the workplace and keep workers enthusiastic about their jobs (Box 10-2).

Nurse leaders who act as giant shock absorbers of uncertainty in an organization can refuel their energy and continue to be empathic by staying in touch with nurses who have direct client contact and listening to their stories of connection (Kerfoot, 2002). Empathy, defined as the ability to understand and interact based on the emotional makeup of others, is one of the key personality traits of emotional intelligence recommended for consideration in hiring employees, along with self-awareness, the ability to recognize one's own emotions and motivation and their effect on others; self-regulation, the ability to control or redirect problematic impulses or moods; motivation, a passion for work and pursuit of goals with energy and persistence; and social skills, proficiency in building relationships and networks (Connolly, 2002).

Box 10-2 | *Empathy Is Not Just for Students*

The following are responses from nurses at an ambulatory surgical nursing conference to these two questions:

1. What would you be willing to do to add joy to the workplace?
2. What behavior would you like from colleagues to help you look forward to coming to work?

Of the workshop participants, 98% chose to respond in writing to these questions. Answers have been combined because the lists were similar.

- Smile.
- Acknowledge each other.
- Focus on the positive.
- Say thanks for a job well done.
- Pitch in and help.
- Avoid listening to gossip.
- Avoid gossiping.
- Tell people how negative comments affect the recipient.
- Listen more.
- Beware of interrupting colleagues when unnecessary.
- Be pleasant even if you are not a morning person.
- Be more positive with new colleagues.
- Do not complain about changes in the schedule.
- End the morning report on a humorous or positive note.
- Appreciate and accept differences in colleagues.
- Send notes to say thank you.

Copyright © 1995 by Julia W. Balzer Riley.

How Empathy Benefits the Nurse

The preceding points clarify how your use of empathy can benefit your clients and colleagues. Empathy also benefits you, the nurse. The most obvious payoff is the warm feeling of compassion you get when you help others feel understood and accepted. Knowing that you have taken the opportunity to make your clients or colleagues feel better provides immense satisfaction and can augment your feelings of competence.

Nurses want to collect enough information from their clients to assess their concerns accurately and to develop the best nursing care plan for treating their health problems. When clients feel accepted, their trust allows them to open up and provide the information necessary for accurate assessment of their situations. Obtaining sufficient data to make a correct nursing diagnosis is the first and most important step in the systematic problem-solving approach to nursing care. Whether clients' problems are physical, emotional, or a combination of both, empathy can be used to acquire sufficient and comprehensive data.

Moments of Connection . . .
When the Tears Come

"I'm a pediatric nurse, a sensitive one. I have always worried about crying too much. I was with a small child who was dying. I was able to do all the nursing care for her, but all the while, tears ran down my face. After she died, the family came to me and told me how much it meant to them that I cried, because they did not have a sense of caring from other staff. I no longer worry about my sensitivity to my work!"

Empathy can be shown at all stages of the problem-solving process. When you are developing a plan of care, it is essential to determine how your clients feel about the proposed treatment schedule and to empathically reflect your understanding. Acknowledging clients' reactions to treatment regimens and, when possible, adjusting plans accordingly are likely to increase compliance behavior.

As a nurse you want to know if your nursing care has been effective. Many objective measures of success exist, but one important yardstick is how your clients feel about their treatment outcome. Clients may be sufficiently satisfied and wish to terminate treatment, or they may want to try an alternative plan to achieve their desired outcome. Clients' input has implications for how to proceed in the client–nurse relationship. Showing empathy lets your clients know that you understand and acknowledge their evaluation of progress.

In your working relationships, being empathic with colleagues augments cohesiveness. Showing that you understand your colleagues not only makes working together more enjoyable, but it helps you prevent and work out difficulties in your relationships.

How to Overcome Blocks to Empathy

Clearly, empathy has many positive benefits for our clients and colleagues and also has a payoff for ourselves. If we are not conveying empathy at appropriate opportunities in our relationships with clients and colleagues, then it is likely we are relating in ways that are not helpful. What are we doing if we are not communicating empathically when it is warranted, and how can we switch to communication that is more caring?

Several activities may result in a failure to express empathy. Be careful not to judge clients or colleagues. If we question the appropriateness of their thoughts and feelings, then we effectively shut off the unbiased and accepting part of our communication. Being truly empathic means being able to put aside our opinions and tune into how the other person is feeling.

To suggest that we should cancel all judgmental thoughts would be absurd. It is only human to have preferences and opinions. We are taught throughout life to be selective in our tastes for food, art, clothing, and people. This discriminating behavior is second nature to most of us. We use it every moment of our lives, such as in deciding what to wear in the morning,

selecting which strategy to use to solve a work problem, or choosing what to eat for dinner. It is highly likely that most of us cannot turn off this judgmental thinking in our interpersonal relationships.

Most times our judgments serve a useful purpose in our lives. When we verbalize our judgments about other people's thoughts and feelings, however, we only make them feel criticized and labeled. Clients and colleagues can feel shut out when they have been judged; they may think that acceptance is impossible. Being judged engenders feelings of rejection and defensiveness. Clients and colleagues tend either to withdraw from us to protect themselves from further pronouncements or to aggressively challenge us in an attempt to defend their thoughts and feelings. Whichever response occurs, the verbalized judgment has served to arrest any therapeutic communication.

The following example illustrates the benefits of empathic communication and the detrimental effects of being judgmental.

Your client has come to the physician's office for a colposcopic examination and says to you:

> I'm scared to death of this copos . . . how do you say it? . . . exam . . . the whole idea spooks me.

You could respond as follows:

> *Nonempathic response:* "Oh! It's nothing to worry about. You'll be just fine. Lots of our patients have one. By the way, it's pronounced *colposcopy*."

This response negates your client's fear and belittles her anxieties about this unknown procedure. This response is unlikely to make your client believe that you take her feelings seriously. Instead of feeling acknowledged, she likely feels misunderstood and put down by your judgmental reply.

You might have responded as follows:

> *Empathic response:* "The thought of having a colposcopic exam is really frightening for you. What can I do to relieve some of your fears about it?"

This empathic opening acknowledges the client's fears about the test, and the accompanying offer demonstrates your desire to help alleviate her fears. She likely will be relieved by this nonjudgmental acceptance of her feelings. Your empathy makes it safe for her to trust you further by asking questions or revealing more of her feelings. Whereas a judgmental response closes lines of communication, an empathic reply opens them.

An example involving a colleague may illustrate this further.

You have just started the evening shift on your unit after several days off, and the nurse manager on the day shift remarks:

Boy! Count yourself lucky to have been off for the past 3 days. It's been like a zoo here! We've had two deaths and five admissions, and we've been short-staffed the whole time. I'm wiped out!

You could respond as follows:

Nonempathic response: "Well, the time passes quickly when you're busy, and after all, you've been trained to handle hectic situations . . . That's what they pay us for."

This reply undermines your colleague's feelings. Your judgment that she should be coping dismisses her feelings as inconsequential and even inappropriate. An uncaring response such as this would only serve to make your colleague hostile and defensive, and would certainly lead to a strained working relationship.

A more understanding response would be the following:

Empathic response: "No wonder you're tired. It sounds like you've had to handle three times the usual workload with the admissions and deaths . . . and all without enough help. When's your well-deserved time off coming?"

This empathic reply makes your colleague feel that she has been heard. There is no doubt that you understand what she has been coping with while you were away. All she desired was for you to register how it has been for her. This response fits that bill.

When we judge others, we effectively ignore their points of view. Instead we shift the focus to what we feel or think and emphasize our perspective. As helping professionals we feel sad when we hurt clients or colleagues by ignoring or upstaging them. The desire to communicate in a caring way is motivation to use empathy. Being nonjudgmentally empathic requires the desire to show acceptance and the will to focus and concentrate on the concerns of others.

Remember this idea so that as a helping professional you can take care of yourself. It takes courage to be empathic (Pike, 1990): "Entering into a patient's world as if it were his own exposes the nurse to the possibility of pain, despair, anger, fear and hopelessness. Courage is especially called for in situations where the nurse is powerless to cure the patient's distress, pain, or suffering."

The greater the maturity and experience of nurses, the greater is their usable vault of knowledge, attitudes, and learning for enhancing their empathy. But all nurses need one important key to open the vault: access to feelings (Pike, 1990).

Empathy is assertive because it takes into account others' thoughts and feelings and protects your right to communicate in a caring way. It is responsible to be empathic because it ensures that your clients feel acknowledged enough to engage in all aspects of the nursing process.

Six Steps to Help You Communicate More Empathically

How can we nurture our ability to reliably convey empathy on a consistent basis? The following guidelines are based on a systematic problem-solving approach. If you truly want to be empathic, then these six steps can be helpful.

1. *Clear your head of distracting agendas.* In your busy life you will have many thoughts going through your head, such as personal worries, pressure from expanding work, or perhaps feelings of discomfort related to talking with a client or colleague. To the extent that you can put these aside, do so. If you are able to focus on the person you are with, you will streamline communication. Paying attention to other speakers increases the chances that you will deal with their situations more thoroughly and more effectively. Listening empathically means not having to return time and time again to get complete information, and that means one less item on your long list of things to do. Teach yourself to concentrate (Raudsepp, 1990).

2. *Remind yourself to focus on the speaker.* Remember that your priority is to listen and hear your clients or colleagues so that you can verbally convey your understanding. Remind yourself that your purpose is to tune in to what a speaker is saying. Some people find that a physical gesture, such as removing their glasses or adopting a definite listening stance, reminds them to focus. "Don't interrupt," reminds Raudsepp (1990).

3. *Attend to your clients' and colleagues' verbal and nonverbal messages.* Hear the words that speakers are using to describe how they are feeling and the reasons for their reaction. Look for what your speakers are also saying nonverbally. Take in the whole message that your clients and colleagues are sending you.

4. *Ask yourself, "What does this person want me to hear?"* Attempt to pick out the most important message being delivered. What is the predominant theme? Is anguish the strongest feeling? Is joy the prevailing emotion? Your answer should be what the speaker wants you to hear, and that very seed is the embryo for your empathic response.

5. *Convey an empathic response.* Verbally reflect the speaker's feelings and the reason for them, ensuring that your response meets the criteria of accuracy and specificity. Pay attention to your nonverbal communication. Convey the amount of warmth you deem appropriate and ensure that the expression is congruent with your intentions to be understanding and accepting.

6. *Check to see if your empathic response was effective.* The purpose of being empathic is to make others feel relieved (that we understand them) and cared for (because of our genuine interest in their situation). Check it out. Do the speakers nod their heads? Do they smile or tell you in other ways that they are delighted you have understood them? Do they visibly relax by letting go of tension or by engaging you in further conversation? These clues let you know that you have been successful.

If your attempt to be empathic has missed the mark, a speaker will let you know in several ways. More assertive clients or colleagues will tell you outright: "No, that's not quite how I'm feeling . . . It's more like this . . . " Others may just slowly withdraw from opening up anymore with you. It is acceptable most times to explicitly ask your speaker if your empathy is on target. Try "Is that how you are feeling?" or "Have I understood how it is for you?" or "Let me see if I have this right."

How to Break Bad News

Nurses are often in a position to reinforce and provide clarification when the client and family have received bad news, especially when they work with a

---

Box 10-3 | *Breaking Bad News*

1. Plan what is to be said ahead of time and organize your thoughts. Anticipate questions family members may ask. Knowledge of previous family coping mechanisms is helpful in planning the team response.
2. Establish rapport. If this has not occurred, ask team members who have established rapport with the family to attend.
3. Control the environment as much as possible. Set aside appropriate time; turn off pagers, cell phones, and televisions; take the phone off the hook. Sit down and listen.
4. Find out what the client and family already know.
5. Find out how much given individuals want to know. Don't make assumptions about this.
6. Use language the client and family will understand. Be sensitive and respectful of cultural issues.
7. Respond to the reactions of the client and family, using an empathic approach. Continually assess and reassess the client's and family's understanding of the information.
8. When appropriate, explain the treatment plan and prognosis, and summarize.

Modified from American Association of Colleges of Nursing and City of Hope National Medical Center: *Training program facility guide*, Duarte, Calif, 2000, End-of-Life Nursing Education Consortium (ELNEC); Matzo ML, Sherman DW: *Palliative care nursing: quality care to the end of life*, New York, 2001, Springer Publishing; and Buckman R: *How to break bad news: a guide for health professionals*, Baltimore, 1992, Johns Hopkins Press.

---

dying client. Talking about death may be a difficult task. Although physicians usually break the initial bad news, the nurse can offer support. The actions outlined in Box 10-3 should be taken when breaking bad news.

How to Center Yourself

The demands of the work of nurses are many and complex. Practice a brief centering technique throughout the day to refocus and bring yourself, fully present, to the people entrusted to your care and those with whom you work. See Box 10-4 for an example.

Box 10-4 — *A Centering Technique to Set the Intention of Being Fully Present with Clients, Family, and Colleagues*

Honor the sacred nature of your work. Take time each day to connect with your own purpose in your work.

1. Before you interact with a client, family member, or colleague, pause.
2. Let go of any distractions or worries just now.
3. Close your eyes briefly and take a deep breath.
4. Say silently to yourself, "I am here for the greater good of all people involved and will give my full attention to this moment."
5. Bring to mind someone or something that evokes love and compassion.
6. Hold that feeling of love and compassion, repeating to yourself, "I am present in this moment."

(This whole process should take only 5 to 10 seconds.)

Adapted from Dossey BM, Keegan LC: *Holistic nursing: a handbook for practice*, ed 5, Sudbury, Mass, 2008, Jones Bartlett Publishers.

Moments of Connection...
Keep on Trying ... Empathy is a Life-long Journey

"This man was such a special person, a quadriplegic for over 30 years who wrote poetry to soothe his spirit and express his deepest feelings. He talked about being able to tell when people who entered his room stopped listening. He said their eyes would just 'glaze over,' and so he would talk 'gobbledygook,' and they never noticed. When I think of empathy, I think of this man. How could we as nurses ever really understand? But knowing him makes me keep trying."

Over time as you see the positive effects of your empathetic response to clients, families, and colleagues, empathy may become a way of being. When describing their work, some nurses say, "It's just the way I am" (Wiseman, 2007).

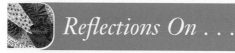

Reflections On . . .

Empathy

Consider what you read about empathy. How would you evaluate your ability to be empathic?

What? . . .
Write one thing you learned from this chapter.

So what? . . .
How will this affect your nursing practice?

Now what? . . .
How will you implement this new knowledge or skill?

Think about it . . .

Practicing Empathy

Exercise 1

This exercise provides you with several hypothetical situations in which clients or colleagues express thoughts and feelings to you. On your own, write down an empathic response to each of the examples. Remember to meet the criteria of being accurate and specific.

After you have written your initial empathic response, critique it and suggest alternative ways of phrasing your first try to make it more empathic. In your improved response, try to convey complete understanding and phrase it in your natural way of speaking.

Example 1. A nurse colleague says: "I'm not going to be able to get through that job interview with Mrs. Jones for the position of assistant head nurse. I just know I'll be so uptight that I'll blow it like I did the last time."

First attempt at empathy: "You're feeling pretty nervous about that interview."

Critique: This reply lacks specificity. Including a reference to the fact that it is a job interview would have acknowledged the importance of the event for your colleague. Referring to the reason for her worry about the interview would have made a more complete and accurate empathic response.

Continued

Suggested alternative: "You're feeling pretty nervous about your job interview for the assistant head nurse position and worried that you might botch it like you feel you have before."

Example 2. A client says: "My first child is retarded. I'd like to have another child . . . but . . . what if that child turns out to be retarded too?"

First attempt at empathy: "Yeah, it's a big chance to take, isn't it—getting pregnant, I mean."

Critique: This is more an opinion than an empathic response, and it might feed her worry. Being more accurate by including a reference to her feelings would make this reply more empathic. Verbalizing her reasons would meet the criteria for specificity.

Suggested alternative: "You have mixed feelings about having another child. On the one hand, you'd like another baby, but on the other, you're frightened that you may have another mentally impaired child."

Example 3. A client tells you: "I didn't have to take any pain medication last night for my injured back . . . and I slept right through the night. It was the first good sleep I've had in four nights."

First attempt at empathy: "That's great! I'm glad you're sleeping better!"

Critique: This statement is more a judgment than a reflection of the client's feelings. The implied feelings are relief (at not having to take the medication) and joy (at sleeping well). These feelings, and the reasons for them, need to be included to make the response empathic.

Suggested alternative: "Boy! What a relief for you to have been comfortable enough to do without your pain medication, and you look overjoyed that you slept so well."

Now it is your turn! For each of the following situations attempt a written empathic response. Then critique your attempt and suggest how it could be improved.

Example 4. A client says to you: "My husband died a year ago. It's been the longest and saddest year of my life."

Your first attempt at empathy:
Your critique:
Your suggested alternative:

Example 5. A client says to you: "I had a real scare today. My chest x-ray has a spot on it and my doctor has called in a specialist to see what it is. I'm so worried because she told me that cancer can't be ruled out until I've had further tests."

Your first attempt at empathy:
Your critique:
Your suggested alternative:

Example 6. An 18-year-old client says to you: "I never thought I could be HIV-positive. I'm not gay. I don't use drugs. I've only had sex with one person. My life is over."

Your first attempt at empathy:
Your critique:
Your suggested alternative:

After you have completed the preceding examples on your own, get together with the rest of your class and compare your responses. It will be interesting to see how many different ways an empathic response can be phrased and still meet the criteria of accuracy, specificity, naturalness, warmth, and genuineness.

Exercise 2

This exercise gives you the chance to experience the differences between passive and active listening. Find a partner with whom to work. One of you will be the speaker and the other the listener. The speaker will talk on any subject about which he or she has strong feelings.

In the first part of the exercise the listener listens passively, and in the second part he or she listens actively. For the first part of the exercise the listener displays attentive nonverbal listening and offers encouraging responses such as "uh huh," "yes," "I see," and the like. Continue with the first part of this exercise for 4 minutes and then proceed to the second part.

In the second part the speaker proceeds as in the first part. This time the listener listens actively by responding with empathic statements at every appropriate opportunity. Proceed with this second part of the exercise for 4 minutes.

After completing both parts of the exercise, answer the following questions.

As speaker: What differences did you notice between passive receiving and active listening?
As listener: What differences did you notice between listening passively and listening actively?

Switch roles so that each partner has the chance both to speak and to listen passively and actively. Then, together as a class, pool all the ideas you have gleaned about empathy from doing this exercise.

Exercise 3

This exercise gives you a chance to receive supervised feedback on your ability to be empathic. Work in groups of four. One person takes the role of speaker, one the role of listener, and the other two are observers. The speaker chooses a topic about which he or she has strong feelings.

The listener's task is to demonstrate empathic listening to what the speaker has to say during a conversation lasting 4 minutes. The observers use the Empathy Rating Scale (Figure 10-1) to evaluate the speaker's ability to be empathic. Tape recorders or video monitors, if available, provide a valuable asset for self-observation.

Roles should be rotated so that each person in the group has the chance to be speaker, listener, and observer.

The information on the Empathy Rating Scale you receive as listener will outline areas in which you are strong and others in which you need to improve your ability to communicate empathically. For example, the Empathy Rating Scale may draw your attention to the fact that you neglect to include the rationale for the speaker's feelings, even though you meet the criteria for accuracy, warmth, naturalness, and genuineness. This exercise can be repeated at intervals after practicing empathy so that over time you can see the pattern of improvement.

Exercise 4

Review the centering technique in Box 10-4. For one day in the clinical setting, practice this technique immediately before you work with a client. You will find you may shorten the centering further with practice. Write a brief reflection on your response to the use of this centering technique.

Response No.	Accuracy: matched intensity?	Specificity: rationale included?	Naturalness: own words?	Warmth: verbal? nonverbal?	Genuineness: interest and caring conveyed?
1					
2					
3					
4					
5					
6					
7					

Criteria for Empathy Rating Scale

1. *Accuracy:* Does the intensity of the listener's words match the speaker's intended message?
2. *Specificity:* Does the listener include the rationale for the speaker's feelings?
3. *Naturalness:* Does the listener avoid parroting? Does the listener reflect the speaker's message in a naturally worded style?
4. *Warmth:* Does the listener convey verbal and nonverbal warmth with an empathic response?
5. *Genuineness:* Does the listener convey interest and caring about what the speaker is saying?

FIGURE 10-1 Empathy Rating Scale.

Exercise 5

Consider what clients have to teach us about their experiences. Ask yourself: if I were a quadriplegic . . . or . . . experience any disease or disability . . . how would I feel? What would I think? How would I cope? The poem below was written by a patient who may have been in residence longer than any other veteran at the Bay Pines Veterans Administration Hospital in Florida. He was a quadriplegic for over 40 years and the author of over 100 poems. It was a privilege to meet this poet whose dream was to have his poems published . . . we are making this dream come true. Howard died in 2006. Howard said he has reframed his life as a teacher of nurses and of the nursing students who cared for him during their clinical rotations . . . and so he was.

Social Malignancy

This but one
   of the little horrors
We must learn
   to endure
And never quite do . . .
Quadriplegia is not unlike
   leukemia of the soul
Always under attack
   by that social cancer
Because the severe disability
   breeds a lack
   of our credibility.

Copyright © Howard G. Kirkman. Used with permission.

Exercise 6

How can you, as a nurse, expand your horizons and your ability to be empathetic? Read poetry . . . Listen to music. Read literature. View art . . . all expressions of the human experience. Consider the AIDS memorial quilt. Visit www.aidsquilt.org. Write a poem about a clinical experience that stays on your mind. Perhaps you have a client with whom you have problems connecting or one that touches your heart. You might write a poem that you would share with colleagues. Poetry can help you be more fully present; remind you to listen again to what is being said; increase your ability to tolerate pain, and understand yourself and others; and discover and reflect upon client's feelings to build the skill of empathy (Goldner, 2005; Raingruber, 2004; Akhtar, 2000; Connelly, 1999).

Exercise 7

Here is another process to help you use the arts to support your reflective practice to deepen empathy. Select a client from your current or past clinical experience who touched you emotionally or, perhaps, one who challenges your ability to be empathetic. Find a piece of art or literature that helps you deepen your understanding of what this client might be experiencing. Write a journal entry describing the clinical experience and several paragraphs relating the piece of art or literature to the client (Brown, 2010).

> *The pen of the tongue should be dipped in the ink of the heart.*
>
> **Native American proverb**
>
> **WIT&***Wisdom*

References

Akhtar S: Mental pain and the cultural ointment of poetry, *Int J Psychoanal* 81:229, 2000.

Alligood MR, May BA: A nursing theory of personal system empathy: interpreting a conceptualization of empathy in King's interacting systems, *Nurs Sci Q* 13(3):243, 2000.

Brown DL: Using art and literature in the clinical setting: an innovative assignment, *Nurse Educ* 3(2):53, 2010.

Buber M: *Between man and man*, Boston, 1955, Beacon Press.

Cartwright-Dymond R, Lerner B: Empathy, need to change and improvement with psychotherapy, *J Consult Psychol* 27(2):138, 1963.

Charon R: Connections that heal, *Second Opin* 2(1):38, 1995.

Clark WL: Being there, *Hosp Health Netw* 70(22):28, 1996.

Connelly J: Being in the present moment: developing the capacity for mindfulness in medicine, *Acad Med* 74:420, 1999.

Connolly KH: The new IQ, *Nurs Manage* 33(7):17, 2002.

Curry MC: What it takes to be a nurse, *Nursing* 24(5):33, 1994.

Davis CM: What is empathy, and can empathy be taught? *Phys Ther* 70(11):707, 1990.

Davis M: a perspective on cultivating clinical empathy, *Complement Ther Clin Pract*, 15(2):76, 2009.

Dicers D: Response to: on the nature and place of empathy in clinical nursing practice, *J Prof Nurs* 6(4):240, 1990.

Dunne K: Effective communication in palliative care, *Nurs Stand* 20(13):57, 2005.

Gallagher RS: *How to tell anyone anything: breakthrough techniques for handling difficult conversations at work*, New York, 2009, AMACOM.

Goldner V: The poem as a transformational third, *Psychoanal Dialogues* 15(1):105, 2005.

Guilmartin N: *Healing conversations: what to say when you don't know what to say*, New York, 2010, Jossey-Bass.

Keefe S: Understanding human behavior, *Adv Nurses* 7(5):29, 2006.

Kerfoot K: Warming your heart: the energy solution, *Nurs Econ* (20)2:74, 2002.

Lafferty P, Beutler LE, Crago M: Differences between more and less effective psychotherapists: a study of select therapist variables, *J Consult Clin Psychol* 57(1):76, 1989.

LaRocco SA: Assisting nursing students to develop empathy using a writing assignment, *Nurse Educ* 35(1):10, 2010.

Marsden C: Real presence, *Heart Lung* 19(6):540, 1990.

McCabe C: Nurse–patient communication: an exploration of patients' experiences, *J Clin Nurs* 13(2):41, 2004.

Olsen DP: Empathetic maturity: theory of moral point of view in clinical relations, *ANS Adv Nurs Sci* 24(1):36, 2001.

Ostwald SK: Caregiver exhaustion: caring for the hidden patients, *Adv Pract Nurs Q* 3(2):29, 1997.

Patten CS: Understanding hospitality, *Nurs Manage* 25(3):80A, 1994.

Pike AW: On the nature and place of empathy in clinical nursing practice, *J Prof Nurs* 6(4):135, 1990.

Potter PJ, Frisch N: Holistic assessment and care: presence in the process, *Nurs Clin North Am* 42:213, 2007.

Press Ganey Associates. *Survey: empathy key to patient satisfaction.* http://www.ahanews.com/ahanews_app/jsp/display.jsp?dcrpath=AHA/NewsStory_Article/data/AHANEWS2A3619&domain=AHANEWS. Originally published in South Bend, Ind, 1996. Accessed 8/12/2010.

Raingruber B: Using poetry to discover and share significant meanings in child and adolescent mental health nursing, *J Child Adolesc Psychiatr Nurs* 17(1):13, 2004.

Raudsepp E: Seven ways to cure communication breakdowns, *Nursing* 20(4):132, 1990.

Rogers CR: *A way of being*, Boston, 1980, Houghton Mifflin.

Shapiro JG, Krauss HH, Truax CB: Therapeutic conditions and disclosure beyond the therapeutic encounter, *J Couns Psychol* 16(4):290, 1969.

Truax CB, Wargo DG, Frank JD, et al: Therapist empathy, genuineness, and warmth and patient therapeutic outcome, *J Consult Psychol* 30(5):395, 1966.

Wiseman T: Toward a holistic conceptualization of empathy for nursing practice, *Adv Nurs Sci* 30(3):E61, 2007.

Suggestion for Further Reading

Pardue KT: Aesthetics and empirics: teaching health assessment in an art gallery, *J Nurs Educ* 44(7):334, 2005.

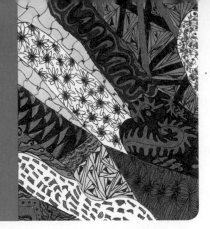

Chapter 11

Self-Disclosure

Objectives

1. Define self-disclosure in the helping relationship
2. Define immediacy in the helping relationship
3. Identify guidelines for appropriate self-disclosure by the nurse
4. Distinguish between helpful and nonhelpful disclosures in selected clinical scenarios
5. Participate in exercises to build skills in appropriate self-disclosure

Self-disclosure is another interpersonal communication behavior that you can use to show your clients and colleagues that you understand them. It can facilitate movement toward a common goal (Grover, 2005). To bring your unique gifts to the creative process of developing a helping relationship is historically referred to as the "therapeutic use of self" (Varcarolis and Halter, 2010). Immediacy is a form of self-disclosure that can facilitate the helping relationship. By the end of this chapter you will understand what is meant by self-disclosure and appreciate how this skill can be used appropriately in your relationships with clients and colleagues. You will have a chance to enhance your self-disclosing skills in the exercises at the end of this chapter.

Self-Disclosure in Personal and Professional Relationships

To disclose means to "unclose" or to open up. To self-disclose, then, means to open up the self to others. When we self-disclose, we reveal our thoughts and feelings and make some of our personal experiences known to others. Throughout your life you have used self-disclosure to let others know about you in an effort to develop closer relationships.

Self-disclosures can take any number of forms: complaining, boasting, gossiping, expressing political or religious views, and sharing endearments, secrets, or dreams. In social relationships self-disclosures are traded back and forth until the partners establish a mutually agreed-upon plateau. Intimate relationships are characterized by more private revelations than those shared between superficial acquaintances. The give and take of self-disclosing can occur with or without formal spoken rules. A specific request for deeper closeness, or an observed withdrawal of the usual pattern of sharing, influences the relationship and readjusts the established level of intimacy. "Nursing is inherently characterized by the desire to be connected to others at a very basic level of human significance . . . in milestone events of birth, death, illness, and growth in the lives of those for whom we care" (Drew, 1997). Nurses are moved to offer self-disclosure where the need for connectedness "transcends theoretical connections. Sharing . . . for the sake of connection and to give the interaction life, meaning and depth" (Drew, 1997). An example of useful information to share with a client with chronic illness and his or her family members is chronic sorrow. A nurse daughter describes it as "a type of lurking presence that periodically engulfs the life of an individual experiencing chronic illness or disability . . . it is an intermittent, bearable sadness that is interspersed with periods of joy and satisfaction" (Rosenberg, 1998). To understand this experience as distinguished from the acute grief of traumatic injury or the chronic despair accompanying depression can be helpful in listening to clients' shared experiences of lifestyle changes.

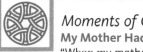

Moments of Connection . . .
My Mother Had Cancer, Too
"When my mother was terminally ill in a nursing home, I was torn between sympathy for her and embarrassment. As a nurse daughter, I worried that my mother's complaints would lead the staff to isolate her. I wished she could be a 'good, compliant patient,' even though I understood that her behavior was a reaction to fear. A nurse took me aside, put her hand on my arm, and said: 'My mother died of cancer a year ago. Your mother is a lovely lady and we will take good care of her.' That nurse's sharing of her experience helped me to know that she understood my pain and my mother's pain."

Immediacy in the Helping Relationship

Immediacy is defined as direct, mutual talk about the interpersonal relationship in a helping relationship. Although immediacy may require more attention in a client–therapist relationship, paying attention to how well you are relating to a client in service of his health may be necessary. When clients contract for therapy

with a counselor they may have interpersonal relationship problems that also surface in the client–therapist relationship. When the therapist recognizes these issues and brings them to the client's attention for validation, the client's examination of the situation may help in skill building with important relationships outside of therapy. Nurses are engaged in mutual problem solving in the service of the client's health, and relationship issues that prevent the client from participating fully in his or her own healthcare and planning may be appropriate topics to be raised by the nurse.

Egan (2002) identifies situations in which immediacy might be helpful. The following are appropriate in the nurse–client relationship:

1. Tension—when you are feeling tension in the conversation with a client, try, "Let's stop a moment so I can determine if you are comfortable with what we are discussing. It seems to me there is some tension between us."

2. Trust—when it seems the client is not trusting in the relationship, try, "It seems to me you are hesitating to answer questions we need to discuss. Are you concerned that what you tell me will not be held in confidence?" It is important to note here that the client needs to understand how information shared will be used. If, for example, the client asks if you will promise not to discuss anything about to be revealed, it is important you let the client know that anything that reveals a danger to the client or to others cannot be kept confidential. This kind of question from a client might precede a client's revealing ideas about suicide, information that must be shared for his or her safety. Often a client would be relieved to know you are concerned and that help is available.

3. Diversity—when there is diversity of culture, age, or gender between you and the client, and you sense that this might be impeding progress in your work with the client, try, "You have had more life experience than I have; is this getting in the way of my being able to help you?" Or a female nurse with a male client: "It seems to me that it is embarrassing for you to talk with a woman about these issues, is that right? . . . This is information we need to discuss for your health and we will get through it the best we can."

4. Dependency—when the client is unable to make decisions and wants advice from the nurse, try, "It seems you want me to give you an answer or direction. I can give you information but the final decision has to be yours."

5. Attraction—when the client is attempting to turn a professional relationship into a social relationship, try, "It is important that our relationship remain a professional one so you can get the best possible care." If this issue persists, or if you find yourself attracted to a client, seek out support and counsel to meet your obligations to keep the relationship professional.

Guidelines for Self-Disclosing in the Helping Relationship

Client–nurse relationships demand special considerations in the use of self-disclosure. A helping relationship is established for the benefit of the client; in other words, this is a client-centered relationship. It follows that anything you reveal about yourself—your thoughts, feelings, and experiences—should be revealed for the benefit of your clients. The focus of the relationship is the client. To continue to maintain healthy boundaries, a characteristic of a professional relationship, you must consider the why, what, when, and how of self-disclosing with your clients (Stuart, 2009).

Why Nurses Should Use Self-Disclosure with Clients

Whereas in a social relationship you might self-disclose to allow others to understand you better, the opposite is true in the professional client–nurse relationship. Self-disclosure is a skill that you can use to show clients how much you understand them because of your similar thoughts, feelings, or experiences, and to increase their comfort with the interaction. When inquiring about breast self-examination practices, for example, a nurse might remark, "Sometimes, as busy as I am, I have difficulty remembering if I examined my breasts that month. Do you have trouble remembering?" The client then feels free to agree. This allows the nurse to introduce information about self-examination reminder systems. The intent of a self-disclosure is to be empathic—to show that you really understand your clients because you have walked a similar path. An effective self-disclosure can transmit all the benefits of empathic responses outlined in the previous chapter.

Because self-disclosure is a sharing of your personal self with your clients, it can deepen the bond between you. Although still within the parameters of a professional helping relationship, your self-disclosure lets your clients know that you are a normal human being and intend to lead the client into an exploration of deeper feelings (Dossey and Keegan, 2008). Such therapeutic self-disclosure may promote comfort, honesty, openness, and risk taking by the client but never burdens clients with your problems (Keltner et al, 1999).

 Moments of Connection...
Making Meaning out of Suffering . . . a Nursing Student's Journey in Use of Self

"A few days ago in my preceptorship at a cancer center, I had a 19-year-old patient, newly diagnosed with osteosarcoma on her first day as an inpatient. She was to begin chemotherapy that night after a port placement. As a cancer survivor myself, I am very careful to share my story only when I believe it will truly be helpful. This young girl was so afraid, curious, and anxious about what lay ahead. Most of the clients here are older and as I walked into her room, I immediately felt myself revisiting my own emotions at 16, newly diagnosed with cancer, with a full head of hair, waiting to have my port placed and begin chemotherapy. Not wanting to cross boundaries, I talked with my preceptor about sharing my own experience with my client and her family. She agreed it would be beneficial. I told her I had cancer 5 years earlier and that I was now doing well. I told her I would be there all day and that if she wanted to talk or ask me questions I would be happy to do that. She asked what it was like when your hair falls out and how it comes back. As I shared my experience, I knew we stood on common ground, something I know is valuable when you have cancer. Her mom told me I had given them hope by sharing my story. I am so thankful to have had this special opportunity."

What Nurses Should Reveal to Clients in Self-Disclosures

As nurses we have to use our judgment about what we reveal to clients. There are two questions to answer before self-disclosing: "Is what I am planning to reveal likely to demonstrate to my clients that I understand them?" and "Do I feel comfortable (safe from repercussions and embarrassment; legally and morally secure) about revealing this information to my clients?" Both questions should receive a solid affirmative response before you self-disclose.

When you self-disclose, it is important to set up a client-wins/nurse-wins situation. If your client wins, your self-disclosure makes the client feel understood. If you win, you feel good that you have been skillful in making your client feel better. If your client loses, it is because your self-disclosure is irrelevant, so that the client is distracted from the major issue of concern and is left feeling misunderstood. If you lose, it is because your self-disclosure leaves you feeling uncomfortably exposed or embarrassed.

When Nurses Should Use Self-Disclosure with Clients

The purpose of a therapeutic self-disclosure is to let your clients know that they have been understood. Self-disclosure augments an empathic reply and deepens the trust between you. When you wish to increase your level of understanding and strengthen that trust, and you feel comfortable revealing the content of your self-disclosure, then self-disclosure is the right choice.

Bateson, a noted anthropologist, wrote a book of stories reflecting her experience in many cultures (Bateson, 1994). "Our species thinks in metaphor and learns through stories." Human beings can join and communicate and learn in spite of profound differences. As we meet people we have never met before, in situations we've never faced, as we try to apply communication skills to real people in real crises, we must "improvise responsibly and with love." This "quality of improvisation characterizes more and more lives today, lived in uncertainty, full of the inklings of alternatives." Consider this as you struggle to choose communication techniques, to say just the right thing, to disclose just the right incident and amount of detail, to be helpful without being self-absorbed. "Rarely is it possible to study all the instructions to a game before beginning to play, or to memorize the manual before turning on the computer. . . . We can carry on the process of learning in everything we do. . . . Ambiguity is the warp of life, not something to be eliminated. . . . [We learn] to savor the vertigo of doing without answers or . . . making do . . . [as we face difficult situations]. We are called to join in a dance whose steps must be learned along the way, so it is important to attend and respond. Even in uncertainty, we are responsible for our steps."

I remember my first communication course in a diploma nursing school, taught from a simplistic text. It all seemed so obvious when I was 17. Not until years later did I realize that clear communication takes work, and the skills to achieve it are anything but obvious.

Take the skills and tools you read about here and practice as much as you can with a serious intent to learn. Communication is a part of your journey and may cause great pain and joy in your personal and professional life as you learn from experience.

How to Self-Disclose in the Helping Relationship

To successfully implement a helpful self-disclosure, you need to follow all the guidelines for conveying empathy outlined in the previous chapter. Here is a concise list of those steps:

1. Clear your head of distracting agendas.
2. Remind yourself to focus on the speaker.
3. Attend to your clients' (and colleagues') verbal and nonverbal messages.
4. Ask yourself: "What does this person want me to hear?"
5. Convey empathy, beginning with an empathic response followed by a self-disclosure. It is usually better to self-disclose after you have made an empathic response. Using an empathic response first keeps the focus on others before shifting it to you. Your self-disclosure enhances and augments your empathic reflection. Beginning with an empathic response and following up with a self-disclosure deepens other people's convictions that they have been understood. As with empathy, the final step is the following:
6. Check to see if your empathic response and self-disclosure were effective.

Moments of Connection . . .
Out of Our Struggle, We Offer Others Our Comfort

"Although I have always known my career was in the Lord's hands, it wasn't until the past 10 years that I realized that my own struggles could help me offer comfort to patients in our chronic pain clinic. My spouse had a kidney transplant and bilateral hip replacements. My mother had fibromyalgia and posttraumatic stress, and had become depressed and inactive. I recently had a herniated disc and needed two epidural steroid injections. My husband is doing fantastically despite his physical trials. My mother is goal-setting and moving off the couch. I am able to calm anxious patients through my experience of epidurals and surgery. I have made a great recovery both spiritually and physically. Through adversity, comfort and connections can heal."

In short, use the following steps for implementing self-disclosure:

1. Listen.
2. Reply empathically.
3. Self-disclose.
4. Check it out.

You may find that you begin to see life as a collection of experiences—your own stories as well as those of others. Listen with the understanding that the experiences of clients, family, or staff members may serve you in the future. These moments can enrich your practice of nursing and your life.

Geriatric clinical practice offers rich opportunities for connections made through self-disclosure (Box 11-1).

Examples of Helpful and Nonhelpful Self-Disclosures

For the following situations, an acceptable empathic reply has been provided. After this example, several ineffective self-disclosures are given, with an explanation of their limitations. Finally, an acceptable complete response is shown.

Situation 1: With a Client

A client, Mrs. Kern, has just relayed the following information to you:

"I was so scared this weekend when I had Jack at home on a pass from the hospital. He started coughing and got all red in the face . . . and then he bent over with this violent chest pain. I thought he was going to die. Luckily his nitroglycerin was right on the windowsill. As soon as I gave it to him, he calmed down. His pain left within minutes, thank goodness!"

1. Listen.

Mrs. Kern wants to hear messages related to the fright she suffered because of her husband's pain and the relief she experienced when he recovered.

2. Reply empathically.

Before using your self-disclosure, you would give an empathic response such as the following:

"Gosh! I guess you were scared that your husband might have a fatal heart attack when he doubled up

---

Box 11-1 | *Recommendations for the Sharing of Self in Geriatric Practice*

- Understand that the connection is dynamic. The client likes and trusts the nurse who shares. The perception of the nurse as a real person aids in establishing the helping relationship. One nurse shared an interest in pottery with the wife of a resident. This topic provided a nonthreatening common ground that established the foundation for the nurse to help the wife cope and grieve.
- Remember that nurses control how much information they want to share. Nurses who use this technique learn how to let the client get to know them without the burden of high levels of intimacy.
- Recognize that the nurse's sharing of self may help decrease the client's level of anxiety and decrease the stress of illness and treatment.
- Although an intuitive sharing of self can be useful, consider the value of self-disclosure as a preplanned intervention chosen with a therapeutic goal in mind.
- Remember that reminiscence is enhanced in elders when they are encouraged to share about specific events. Speak of personal holiday traditions and question clients about theirs.

Modified from Nowak KB, Wandel JC: The sharing of self in geriatric clinical practice: case report and analysis, *Geriatr Nurs* 19(1):34, 1998.

---

like that with his chest pain. It was probably twice as frightening because you were at home without the security of all the hospital emergency equipment. What a relief for you when the nitroglycerin worked."

This satisfactory empathic introduction would be followed up with a self-disclosure.

3. Self-disclose.

The following examples help you differentiate between satisfactory and unsatisfactory ways of implementing self-disclosure.

Unsatisfactory response 1: "I remember hearing about my grandfather having chest pain, and I recall them saying that my grandmother had some hair-raising moments. They lived in the country and even the telephone system was unreliable."

This attempt at self-disclosure is inadequate because it is not your personal experience and the extra details would likely confuse and distract Mrs. Kern.

Self-disclosure should be brief and should be used only if your experience is similar. It is better to choose not to use this technique if you have not had the experience. It is also important to remember that no two people experience things in the same way and that this technique is only one possible way to be supportive.

Unsatisfactory response 2: "Scares like that are really traumatic. I, too, had a frightening situation over the weekend. The fire alarm went off, and I was the only nurse on the floor. I almost panicked, but like you, I remained calm, and luckily it turned out to be a false alarm."

This response competes with Mrs. Kern's. One important feature of a self-disclosure is that the content must be pertinent to the speaker's situation. If your self-disclosure is beside the point or, worse still, unrelated, then the message Mrs. Kern will get is that you do not really understand her situation. This response has little to do with Mrs. Kern's anxious moments with her husband. Shifting gears to talk about your unrelated experience will likely convey the message to Mrs. Kern that you are trying to upstage her. She might be jarred into refocusing on your plight and become the helper instead of the help receiver.

Unsatisfactory response 3: "Yes, I sure know how terrible it can be watching someone suffer excruciating chest pain right before your eyes. Last week there was a woman on the unit who suffered an episode of extreme chest pain, and like you, I was anxious and worried. This lady had three children at home, and you really wondered how they would cope if she died. She was a single parent, so they said . . . Guess her husband left her years ago . . . a drinker, even abused her, I've heard. You know, it makes you wonder . . . "

This response is far too vague and tangential. The material is irrelevant and detracts from any caring intended by the response. The whole purpose of a self-disclosure is to reassure others that you understand their plight because you have had a similar

experience. The self-disclosure should be brief and focused on the important issues pertinent to the situation. For Mrs. Kern, it would be important to relate your understanding of her fear and relief as succinctly as possible. The more focused your self-disclosure, the more clearly your understanding is transmitted.

Satisfactory response: "My dad had severe angina, too, and I had some pretty anxious times when he would turn ashen and look so tortured when his chest pain got excruciating. When all I could do was just stand by and hope that the nitro would work, I used to feel so desperate and helpless. Did you feel that way this weekend?"

This response meets one of the criteria for an effective self-disclosure because it empathically demonstrates that you have had a similar personal experience with a loved one; therefore, your revelation is relevant to Mrs. Kern's. This self-disclosure is brief and focused, so Mrs. Kern perceives immediately that you are absolutely tuned in to how she felt about being alone with her ill husband.

4. Check it out.

The satisfactory response meets an additional criterion for self-disclosure: it is tentative. The question "Did you feel that way this weekend?" invites Mrs. Kern to talk more about her feelings. It refocuses on her and allows her to confirm or expand on how she felt. A question like this helps you check to see whether your self-disclosure has hit the mark. By inviting Mrs. Kern to comment, you appropriately return the focus to her reactions about her situation.

A complete and fully acceptable self-disclosure to Mrs. Kern could be worded this way:

"Gosh! I guess you were scared that your husband might have a fatal heart attack when he doubled up like that with his chest pain. It was probably twice as frightening because you were at home without the security of all the hospital emergency equipment. What a relief for you when the nitroglycerin worked. My dad had severe angina, too, and I had some pretty anxious times when he would turn ashen and look so tortured when his pain got excruciating. When all I could do was just stand by and hope that the nitro would work, I used to feel so desperate and helpless. Did you feel that way this weekend?"

This response integrates the steps of listening, responding empathically, self-disclosing, and checking it out. It is clear that you have understood Mrs. Kern and are interested in discussing her situation with her.

Situation 2: With a Colleague

A fellow nursing student, Joan, says the following to you:

"I'm just thrilled! I've had the most wonderful day on the neuro unit where I'm doing my practicum. I'd been paying close attention to this young client's pupillary response and blood pressure. I kept checking his vital signs, and I was sure I could detect a rising trend in his blood pressure and some sluggishness in his pupillary reflex. I decided to point out my observations to the neurosurgeon who came by on his rounds. He checked out my concerns and promptly arranged for my client to go to surgery. In the operating room they removed a life-threatening hematoma. I felt so pleased that my careful attention helped save his life. Days like this make all the hard work and studying worth it."

1. Listen.

The message your classmate wants you to hear is that she is proud of her astuteness and grateful that her diligence helped save her client's life.

2. Reply empathically.

Before self-disclosing, give an empathic response such as the following:

"Wow! No wonder you're ecstatic! Thanks to your vigilance, your client's life was saved. You look thrilled that your astuteness paid off so dramatically. It was life or death, and you're pleased that you picked up on the subtle changes in his vital signs."

This satisfactory empathic introduction is followed up with a self-disclosure.

3. Self-disclose.

The following examples can help you differentiate between satisfactory and unsatisfactory ways of implementing self-disclosure.

Unsatisfactory response 1: "My sister had the same experience when she was a student nurse. It was

5 years ago, but it meant so much to her that she still talks about how excited she felt. She happened by a client's room and saw him choking. She did the Heimlich maneuver and of course rescued the man."

This attempt at self-disclosure is inadequate because it is not your personal experience and does not demonstrate to Joan that you really understand her moment of achievement. Your story about your sister would not convince Joan that you have been where she is, felt what she is feeling, or experienced what she is experiencing. A personal disclosure of your own is the best way to persuade Joan that you understand her. Joan may interpret this response as a competitive remark, a story to upstage her own.

Unsatisfactory response 2: "I know just how you feel. I had a great day, too. I got my whole assignment finished and all the orders caught up by noon. So then I was able to take the clients out for a walk. They enjoyed the break and the fresh air, so I, too, feel like I accomplished something today."

Your situation is not one of life or death and does not compare with Joan's. The irrelevance of this response would create a gulf between you and Joan, rather than bring you closer together through understanding. Your feeling of accomplishment is not equivalent to Joan's because she was directly responsible for saving a life.

Your self-disclosure must be relevant to the speaker's situation to show that you completely grasp the significance of her reaction. If your self-disclosure is off the mark, as this response is, it tells Joan that you do not really understand what she has told you.

Unsatisfactory response 3: "I know how thrilling it can be to save someone's life. Last summer I saw a boat out on the water in front of our cottage . . . you know the spot, right near the small island . . . Well, it was there a long time. I could see this person waving both arms overhead back and forth. I remembered that Jan had told us that arm waving like that is the international distress signal. It turned out to be two young girls who were joyriding in their parents' motorboat and had run out of gas. They had no paddles and no life jackets. And one of them was quite sick. She was a diabetic, and she'd had some beer and too much sun, and she desperately needed her insulin. We brought them back to shore and got them to safety, so I know what it's like to have saved someone's life."

Instead of feeling understood by this response, Joan will likely feel bored and irritated. It can be exasperating to wade through unimportant details and sift through irrelevant recollections. It is considerate to word your self-disclosure as briefly and clearly as you can. Succinctness causes your speaker to understand your message sooner, not later or never, as in the previous example.

Satisfactory response: "I've had that proud feeling of knowing that if it hadn't been for me, my client might not have lived. When I was on floor 4J, I discovered a client having a myocardial infarction. I called the code and started CPR . . . and he lived! Isn't it reassuring to know that you can remember what you've studied and apply it correctly in the real world?"

This response meets the criteria for an effective self-disclosure because the similarity of your experience makes it relevant. It is brief and focused so that your colleague Joan immediately receives your message that you have understood her.

4. Check it out.

Including the tentative question at the end is an effective technique for checking with Joan as to whether your self-disclosure corresponds to her experience. Your question returns the attention to Joan, where it should be. Joan has the chance to elaborate further on how she is feeling. This response does not upstage her excitement but adds to it. By sharing your relevant experience, you have made her feel understood.

A complete and accurate self-disclosure that includes the four steps could be phrased like this one:

"Wow! No wonder you're ecstatic! Thanks to your vigilance, your client's life was saved. You look thrilled that your astuteness paid off so dramatically. It was life or death, and you're pleased that you picked up on the subtle changes in his vital signs. I've had that proud feeling of knowing that if it weren't for me, my client might not have lived. When I was on floor 4J, I discovered a client having a myocardial infarction. I called the code and started CPR . . . and he lived! Isn't it reassuring to know that you can remember what you've studied and apply it correctly in the real world?"

This response combines the steps of listening, responding empathically, self-disclosing, and checking. Your clients or colleagues feel heard, understood, and respected when you actively listen with empathy and self-disclosure, and then close by turning the conversation back to them. Picard and colleagues (2004) conclude that nurses who are cancer survivors may use compassionate self-disclosure with colleagues and clients to improve clinical practice. Self-disclosure is responsible because you bring your own relevant experiences to the interaction. When you self-disclose you are assertively safeguarding others' rights to be understood and preserving your right to communicate in a caring way.

WIT&*Wisdom*

Self-Disclosure
As I grow older,
Crises I master.
Lessons I've learned.
Growth comes faster.
From my experience
I may offer reflection.
It's not up to me
To offer direction.
When you feel pain
I think I've seen
I can share a few words.
On me you can lean.
I share my path. Was that your view?
I want to understand.
Was it like that for you?

Julia Balzer Riley.

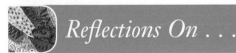

Reflections On . . .

Self-Disclosure

Consider what you read about what it means to share your experience with clients and families. How has this technique worked for you in the past? Has sharing information ever caused a problem for you? Self-disclosure is a communication skill that takes understanding, experience, and purpose.

What? . . .
Write one thing you learned from this chapter.

So what? . . .
How will this affect your nursing practice?

Now what? . . .
How will you implement this new knowledge or skill?

Think about it . . .

Practicing Self-Disclosure

Exercise 1

One of the purposes of self-disclosure in the nurse–client relationship is to demonstrate empathy. As you reflect on your own experiences you can distill the lessons learned, which might be useful in self-disclosure in the clinical setting. Select a chronic illness or disease process or other life experience with which you or someone close to you has personal experience. Write a poem to express what you know about the effects. For example:

Arthritis is stiff mornings and achy days
Arthritis is aging before its time
Arthritis is abandoned wedding rings

Single parenting is all the decisions
Single parenting is being the heavy
Single parenting means pizza for Thanksgiving and a movie on Christmas day . . .

Exercise 2

During the next few days, note when people self-disclose to you. Are these self-disclosures relevant, brief, and personal? Are they conveyed to make you feel understood? Note your reactions to these self-disclosures from colleagues, salespeople, teachers, or friends. Consider what characteristics of their self-disclosures led you to feel cared for and what features jarred you and made you question the genuine interest of the self-disclosure.

After you have done this exercise individually, get together with your classmates and compare your findings about the communication behavior of self-disclosure.

Exercise 3

This time observe your own self-disclosures to others. Note your intentions when you self-disclose to people you contact. Is it for their benefit or yours? Remark on the characteristics of your self-disclosures. Are they your own personal experiences? Are your self-disclosures brief and focused? Do you end them with a tentative question?

From your observations, assess your ability to self-disclose effectively. What are you doing well and what improvements could you strive for in your use of self-disclosure?

Exercise 4

For this exercise, work in groups of three. One of you is the speaker, another is the listener, and the third is the observer. Speakers should choose a topic with which their listeners are familiar. This way it is more likely that they will have had similar experiences so that they can realistically make a self-disclosure.

As speaker your task is to talk for 5 minutes about this topic, conveying your thoughts, feelings, and reactions. The listener's task is to attempt to implement a self-disclosure at every appropriate opportunity. The observer makes note of the listener's self-disclosures and gives feedback about how the self-disclosures meet the following criteria.

Criteria for a Complete Self-Disclosure

- Empathic response: Was an empathic response included before the self-disclosure?
- Self-disclosure: Was the self-disclosure personal? Was it brief, focused, and relevant?
- Checking: Did the listener complete the self-disclosure with a tentative question as a way of validating with the speaker?

After 5 minutes, stop and debrief with these questions:

As listener: How did you feel using the skill of self-disclosure? Which aspects were awkward and which went smoothly for you?

As speaker: How did the listener's self-disclosures make you feel? From your point of view, is there anything the listener might have done differently to make you feel more understood?

As observer: What aspects of the listener's self-disclosures were done well? What suggestions can you make for improvement?

Rotate roles so that each of you has a chance to be speaker, listener, and observer.

This exercise gives you a chance to think about self-disclosures from many different angles. What has your contemplation taught you about the important communication behavior of self-disclosure? Compare your thoughts with those of your colleagues.

Exercise 5

Select a nurse faculty member or a colleague and ask if this person would be willing to share a life story that has increased their personal understanding of the patient or family experience. As we share our own stories, we increase our understanding of the value of self-disclosure and its effects on others.

References

Bateson MC: *Peripheral visions: learning along the way*, New York, 1994, HarperCollins.

Dossey BM, Keegan L: *Holistic nursing: a handbook for practice*, Sudbury, Mass, 2008, Jones and Bartlett.

Drew N: Expanding self-awareness through exploration of meaningful experience, *J Holist Nurs* 15(4):406, 1997.

Egan G: *The skilled helper: a problem-management and opportunity-development approach to helping*, ed 7, Pacific Grove, Calif, 2002, Brooks/Cole.

Grover SM: Shaping effective communication skills and therapeutic relationships at work: the foundation of collaboration, *AAOHN J* 53(4):177, 2005.

Jourard SM: *The transparent self*, New York, 1971, Van Nostrand Reinhold.

Keltner NL, Schwecke LH, Bostrom CE: *Psychiatric nursing*, St. Louis, 1999, Mosby.

Picard C, Agretelis J, DeMarco RF: Nurse experiences as cancer survivors: part II—professional, *Oncol Nurs Forum* 31(3):537, 2004.

Rosenberg CJ: Faculty–student mentoring: a father's chronic sorrow: a daughter's perspective, *J Holist Nurs* 16(3):399, 1998.

Stuart GW: *Principles and practice of psychiatric nursing*, ed 9, St. Louis, 2009, Mosby.

Varcarolis EM, Halter MJ: *Foundations of psychiatric mental health nursing: a clinical approach*, St. Louis, 2010, Saunders.

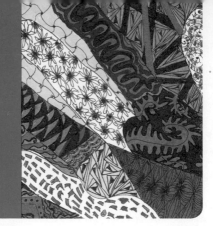

Chapter 12

Specificity

Objectives

1. Define specificity
2. Identify the usefulness of specificity and its effect on communication behavior
3. Identify strategies to communicate with specificity
4. Contrast the placebo effect and the nocebo effect
5. Participate in exercises to build skills in specificity

Recognizing When Specificity Is Useful

Being specific means being detailed and clear in the content of our speech. It means being concrete, so that our communication is focused and logical. In contrast, vagueness can be frustrating, and lack of clarity creates distance between people who are trying to communicate. Miscommunication has been estimated to account for as much as $236 billion in unnecessary healthcare expenses according to the Institute for Healthcare Advancement (2008). A lack of specificity contributes to miscommunication. In addition to clarifying our own speech, the technique of specificity assists clients (or colleagues) in moving from broad, elusive areas of discussion to narrower, more pinpointed areas of concern.

Using concrete communication is especially advantageous in certain interpersonal situations. Being specific is important when we are doing the following:

- Explaining our thoughts and feelings
- Reflecting others' thoughts and feelings
- Asking questions
- Giving information or feedback
- Evaluating

This list covers situations that nurses repeatedly encounter with clients and colleagues. Being specific or concrete benefits communication in three ways (Arnold and Boggs, 2011; Stuart, 2009):

1. The process of communicating is more satisfying when we are "on the same wavelength" as those with whom we are communicating.
2. Communicators achieve clearer comprehension of their own thoughts and full understanding of others' thoughts.

3. The foundation for problem solving is complete and accurate, which enhances the success of further communications in our relationships with clients and colleagues.

Being Specific When Explaining Your Thoughts and Feelings

Gradients exist to any emotion, and it is important to choose the descriptor that says exactly what you want to convey to your listener. In the anger category, for example, you might be feeling enraged, frustrated, furious, annoyed, or irritated. Each subtle variation conveys a slightly different mood. Hitting the mark by expressing exactly the right flavor of emotion ensures that your meaning is completely clear.

If you tell clients that you are enraged with them for being late for their clinic appointments when you are really only mildly irritated, you may create a gulf between you by overstating your case.

With the emotion of sadness, you might feel "blue," depressed, hopeless, or discouraged. If you tell your co-workers that you are merely out of sorts when you are really in despair because your child support check has not arrived and your taxes are due, such minimizing of your feelings risks diminishing the intimacy and trust between you.

When we are not specific in describing our thoughts and feelings, we invite misunderstanding. Because the purpose of communicating is to enhance the understanding between two people, being indirect or unclear is unproductive.

In addition to hitting the mark about the quality of emotion, saying specifically what makes you feel a certain way clarifies your feelings further. For example, you are happy that your client has initiated a reduced-calorie diet and has begun to walk 2 miles a day. You convey your pleasure by saying the following:

> Mr. Weller, I'm pleased that you are working to improve your health with diet and exercise. I know it can be a challenge, but you will find that you have more energy when you take time for yourself.

Being specific by adding a rationale for your feelings enhances the sincerity of your message. Your explanation has built-in rewards for Mr. Weller. Such a response would make a lot more sense to him than the following:

> That's great, Mr. Weller. Glad to see you are doing well.

In this example, it is unclear why you are pleased: because he is a dutiful client? Because you will not have to spend time reminding him to eat well and exercise?

Here is another example from the workplace. You are grateful that your colleague on the night shift has highlighted all abnormal laboratory results and displayed them clearly for your inspection when you arrive for the day shift. You tell her:

> I'm thrilled with this chart you prepared, Jo, and grateful for the time it'll save us on the day shift. Your highlighting will streamline our alerting the physicians and indicate at a glance which patients need temperatures taken or repeat laboratory work. Thank you.

This specific articulation about why you feel grateful adds depth and conviction to your feelings. It respectfully conveys your appreciation, more than a glib "Great" or "Thanks" would have.

Some nurses, clients, families, and colleagues prefer logical, rational thinking processes; they are proficient at appreciating, and being specific about, facts. They may not readily consider feelings or be comfortable dealing with them. Because their strength lies in logical, objective thinking, they may lack the vocabulary to be specific when discussing feelings. Those who prefer thinking over feeling tend to decide things impersonally, are more analytical, and respond more easily to others' thoughts. Nurses, clients, families, and colleagues who prefer to make decisions on the basis of personal feelings and human values are more attuned to others' feelings and likely have more vocabulary and the comfort to talk about feelings. They tend to be more concerned about the human feelings and values in communication than with factual, objective information (Myers and Myers, 1995).

You can learn more about specificity in relation to expressing your thoughts and feelings in Chapter 11.

WIT&*Wisdom*

Be specific and precise about what you want. Some people hold an entire conversation without saying what they want while others can be too blunt. Say what you want and say it in a way that is appropriate for the conversation (Sherrod et al, 2009).

Being Specific When Reflecting Others' Thoughts and Feelings

Listening is not a silent pastime. It is active and vocal. Through your warmth and respect you can show that you are attending to what your clients or colleagues are saying. By being specific, you can convince them that you have heard and understood the meaning of their dialogue.

When you reflect others' thoughts and feelings, you are like a recording, giving them a chance to hear what they are really saying. When helpers respond with clear, concise, detailed statements about others' concerns, it helps the people with problems to clarify them.

For example, one of your clients has given you a lengthy description of her son's epilepsy:

Mrs. Cant: "I'm so frightened he'll forget to take his medication that I often call the school nurse to check that he's taken it. And when he's late getting home from school, I worry to death that he's lying on a sidewalk somewhere having a seizure. When he plays soccer I'm right there on the sidelines— not so much cheering as praying that all that running won't fire off a seizure. My Lord, will it always be like this?"

Here is an example of a specific reflection:

Specific response: "You're wondering if your son will be able to live a normal life, and whether you'll ever be free from worrying about his health and safety."

You can pinpoint the essence of other people's meanings by being specific when they become engrossed in relating their thoughts and feelings. This tactic helps them grasp more fully both the sense and the significance of what they are saying.

Contrast the clarity of this response with these nonspecific alternatives:

Nonspecific response 1: "You must be very tense, fretting about your son."
   Nonspecific response 2: "It sounds like you spend a lot of time worrying."

Neither of these statements captures the exact meaning that Mrs. Cant was trying to convey. Replying accurately and specifically demonstrates that you fully understand your listener. Chapter 10 provides more detail about the communication behavior of reflecting others' thoughts and feelings in a concrete way.

Being Specific When Asking Questions

As an interviewer, at times you might wish purposefully not to be specific so that the interviewee takes the lead. This open-ended strategy generally is used at the beginning of an interview ("How may I be of help to you?" or "What is the pain like?") or at a point in an interview at which you want more information ("Could you tell me more about your family?" or "Could you describe your exercise habits?").

As clinicians, we often want specific information from our clients. To get exactly what we want, we must specifically ask for it. You may wish to know more about a client's family health history, for example. If you ask, "Tell me more about your family's health," you might get everything from "It's fine!" to "Well, let me see, in 1901 my great-grandfather was ill on his sailing venture." A brief response provides you with no information, and a lengthy response requires sifting through to glean the essential details.

Occasionally clients' historical recountings may be jumbled or confused, either because they are unsure of dates and details or because their emotional reactions to their changed health status are interfering with their clarity. When this occurs, it is helpful to stop undirected digressions, backtrack, and reestablish specific points. This process helps clients' thinking to become clearer and more focused.

You likely will need to know specific aspects of your clients' family history: history of cancer, history of cardiovascular diseases, and so on. Getting to the point and asking for specific information simplifies what you want and increases your chances of getting it from your clients. Using the skill of specificity, you can prevent frustration or fruitlessness in the communication encounter. As nurses, if we fail to achieve clarity, our clients may be left feeling confused and may even doubt our ability to contribute to the interaction. Phrases such as "I'm not sure I understand that" or "Would you go over that again?" let our clients know we are interested and that we need help in understanding what they want us to know (Sundeen et al, 1998).

Being Specific When Giving Information or Feedback

As nurses, we are often involved in teaching clients about their treatments, tests, medications, and health behaviors. To provide clients with material that is new to them and to avoid the disrespect of boring them, it is important to focus on the aspects that they particularly want to know. A good general screening question for clients is, "What would you like to know about your treatment (test, medication, diet)?" Posed in an inviting way, this question makes your clients delineate the most important areas for them. Jumping right in with a complete and chronological explanation wastes time, might be irrelevant, and may even focus on material that is too frightening to them.

The same approach can be used with clients or colleagues who want feedback from you. Clarifying the nature of their request at the outset ensures that your feedback is focused on the area that is important to them.

Imagine, for example, a situation in which a newly hired nurse with 6 months of postgraduate experience asks you for feedback on her performance as a team leader during the past five shifts. At this point you could enthusiastically jump in with praise and advice, but you pause before bombarding her. Instead you respond to her request for feedback with, "I'd love to comment on your team leadership abilities. What specific areas would you like me to focus on?" This approach allows her to clarify that her abilities to delegate and to handle unforeseen crises are what she wants you to address. Requesting specificity allows you to focus your feedback so that it is helpful to the other person.

Moments of Connection . . .
Never Assume, Clarify!
"I was working with a 16-year-old young man with Hodgkin's disease who had just been told by his doctor that he would be 'infertile.' After the doctor left the room, the look on the man's face told me he was devastated. I asked if he knew what the word infertile meant, and he replied, 'I won't be able to have sex.' I was able to clarify what the term meant and put his mind somewhat at ease. He did well, had a complete remission, and went off to college. We need to be specific in the use of language."

Moments of Connection . . .
To Reduce Anxiety, Provide Information
"One of my patients had been having extreme pain from postherpetic neuralgia and was not able to sit or lie still at all for about 6 weeks. She was exhausted and scared. I went to see her 4 days in a row to explain how epidurals are done and how they can help to control pain. She said she finally understood, believed it would help, and agreed to have the medication. About 5 minutes after the medication was injected, she fell asleep. When she awoke, she said she had never slept so deeply, hugged me, and thanked me for making a difference in the quality of her life. She received two injections and needed no more."

Being Specific When Evaluating

After you have implemented any nursing action, it is important to evaluate its success. Whether you have led a training session or carried out a treatment, it is important to find out if you have accomplished your goals. Your evaluation questions can be phrased specifically. Instead of asking a vague question such as "How was that?" or "Have you got the hang of it now?" you can phrase your questions to reflect the objectives that necessitated your nursing action.

For example, you could ask your colleague who wants feedback on her team leadership: "Has my feedback on your abilities to delegate and to handle crises been helpful to you?" To the client who wants to know what would be facing him in the week after surgery, you could say, "Did I cover all the points you wanted to know about the recovery phase after your open-heart surgery?" You could ask the first-time father who feels awkward and nervous about bathing his baby, "Has my demonstration on how to bathe your son improved your confidence?" These specifically focused questions assist nurses in evaluating whether they have been helpful. Asking these follow-up questions completes the nursing process.

Providing Specific Documentation

The use of specificity to collect information from clients needs to be complemented by systematic recording of the data. Clear documentation increases the likelihood that clients will receive the best care. Today, when the courts are holding nurses liable for their own actions, as many as one of four malpractice suits is decided from nursing documentation in clients' charts. Obviously, good care and avoidance of a malpractice suit are two solid reasons for completing the nursing record in a clear and logical manner (Mosby's Surefire Documentation, 2007). Your nursing records should follow the care plans and indicate that the care you provided responded to specific client needs and was appropriate for specific nursing and medical diagnoses. When nursing documentation is written with specific problems and outcomes in mind, the nurses' notes provide a concise, chronological, factual, and easy-to-audit record of clients' progress (Mosby's Surefire Documentation, 2007). Careful documentation affects the ability of a healthcare agency to be reimbursed for services. Greater precision and detail are being demanded to offer legal protection (Krantz, 1998). There is an old adage, "If it isn't documented, it wasn't done." Although this may not be literally true, an agency's documentation procedures must be followed to ensure a complete representation of the care given and assessments completed. Review the documentation procedures of the organization where you work to make sure you are being as specific as is required.

Philpott (1985) outlines 22 reasonable and prudent nursing recording policies, practices, and systems. A few of Philpott's key points pertinent to the skill of specificity follow:

- The complexity of the health problems and the level of risk posed by clients themselves, by their condition, or by the use of medical, nursing, or other therapies dictate the detail and frequency of documentation.
- The higher the risk to which a particular client is exposed, the more comprehensive, in depth, and frequent should be the nursing recordings.
- Effective nursing recording is factual, honest, and based on accurate data taken directly from visual, verbal, and/or olfactory cues and palpation.
- Effective recording shuns bias, avoiding tendencies to prejudge or label patients.
- Effective documentation tends toward quantitative expression, avoiding vague generalizations. For example, with a client who is experiencing a sleeping problem, recordings such as "usual night" or "fair night" offer no useful understanding, waste charting space and nursing time, and may mask a serious

problem. Specific documentation such as "slept from 0200 hours to 0300 and states she slept soundly and feels refreshed" provides a clear, accurate, and concise picture of the client's situation; it also enhances credibility for the nurse writer.

Understanding the Power of the Placebo Effect and the Nocebo Effect

Consider the power of the choice of language in supporting or undermining your client's healing. You may have heard of the *placebo effect*, language or expectations of a clinician that positively affect the course of the client's illness by suggestibility. The *nocebo effect* produces negative responses. Both the placebo and nocebo effects are "clinical outcomes . . . not attributable to the actual pharmacological or physiotherapeutic intervention and are susceptible to attention, expectation, suggestion, and conditioning" (Lang, 2005, in Schenk, 2008, p. 57). The nocebo effect can occur when a nurse or other healthcare provider sends a negative message through choice of language, words, or tone of voice.

Examples of language choices include some of the following:

> *Rather than:* "Here's your pill for pain" (suggesting that pain is expected), say: "This medicine will help you be more comfortable" (suggesting the medication will increase comfort).
>
> *Rather than:* "Try not to miss a dose of this medication" (suggesting the client is likely to miss a dose), say: "It is important to take this medicine regularly and at the times it is prescribed" (suggesting that the client will comply).
>
> *Rather than speculating or carelessly thinking aloud:* "Sometimes people have terrible scars from plastic surgery," say, "Your surgeon has prescribed a cream you can use to promote healing" (Schenk, 2008).

More extreme examples of careless or just-thinking-out-loud language are actually inflammatory or alarming. A cardiac surgeon, after performing a quadruple coronary bypass, speculated at the client's bedside, "There was one vessel we just couldn't get . . . we try to do no harm you know! . . . but it probably won't make a difference." This no doubt conscientious physician was reviewing the procedure in his mind but was giving the client more information than was needed. Later, this same patient had an initial visit with a new primary physician who commented about the surgery, "Well, bypass surgery is a good thing unless the grafts fail and you bleed out." Perhaps, the physician's comment came from a painful memory of the death of another client, but this client would have been better served to have reinforcement of positive eating habits and regular exercise.

Healthcare providers may be seen as experts by the client, who trusts that what they say is to be taken literally. A client, normally anxious in a situation in which personal health is threatened, may be hypervigilant, paying attention to nuances of nonverbal behavior from the healthcare provider. Remember to remain matter of fact when you first see an incision or wound or when the client's symptoms alarm you. A calm approach and appropriate intervention are supportive of the client.

WIT&*Wisdom*

TMI!

TMI, a common expression meaning Too Much Information, is a light way of saying spare the graphic details . . . good advice in our professional and personal lives.

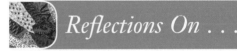

Reflections On . . .

Specificity

Consider what you read about being specific in communication with clients, families, and colleagues. Clarity and accuracy in communication are necessary for successful relationships.

What? . . .

Write one thing you learned from this chapter.

So what? . . .

How will this affect your nursing practice?

Now what? . . .

How will you implement this new knowledge or skill?

Think about it . . .

Practicing Specificity

Exercise 1   `QSEN`

When communicating with other team members, it is important to be concise, clear, and to the point, yet convey critical information accurately and clearly. Standardized communication strategies are one way to ensure that you are effectively conveying information. The SBAR (Situation, Background, Assessment, and Recommendation) technique is widely used to improve safe, team-based communication. Practice SBAR by recalling a recent client. Record how you would place a call to a physician to request assistance or intervention.

Situation: Describe the situation; what is going on. (I am calling about Mr. Smith, a 45-year-old . . .)

Background: Describe the clinical background to provide a relevant context. (His blood pressure has been dropping, from 140/90 to . . .)

Assessment: State the problem of what you think may be going on, your conclusion. (I think he may be . . .)

Recommendation: State the recommendation or the assistance needed. (I need a physician to check . . .)

QSEN Competencies: Patient-centered Care; Teamwork and Collaboration; Evidence-based Care; Safety

Exercise 2

Here's an exercise that is fun and nutritious, and sets the tone for practicing skills of specificity. This activity is a good ice breaker for work teams, too.

Bring enough apples to class so that each person in your group can have one. Have each student select an apple and observe it. Write down specific details about your apple. Return the apples to a container. Mix them and have each one in the group try to find the apple they observed. Discuss the role of attention to detail in communicating with clients and colleagues. Improving your powers of observation can improve skills of specificity.

Exercises 3 through 5

One way to really understand the benefits of an interpersonal skill is to experience the negative reactions in a situation in which the skill is not being used. The first phase of each of the following exercises provides that opportunity.

Exercise 3

Find a partner with whom to work. One of you role-plays a nurse and the other a client. As the client, you want specific information from the nurse. Decide in advance exactly what information you want and why you want it. During the interview, attempt to be as specific as you can. As the nurse in this role play, do not make any efforts to determine the exact nature of what the client wants to know or why he or she wants the information; also, be unfocused, vague, and unclear. Proceed with a discussion for 4 minutes and then pause to debrief using these questions as guidelines:

As the client: How did you feel when the nurse neglected to determine what you specifically wanted to know or the reasons you had for wanting the information?

As the nurse: How did you feel when you neglected to determine what your client wanted?

Switch roles so that each of you has the chance to give and receive vague, unspecific communication.

Exercise 4

Find a partner with whom to role-play. One of you acts as a home health nurse and the other as a physician. The nurse telephones the physician to obtain orders for a client. The nurse uses vague language when describing the client's condition. The physician must either ask many questions or risk making a decision based on inadequate data. After a 4-minute discussion, debrief using these questions as guidelines:

As the physician: What thoughts were you having about the nurse and her skills? How did this affect the way you responded to this nurse's questions?

As the nurse: How effective were you at getting what you needed for the client?

Replay the exercise with the nurse giving the physician clear, specific information. After a 4-minute discussion, debrief using these questions as guidelines:

As the physician: What thoughts did you have about the nurse's skills? How did this affect the way you responded to the nurse?

As the nurse: How effective were you at getting what you needed for the client?

Exercise 5

"I just want the facts, ma'am, just the facts." This is a quote from detective Joe Friday on an old television show, *Dragnet*. A psychiatric nurse consultant was called into a critical care unit to facilitate communication between a nurse manager and a physician. The physician was busy and wanted brief, specific communication about unit problems. The nurse manager tended to want to give all the extra details, which led to the physician limiting access to the manager, compromising communication. The consultant suggested the manager use a $3'' \times 5''$ index card to list a few specific points to be made. Preparing this card helped streamline the issues. Being specific can be useful when a nurse needs to call a physician in the middle of the night. Identify a clinical situation that you need to summarize to be more brief and concise. Using an index card, list the few important points to practice specificity in communication.

References

Arnold E, Boggs KU: *Interpersonal relationships: professional communication for nurses*, ed 6, Philadelphia, 2011, Saunders.

Institute for Healthcare Advancement: News, notes and tips, 10 common errors healthcare professionals make with their patients, *Nurse Educ* 33(6):240, 2008.

Krantz J: Taming the new E&M guidelines, *Physicians Manage* 38(3):41, 1998.

Lang EV, Hatsiopoulou O, Koch T, et al: Can words hurt? Patient–provider interactions during invasive procedures, *Pain* 114 (1–2):303, 2005.

Mosby's surefire documentation: how, what, and when nurses need to document, St. Louis, 2007, Mosby.

Myers IB, Myers P: *Gifts differing*, Palo Alto, Calif, 1995, Consulting Psychologists Press.

Philpott M: *Legal liability and the nursing process*, Philadelphia, 1985, WB Saunders.

Schenk PW: "Just breathe normally": word choices that trigger nocebo responses in patients, *Am J Nurs* 108(3):52, 2008.

Sherrod D, Sherrod, B, Sherrod, T: Expand your communication style, *Men in Nursing* 39(3)18, 2009.

Stuart GW: *Principles and practice of psychiatric nursing*, ed 9, St. Louis, 2009, Mosby.

Sundeen SJ, Rankin EAD, Stuart GW, et al: *Nurse–client interaction: implementing the nursing process*, ed 6, St. Louis, 1998, Mosby.

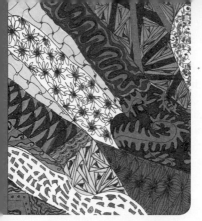

Chapter 13

Asking Questions

Objectives

1. Discuss the importance of the skill of asking effective questions
2. Identify six points to keep in mind when asking questions
3. Identify common errors in asking questions and strategies to avoid them
4. Participate in exercises to assess and build skills in asking questions

Importance of Asking Questions Effectively in Nursing

The word *question* is derived from the Latin *quaerere* (to seek), and this is the very power of good questions. When you take the time to ask questions you demonstrate interest and respect (Gallagher, 2009). Asking questions effectively is fundamental to nursing assessment and to building the helping relationship. For example, if you ask a client if he has chest pain, a closed question, you will receive less data than if you ask him to describe any discomfort he is experiencing (Kleiman, 2002). As you make initial contacts with clients, consider that they are performing their own assessments to see if you measure up to their expectations (Sundeen et al, 1998). Illness often makes clients feel vulnerable; they are forced to depend on an unfamiliar person to initiate the process of sustaining themselves through a frightening life experience on the journey to healing. The client needs to trust that information you seek will be used appropriately and with discernment for promotion of health, dignity, and privacy (Carter, 2009; Matiti and Trorey, 2008). As a professional nurse, you will spend about half of your working time asking questions of clients and colleagues. Pay careful attention to building this skill. Remember to listen for what is said and what is left unspoken.

Adeptness at asking questions is a fundamental requirement for competent and considerate nursing. The more effective you are in asking questions, the more time you save yourself and others, the more pertinent and useful the information you collect, and the more effective your interviewing experience. Effective questioning ensures that you collect the data you need to provide quality nursing care. As you become accustomed to asking questions about nursing practice, you build a foundation for contributing to the profession by posing the questions that stimulate research to support evidence-based practice (Knoll and Leifso, 2009).

Moments of Connection . . .
Questions to Help Move beyond the Obvious

"I was working with a 31-year-old woman with myelitis who was in tremendous pain. As I was doing the morning assessment and we were discussing her pain, she began to cry. Upon further exploration, the client revealed that it was not the pain that was her worst concern. With support, she began to tell me about her grandfather, who was dying, and her grandmother, whose cancer was no longer in remission. She was afraid she would never see her grandfather again to be able to tell him what he had meant to her. She touched me deeply because I had had a similar experience. To help her regain some control of her situation, I helped her place a call to her grandfather, and she was able to find closure."

From the time your clients enter your care until the completion of your helping relationship, you will be asking them questions. You will ask them about the nature of their concerns so that you can agree on a nursing diagnosis. Finding out what they hope to achieve with the help of your nursing services requires effective questioning. You will discover their preferences for a treatment plan and frequently check with them about its effectiveness. Determining their readiness for the termination of your relationship and their readiness to take care of their own health concerns after discharge demands that your questioning skills be clear and focused. Remember, too, that helping clients learn how to ask questions of you, their physicians, and other healthcare team members is an essential part of being an active part of their own team (Sobczyk and Shulman, 2002). A study on how clients' communication styles affect physicians' communication concluded that physicians engaged in significantly more client-centered communication when interacting with clients who actively participated in their care by asking questions and providing information (Cegala and Post, 2009).

You might be thinking that the client–nurse relationship is composed primarily of questioning. Well, to a great extent it is. Therefore, it is crucial that you attain proficiency in this fundamental nursing communication behavior.

In your role as a nurse, the main reason for asking questions is to secure data that are essential to providing quality care to your clients. Six questions need to be answered to ensure that you obtain the facts you need.

> **WIT&***Wisdom***
>
> When you have asked all the questions you need to ask, pause, and ask, "Are there any other questions I should be asking at this time?" You might be surprised at how much additional information you might acquire.

Why, What, How, Who, When, and Where of Asking Questions

If obtaining the information you want is important, then it is worthwhile to spend the time planning the strategy that is most likely to secure these facts.

Why of Asking Questions

Before you make any inquiries, you should be sure about why you need the information. Irrelevant questions send the message that you are unfocused (Gallagher, 2009). Questions rooted in personal curiosity may offend your clients. Before you speak, silently answer this question: "How will the information I am seeking direct me in helping my clients?" If you can justify the question, then ask it!

If there is any doubt as to whether your clients will understand your reasons for asking, then explain those reasons in advance. Consider this example.

In your investigations of your client's fall off a ladder, you want to learn about his safety habits in general to determine if he is in danger of future home accidents. Before barraging him with what might seem to be unrelated or even nosy questions, you can clarify your objective by saying something like the following:

> I'd like to ask you some questions about your safety precautions with the ladder and about your home

safety measures in general. About 80% of accidents occur in the home. My questions might trigger some ideas that could make your home a safer place in which to work and live. Are you agreeable to exploring this area with me?

Here is another example:

Within the past year, your 79-year-old client has been brought to the emergency department three times after fainting. The cause of the fainting has not been discovered, and your observations about her thinness and lack of vitality make you wonder whether inadequate nutrition might be at the root of her fainting. The following statement can clarify the purpose of your questions:

> We still don't know what is causing your fainting, Mrs. Jones, and we want to investigate every likely source. One possible cause could be a lack of the nutrients essential to keep you going. I'd like to ask you some questions about your diet to determine whether you are getting all you need from the foods you eat. Is that OK with you?

Both of these examples illustrate how you can prepare your clients for your line of questioning. When clients understand your purpose, they are more likely to be open and to reveal information, rather than being guarded because they are uneasy about your intentions.

What and How of Asking Questions

What you ask and how you ask it are the next considerations in your strategy. When you have determined why you require the information, then you must plan what to ask to ensure that you are clear in your intentions and know how to phrase your question in a way that invites your client to respond.

What you say must be phrased clearly, and a logical progression to your questions is helpful. They should be worded in a way that shows your respect for your clients' privacy and personal information. Any judgments you have about the responses should remain unspoken.

For example, imagine that you require some information about a client's overall activity level and day-to-day schedule to help him fit in his colostomy hygienic care. Having explained your purpose and secured his permission, your next step is to proceed with your inquiry. You choose to proceed in a systematic order starting with the following:

> Let's begin with your mornings. Could you outline what you do, hour by hour, on a typical weekday morning, from the time you get up until lunchtime?

This question outlines for your client exactly what you want to know. He can focus on the mornings, and it is apparent that you will proceed to other times in his weekly schedule.

Consider another example:

You are completing a health history on a client who has just arrived in an outpatient surgical center. He will be receiving an anesthetic, and you need information about his past health status, past illnesses, and family health history. Your facility employs a concise preoperative assessment tool to efficiently obtain this extensive material from clients. Having secured your client's permission, after explaining the purpose of your line of questioning, you proceed with the following:

> As you know, this is a lot of material to cover. To streamline things I'm going to use this guideline our unit has developed. It's a good checklist to ensure that we cover everything. Please ask me if there's anything I say that isn't clear to you. Beginning with your childhood, did you ever have diphtheria? . . . or whooping cough? . . . or rheumatic fever?

Explaining your format helps clients accept what might otherwise seem like a barrage of unrelated questions.

Any material that clients provide is of a personal nature, and some areas are more sensitive than others. For some clients, talking about sexual activity or birth control practices may be difficult. For others, talking about personal hygiene or alcohol consumption may be embarrassing. Some clients do not feel comfortable revealing their self-care practices. Others hesitate to reveal family issues or job-related information. You cannot know in advance which topics might be difficult for your clients, so you must keep in mind that any information clients reveal about themselves, their significant others, or their healthcare practices might be sensitive for them.

As a nurse you can take certain steps to put your clients at ease and to make them feel more comfortable in revealing this information. One thing you can do is to reassure them about the confidentiality of your relationship. This step should be taken at the beginning of an interview or at the earliest point possible in your relationship. If you wait until later, you may lose opportunities for uncovering important information.

Confidentiality has a wide range of meanings, and you must be honest and clear with all your clients so that they understand exactly what the parameters are. Does confidentiality mean that you will not repeat what your clients have said? Does it mean that you will verbally pass the information along to a trustworthy colleague but not put it in writing? Does it mean that you will convey information to team colleagues at client-care conferences? Or does it mean that confidential information will be written on a chart for other team members to read? Exactly what your clients reveal will likely be determined by what you intend to do with the information they contemplate telling you.

It is essential that you and your clients have an identical understanding of the meaning of confidentiality. Sundeen and colleagues (1998) remind us that clients may feel betrayed if they have been under the impression that client–nurse relationships are confidential and then discover that you have revealed what they consider personal information to another health team member or have written it on their charts.

Another way you can increase your clients' comfort is to treat all areas you discuss respectfully and professionally. Making the effort to ensure that your clients have privacy and the time to respond unhurriedly facilitates their replying openly and fully. Being equally relaxed and straightforward, whether you are discussing sexual matters, family health history, bowel habits, or exercise patterns, contributes to putting your clients at ease. If you flush, wriggle in your chair, lose eye contact, or lower your voice, your clients quickly get the message that this topic is a sensitive one for you, and they may feel even more embarrassed. To improve your ability to be at ease when asking questions in a variety of areas, you may find rehearsal with friends or colleagues helpful.

Who of Asking Questions

Whom to ask is another important consideration. If your clients are able to speak for themselves, then they are the ones to approach. Occasions may arise, however, when you need information that your clients might not be able to provide. There are times when the observations of significant others can shed light on a client's situation, and this perspective is also valuable to have. For example, if your client has been on a mood-elevating medication, you may wish to have his wife's observations of any changes, in addition to your client's sense of the effectiveness of the drug. Or, on one of your home health visits to a client with multiple sclerosis, you may wish to obtain family members' perspectives on the client's ability to manage at home. Whenever you consult family members or friends, it is courteous and respectful if you do so with the knowledge of and, when possible, in the presence of your client. In some agencies it is the policy to secure written consent from clients before questioning significant others and previous or concurrent healthcare providers. To respect client confidentiality and protect the legality of your actions, it is important that you make yourself aware of such policies.

There are times when clients cannot answer questions. For example, unconscious, aphasic, or psychotic clients are not able to provide information that might be important in their recovery. In these instances you must do some detective work to discover the essential people from whom to obtain this information.

When and Where of Asking Questions

When and where to carry out your questioning is your next consideration. The physical setup of many hospitals and clinics makes it difficult to secure a completely private place to interview your client. You should make every effort, however, to arrange for a time and place in which you will not be interrupted by telephone calls, noise, other clients, agency activity, or visitors. Arranging such a time and place may require patience, as both you and your client have days filled with scheduled and unscheduled activities. It does not usually pay to rush an interview or talk about sensitive issues in an open ward area. Clients have every right to privacy and a sense of unhurried attention from you.

Keeping in mind these six aspects of asking questions will improve your effectiveness by making you a systematic and sensitive interviewer.

Common Tactical Errors in Asking Questions and What to Do about Them

The broad strategies outlined in the preceding section are valuable in guiding your inquiries in a general way. When it comes to the nitty-gritty of speaking, the following suggestions about avoiding or overcoming poor techniques provide a helpful reference.

Long-winded Build-Up

In efforts to explain the purpose of our line of questioning to our clients and colleagues, we sometimes go overboard. When we provide a rambling, detailed introduction, we run the risk of confusing or boring the other person. When we are providing an explanation of the rationale for our questions, the KISS principle is best: Keep It Short and Simple!

The wrong way would be as follows:

Long-winded approach: "Mr. Haddon, I'd like to ask you some questions about your allergies so that we can eventually work out a lifestyle plan that will allow you to avoid or minimize the stressful reactions you suffer from the various things that irritate you. As you know, repeated allergic reactions can be stressful for the body when it has to constantly fight to return bodily functions to normal. When you are in an allergic reactive state, your body is in the alarm phase and is working overtime trying to return things to normal. When you feel miserable because of the allergies, you also feel tense and anxious, and maybe even at times frightened that your allergic reactions will get out of control. It's only when we have all the information that we can help you plan the best ways to avoid your irritants. Shall we begin?"

A long-winded build-up such as this can put off the client who understands the purpose and wants to get down to the business of the task. Openers that are redundant, wordy, and too detailed are diversions that detract from the task.

The right way would be as follows:

Focused approach: "Mr. Haddon, I'd like to ask you some questions about your allergies so we can eventually work out a lifestyle plan that will allow you to avoid or minimize your stressful reactions to the various things that irritate you. Your chart indicates you have both food and environmental allergies. To begin, could you tell me to which foods you are allergic?"

This concise opening spells out your purpose and how and why you are asking this client your particular questions. The clarity and brevity of this statement will not bore, frighten, insult, or confuse him.

Thunder Stealer

Our questions sometimes take the form of asking clients their opinions about the cause of their health problems, their preferences for effective treatment, or the degree of cure or alleviation of the problem they think should be sought. It is respectful to give our clients the opportunity to offer their ideas, especially when we have requested their perspective. In our enthusiasm we sometimes jump in with our views and opinions before giving our clients a chance to speak. This zealousness on our part can be intimidating for clients and prevent them from expressing their real views. Jumping in and upstaging clients can anger some of them. Many clients feel hurt that we would barge ahead, expounding our beliefs, without extending them the courtesy of listening to their point of view about their own healthcare situation.

The wrong way would be as follows:

Upstaging approach: "Well, Miss Ricco, together we have agreed on six possible steps you could take to minimize your facial blemishes. I'm interested in knowing what you think of each of these options. I know which I would recommend. Definitely get rid of any oil-based skin care products you have and start using oil-free products. Don't you agree that this change would prevent your pores from clogging up? And you likely agree that you should buy the special soap Dr. Best recommended, don't you? I think you should go for our second option too."

Miss Ricco would soon get the message that you are not interested in her views. Usurping every opportunity for your client to speak is frustrating and demeaning. Stealing our clients' thunder gives them the message that we think that what we have to say is more important and that they should depend on us for direction. This picture is out of line with today's well-informed health consumer and a healthcare system that is striving to get people to assume their healthcare responsibilities.

The right way would be as follows:

Considerate approach: "Well, Miss Ricco, together we have agreed upon six possible steps you could take to minimize your facial blemishes. I'm interested in knowing what you think of each of the options we've talked about."

The nurse who is genuinely interested in discovering what Miss Ricco really thinks about the treatment options would stop here and let the client proceed. Clients have preferences that motivate them to choose certain health behaviors, as well as barriers—such as cost and time—that work against other treatment choices. Clients have a responsibility for their own healthcare, and as nurses we can encourage their participation by giving them a chance to speak and by listening to them when they answer our questions.

Multiple Choice Mix-Ups

As interviewers we sometimes get carried away and assault our clients with a barrage of questions. After receiving a string of questions, our clients become confused and do not know what information we are looking for or where to begin answering.

The wrong way would be as follows:

Bombarding approach: "Mrs. Parker, there are some things we need to know to help you through your labor, delivery, and postpartum stay. Have you discussed what kind of delivery you prefer? Have you and your husband met with your physician and gone over all the options? What I mean is, have you decided on whether you will receive analgesics and/ or any type of anesthetic during labor? Do you know the various types—general, spinal, perineal block? And next we need to know your plans for breast-feeding. Have you decided on that yet?"

Whew! Mrs. Parker's head would be spinning as she tried to keep pace with this bombardment. Just as she would have formulated a response to one question, you were off to the next, probably making her feel distracted, confused, and irritated.

The right way would be as follows:

Clear approach: "Mrs. Parker, there are some things we need to know to help you through your labor, delivery, and stay afterward. I'd like to review your plans for pain management during labor and for feeding your baby. Are you comfortable enough to go over these two areas now?" You pause to check out her readiness. "First, are you planning to use any type of pain medication during your labor and delivery?"

Mrs. Parker has been given one question to answer in this example. She knows that more questions are forthcoming, but she knows exactly what you are seeking when a single, clearly worded question is posed.

Incomprehensible and Cryptic Codes

As nurses, we become accustomed to medical terminology and develop our own shorthand to abbreviate long, unwieldy medical terms. Using this jargon among professionals is fine, but using it with clients only adds to their confusion. Clients have a right to be asked questions that are worded clearly in language they can understand.

The wrong way would be as follows:

Cryptic approach: "I've come with your digoxin, Mr. Winters. Before I give it I need to check out your apical and radial pulses and estimate your edema. Have you had any angina, palpitations, or SOB this morning? We want to prevent chemotoxicity."

Mr. Winters would almost need a medical dictionary or decoder to decipher your questions! Your use of medical jargon might make him feel stupid or uncomfortable. Just as bad, you might receive incorrect information from clients who give answers to questions they do not understand because they are embarrassed or confused.

The right way would be as follows:

Clear approach: "Mr. Winters, I've come with your heart medication—digoxin. Before I give it to you I need to check your heart rate over your heart with my stethoscope and at your wrist. Have you had any chest pain this morning?" After pausing for an answer, you ask, "Have you noticed any fluttering or fast beating of your heart this morning?" After receiving his answer, you ask, "Have you had any shortness of breath at any time this morning?"

Asking questions in plain English increases the probability that clients will understand what you are asking and, in turn, give appropriate responses.

Offensive Misuse of "Why"

As nurses we do a lot of detective work in trying to determine why our clients are sick, why they are upset, why they do not follow their treatment regimen, and so on. These "whys" are all legitimate questions, but when it comes to asking, it is usually best to refrain from using "why" too frequently with clients because doing so tends to make them feel threatened. To avoid such an aggressive tactic, it is better to rephrase the question so it is softer and more receivable.

The wrong way would be as follows:

Threatening approach: A client is slamming his pillow against his bed frame: "Why are you doing that, Mr. Kent?"

A teenager is using his crutches incorrectly: "Why aren't you weight bearing more?"

A diabetic woman is having three toes on her left foot amputated: "Why don't you take better care of your feet?"

An elderly widower is sad: "Why are you letting life slip by you instead of getting back into things?"

Each of these "why" questions is aggressive and blunt. Each one might force the client to become defensive, curt, or protective in some other way. Withdrawal or hostility diminishes the chances for an open and honest response.

The right way would be as follows:

Gentle approach: To the client who is slamming his pillow against his bed frame: "Will you tell me what's wrong, Mr. Kent?"

To the teenager who is using his crutches incorrectly: "What is it that prevents you from weight bearing more?"

To the diabetic woman who is having three toes on her left foot amputated: "What factors make it difficult for you to take better care of your feet?"

To the elderly widower who is sad: "What are some of the things that keep you sad and prevent you from getting involved in things you used to enjoy?"

Each of these questions seeks the same information as the earlier questions, but they are less aggressively phrased. These questions do not put the client on the spot; rather, they invite the client to respond.

Misuse of Open and Closed Questions

Closed questions are focused and posed to elicit specific and brief responses from clients. Open questions invite respondents to elaborate in whatever direction they choose. Skilled interviewers know when to use each type of question.

The wrong way would be as follows:

Closed approach: A client has just returned from the radiology department, where he underwent a barium enema, a procedure he was dreading. You ask, "Did your barium enema procedure go OK?"

This question requires only a yes or no and does not invite your client to elaborate further about his experience.

In taking an initial health history, you ask your client, "Do you eat a well-balanced diet?"

The yes or no response to this type of question will tell you little about the client's nutritional intake.

Your 63-year-old client is going to be transferred to an extended care facility. You ask, "Are you looking forward to going to Haven's Point?"

This approach gives your client little choice about how to answer.

The right way would be as follows:

Interested approach: A client has just returned from the radiology department, where he underwent a barium enema, a procedure he was dreading. You say, "Tell me how the procedure went for you."

In taking an initial health history, you ask your client, "What did you eat for breakfast today?"

Your 63-year-old client is going to be transferred to an extended care facility. You ask, "How do you feel about leaving here and going to live at Haven's Point?"

These three examples are open-ended questions that require your client's elaboration. The information obtained by asking these questions provides you with a better understanding of your client's perspective.

In nursing practice, we err more frequently on the side of posing closed questions when open-ended ones would provide more useful information. However, we are sometimes too general when we should be more focused in our question asking. Therefore, it is worthwhile to examine your question-asking practices to see if there are times when you might make your questions more focused.

Mystery Interview

When we ask questions of our clients, they respond with the belief that as skilled clinicians, we are sorting, sifting, and analyzing their data to contribute to their nursing care plan. It makes our clients feel connected and respected when we give them feedback on the problem-solving process.

The wrong way would be as follows:

Abrupt approach: You have been doing an initial health assessment with a client admitted for extreme and rapid weight loss. The time allotted for the interview is over, and you say to your client: "I've got to go now. I'll see you later, and we can continue our interview then."

Clients feel left out when we end an interview without giving them any indication of our assessment.

The right way would be as follows:

Clear approach: If you must end an interview before you can complete your assessment, you can say something like: "We've talked about your weight loss problem a fair amount today. To determine all the factors that might be contributing to your weight loss, I need to obtain more information from you at our next interview. Until we meet again this afternoon, could you think about anything you can recall, anything unusual that happened to you at the time you first started losing weight?"

Even though this closing remark does not offer a definite summary, it does show that you are up to date with your clinical assessment of the problem. Informing our clients of what is happening, including your plans and what clients can expect next, provides helpful transitions so that they can map their progress, feel included, and minimize worrying about erroneous assumptions.

Continuing to Build Your Skills in Asking Questions

As you become more comfortable with asking questions of clients and families, consider these lessons learned over time:

End with a question that invites further disclosure. "What other questions should I be asking; is there anything else that would be helpful for me to know?" (This question is also useful in consumer situations when you are contracting for a service or purchasing a product.)

At times *"silence is golden."* Take a moment to pause to give yourself and the other person time to think more critically, to process information, and to remember details lost in an anxious moment. Take a breath to center yourself and communicate your willingness to be responsive to the other's genuine concerns. When you are quiet and the other person is deciding whether to reveal important sensitive information or ask questions that might be troubling, you create sacred space by inviting deeper communication.

If you use the suggestions in this chapter, your question asking will be assertive and responsible. You will respect your right to secure the information you need to complete the nursing process yet maintain the dignity of your clients. Reflect on the questions in Box 13-1 and find your own words to help clients actively participate in their own healing journeys. Remember that clients and families will ask you questions, too. Sometimes you may need to answer the same questions and provide the same answers over and over, especially in times of high anxiety or when you work with the family of a dying person (American Association of Colleges of Nursing, 2000). You ask questions with respect, and you answer questions with respect.

> *Notice the word "communion" in communication; the two-way exchange of words, thoughts, energy, and the unspoken.*
> **Guilmartin (2010, p. 40)**
>
> **WIT&** *Wisdom*

Box 13-1 | *Questions to Deepen Healing Relationships*

1. What can we do to help you?
2. Tell me what's on your mind just now.
3. You look uncertain. What is that about?
4. I might be wrong, but you look like you are worried. What's bothering you?
5. What questions do you have for me?
6. What do you need to feel better?
7. What have you already done to help yourself feel better?
8. What have you found helpful to make you feel more comfortable?
9. For the nurse working with the terminally ill: consider the need of this client to talk intimately. What do you allow your client to tell you? If someone you know and love were dying, what care would you want for her or him?

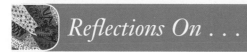
Reflections On . . .

Asking Questions

Consider what you read about asking questions and the importance of question-asking skills. Consider how asking questions in a professional relationship is different from asking questions in a personal relationship.

What? . . .

Write one thing you learned from this chapter.

So what? . . .

How will this affect your nursing practice?

Now what? . . .

How will you implement this new knowledge or skill?

Think about it . . .

Practicing Asking Questions

Exercise 1

For this exercise, work in groups of three. One person acts as the interviewer, one as the interviewee, and one as the observer. The interviewee chooses a topic on which to be interviewed; for example, an interest such as music, windsurfing, or skiing; the latest paper he or she is writing for a course; or a new product he or she is planning to buy. The interviewee must let the interviewer know what the topic is before the interview begins.

For 8 minutes the interviewer asks questions about the topic the interviewee has chosen. During the exchange the observer makes note of how effectively the interviewer asks questions. At the end of 8 minutes the observer provides feedback on the strengths of the interviewer and ways in which the interviewer could improve.

- Tape recording this exercise can give you a chance to review your work more thoroughly.
- The members of the group should exchange roles so that each gets the chance to try all roles.
- What has this exercise taught you about the skill of asking questions?

Exercise 2

Using Box 13-1, Questions to Deepen Healing Relationships, work with one other student. One student assumes the role of a client with whatever condition/challenge the student chooses. The other student uses questions from Box 13-1 to elicit information. Discuss what it was like to ask and to be asked these questions. Then switch roles.

Exercise 3

As a nurse working on an orthopedic unit, you are nursing a newly admitted, elderly female client, Mrs. Haley, diagnosed with Alzheimer's disease and a broken left hip. This evening her son and daughter-in-law and her frail, elderly husband, with whom she lived before her recent admission, have come to the unit to visit your client. It is your responsibility to determine how your client fell and broke her hip.

Working on your own, choose and write down what your first three questions would be. Be able to defend them by describing the following:

- Why you chose to ask those questions
- What exactly you would ask
- How you would ask the questions
- Whom you would ask
- When you would pose your questions
- Where you would ask your questions

When you have finished writing down your three questions, compare the similarities and differences between your approach and the approaches of your classmates. This exercise focuses on your question-asking and problem-solving skills. What has this exercise taught you about the relationship between question asking and problem solving?

Exercise 4

You can increase your own self-awareness, an important part of caring communication with others, by keeping a journal. Posing questions for reflection is a useful strategy for journal writing. Answer some of these questions and create your own.

- What are some of my basic assumptions in life?
- Who are the caring people in my life?
- What are my dreams in life?
- What fears do I have that get in my way?
- What lessons have I learned in my life?
- What are my strengths? What are my areas for growth? (Jacobs, 2001)

Exercise 5

QSEN

Reflective practice is the art of constantly asking yourself, Why did I do what I did, applying what you know from multiple perspectives, and concluding the best action to take in similar situations in the future. Applied to quality and safety competencies, reflective questioning is the basis for a spirit of inquiry that can improve practice. This constant learning from asking questions about your experience is critical in moving from novice to expert. Focus on the following reflective questions as you care for your patients. How can this help focus the questions you ask them?

1. Patient-centered Care: What is the most important thing I can do right now for my patient?
2. Teamwork and Collaboration: Who needs to know the information I have about my patient?
3. Evidence-based Practice: What is the basis for my actions in caring for this patient?
4. Quality Improvement: How can I improve the outcomes of my care?
5. Safety: Where are potential safety hazards that could lead to errors?
6. Informatics: How can technology improve how I manage care?

QSEN Competencies: Patient-centered Care; Teamwork and Collaboration; Evidence-based Practice; Quality Improvement; Safety; Informatics

References

American Association of Colleges of Nursing, City of Hope National Medical Center: *The-End-of-Life Nursing Education Consortium (ELNEC) faculty guide*, Module 9: *Preparation and care for the time of death*, Duarte, Calif, 2000, The Medical Center.

Carter MA: Trust, power, and vulnerability: a discourse on helping in nursing, *Nurs Clin North Am*, 44(4):393, 2009.

Cegala DJ, Post DM: The impact of patients' participation on physicians' patient-centered communication, *Patient Educ Couns* 77(2):202, 2009.

Gallagher RS: *How to tell anyone anything: breakthrough techniques for handling difficult conversations at work*, New York, 2009, AMACOM.

Guilmartin N: *The power of pause: how to be more effective in a demanding, 24/7 world*, San Francisco, 2010, Jossey-Bass.

Jacobs RD: *The way in: journal writing for self-discovery*. New York, 2001, Stewart, Tabori & Chang.

Kleiman N: Asking the right questions is the key to proper diagnosis, *Buffalo News*, final edition (My View column), p. C4, May 1, 2002.

Knoll S, Leifso G: Asking questions—improving practice, *Can Oper Room Nurs J* 27(3):6, 2009.

Matiti MR, Trorey GM: Patients' expectations of the maintenance of their dignity, *J Clin Nurs* 17:2709, 2008.

Sobczyk R, Shulman NB: *Your body, your health: how to ask questions, find answers, and work with your doctor*, Amherst, NY, 2002, Prometheus Books.

Sundeen SJ, Rankin EAD, Stuart GW, et al: *Nurse–client interaction: implementing the nursing process*, ed 6, St. Louis, 1998, Mosby.

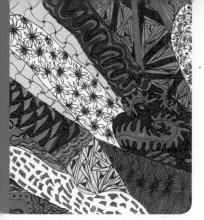

Chapter 14

Expressing Opinions

Objectives

1. Distinguish between giving advice and expressing opinions

2. Identify strategies to express opinions in an assertive way

3. Discuss examples of sharing positive regard for others

4. Identify the effects on empowerment of expressing opinions

5. Participate in exercises to build skills in expressing opinions

How to Differentiate between Giving Advice and Expressing Opinions

Expressing opinions as a nurse refers to the act of disclosing what you think or feel about healthcare situations affecting your clients or colleagues. Expressing opinions or offering recommendations is an assertive behavior. Having confidence in your ability to communicate, self-efficacy, can help prevent miscommunication, a significant threat to the safety of hospitalized clients (Raica, 2009). The Joint Commission and Institute for Healthcare Improvement mandate healthcare organizations' work to improve professional communication (Thomas et al, 2009). In a professional setting, your opinions are offered as additional information for clients' and colleagues' problem-solving and decision-making processes. In contrast, giving advice is a unilateral process of solving problems or making decisions for others. Offering advice prevents clients from becoming independent and gives colleagues the idea that you might think they are incapable of self-direction.

Expressing opinions can be part of providing clients with a fuller picture to make choices about their health and treatment plans. Clients have a moral right to information, and you as a nurse have a duty to provide information. Expressing opinions is not telling others what to do, but giving them the benefit of your point of view. It assists clients in their health decision making and avoids both the dependency when clients rely on their nurses and the anger and blame when the nurses' advice is rejected at some point.

When to Express Your Opinions as a Nurse

Clients and colleagues may seek your nursing counsel when they are at a point at which they must make a decision about any of the following.

Whether to provide or withhold information: For example, clients may wonder whether they should expose information about their condition to a physician or to another family member. Colleagues may be in a quandary about whether to reveal information to clients and/or their families or to colleagues or supervisors. Fellow students may be undecided about whether to confide in their nursing instructors about personal problems.

Whether to comply with a treatment plan or resist it: Some clients may have conflicting doubts and hopes about their health problems and might be unsettled about whether to follow a treatment plan or attempt to survive without it. Fellow nurses may have mixed feelings about adhering to restrictions imposed on tasks they can perform while making a home visit. Student colleagues may face a dilemma about whether to report an honors violation.

Which strategies to implement to achieve the desired outcomes: Clients who know what expected health status they are aiming for may not be able to decide which treatment plan to follow. Colleagues at work may know exactly what outcomes they want but need help in deciding what actions they can take to most likely ensure that they reach their goals. Classmates may be lost about what approach to take to ensure that they receive a high grade on their next assignment.

Your views may be sought by clients or colleagues at any one of these decision points. Your opinions provide others with information that can be incorporated into their decision making.

Although they are referring to the psychotherapeutic helping relationship, Jensen and colleagues (1989) have several pointers about sharing information with clients that also apply to the client–nurse helping relationship. Nurses might share their opinions about any of the preceding situations when uncertainty exists about outcome, when the options have both negative and positive effects, or when one course of action is not necessarily superior to the other. Giving your opinions as a nurse can create an environment for discussing any one of these decision points and can provide an opportunity to collaborate in the healthcare of your clients. Both of these mutual acts strengthen your relationships.

Your Feelings about Expressing Opinions

Before proceeding any further, take a pencil and jot down your responses to the following questions:

1. How do you feel when others express their opinions to you without your seeking them?
2. How do you feel when others refrain from giving you their opinions when you have sought their counsel?

After you have expressed your feelings about these questions, compare your reactions with those of colleagues in your class.

Many of us feel differently about opinions we have sought than about viewpoints we did not seek. In our culture, in which we place a high value on liberty and the freedom to act as we choose within the limits of the law, many of us likely feel some resentment when others take it upon themselves to try to influence us without our consent. We are usually more willing to consider opinions that we have agreed to receive. This knowledge of our nature suggests a principle for expressing opinions: whenever possible, find out if your opinion is wanted. You may have strong opinions about what decision a person should make, but you are wasting your time and may be jeopardizing the relationship if you persist in expressing them without the person's consent.

In response to the previous questions, many of you will have indicated that you expect to be given opinions from someone whose counsel you have sought and that you feel cheated when denied such counsel. When we ask lawyers, physicians, and teachers for their professional opinions, we expect them to provide us with guidance. So it is with our clients and colleagues who seek our points of view in our professional capacity as nurses. Remember that people sometimes have the right to learn from their own mistakes. It could be possible that your answer is not the best one for them anyway. When others make their own decisions, the blame or the glory is their own.

> *Sometimes not to decide is to decide.*
> **Author unknown**
>
> **WIT&***Wisdom*

Here are two more questions about expressing opinions:

1. How do you feel when clients (or friends, family members, or work colleagues) who have asked for your opinion do not act on the views you express?
2. How do you feel when clients (or friends, family members, or work colleagues) incorporate your opinions into their actions?

You may have no strong feelings about whether other people act on your opinions. On the other hand, you may experience pride or relief that others follow your counsel, or you may feel hurt or disappointment when they do not. The strength of your feelings may be related to how much you derive a sense of power or control over other people's actions. Consider to what extent your self-esteem as a nurse depends on your clients or colleagues doing things your way versus knowing you offered them your wisest counsel so that they had adequate information on which to base their decisions.

The degree to which we allow others the freedom to make their own decisions depends on the degree to which we value their autonomy and well-being more than we care that our opinions are revered. As nurses, we must keep in mind what expectations our clients have about seeking opinions and, more important, what agendas we carry around about offering others our viewpoints.

How to Express Your Opinions in an Assertive Way

As a nurse you will be called upon to express healthcare opinions in your professional life by your clients and colleagues, and in your personal life by friends, family, and even perfect strangers. Because you are an educated, professional nurse, there will be innumerable times when you will be tempted to express opinions to clients, friends, or family about their healthcare. You will feel more confident about handling these situations if you have worked out some principles to follow in expressing opinions. The following sections provide some guidelines.

Get the Consent of Your Receiver before Expressing Your Opinions

To avoid generating feelings of hostility or resentment in your clients or colleagues, ask if they are interested in hearing your viewpoint. To complete this courteous step, here are several phrases you can use that can flow naturally into your conversation:

"A former client told me a good way to get around a situation like yours. Would you like to hear that suggestion?"

"I've just read an article that had some excellent ideas on how to solve your problem. Do you want to hear what it had to say?"

"Last year I had the same difficulties you are now having. By trial and error, I learned some great ways to get rid of the problem. Would you be interested in hearing how I worked things out?"

"I've seen many people with a problem similar to yours. I have some recommendations for you that have come from those experiences. Would you like to hear them?"

"I've thought about this issue for a long time, and I have some opinions I'd like to express to the team if you'd like to hear them."

Although you think you may have helpful information, the other person may not necessarily want to hear it. As one friend of a psychiatric nurse once remarked, "If you know of any other developmental crisis I'm about due for, just keep it to yourself!"

Clients or colleagues from whom you are requesting permission to proceed will let you know whether they want to hear your ideas. Those who are verbal and direct will reply with a definite yes or no. Those who are less direct will send you nonverbal signals that will tell you whether to proceed or refrain from sharing your conclusions. If they look away, change the subject, or argue that their situation is unique, they are warning you to back off and keep your opinions to yourself. If they give interested gestures, that is your cue to continue.

Make Allowances for the Uniqueness of Your Client or Colleague

We give opinions based on the knowledge that our ideas have worked in similar situations with like people and circumstances. However, it is impossible for us to know all the circumstances and personal factors that affect everyone with whom we deal. Consequently, we should avoid being dogmatic when expressing our opinions. We should be tentative about offering our persuasions to show our consideration of others' special circumstances.

Avoiding strong phrases such as "I really think you should . . . ," "You really ought to . . . ," or "It should be clear to you that this is the direction to take" makes your views more receivable so that they can be incorporated into other people's problem-solving processes.

When offering your opinion, you can include one of the following phrases, which gives others a fair chance to accept or reject your ideas:

"Do you think this idea will help in your situation?"
"What do you think about these recommendations?"
"How do you think this suggestion will fit your lifestyle?"
"How does my slant on your situation strike you?"
"Can you adapt any of these ideas to your situation?"

Include the Rationale for Your Viewpoint

Your clients and colleagues expect you to have opinions about healthcare and work- or school-related issues. Giving your rationale is a responsible way to defend your position. It ensures that sufficient information is available for clients and colleagues to make the final decision.

Here are some phrases that you might use to include your rationale with your opinions to clients:

"In my view, options 2 and 4 would be the most likely to get the results you are looking for. Which options do you favor?"

"If you have the money, I think the clinic in Healthtown is the best resource for you. If finances are strained, you might wish to consider one of the self-help groups here in town. What do you think?"

"If I were feeling as desperate as you seem to be, I think I would go for the quick-start option rather than the slower one. After you get some relief from your symptoms, you can shift over to the regular stream. How does that plan sound to you?"

"I hesitate to suggest plan A because all your social supports and family are out of town. Plan B would ensure that you get some regular supervision while you are learning the technique. What are your preferences?"

"In my clinical experience, using the prepared formula has proven to be more successful than using the one clients have to mix from scratch. That's my recommendation. Does that help you make a decision?"

"I really don't know which way would be better for you. In my experience, there have been clients who have been happy with both treatment choices. The final decision gets down to personal preference since both options are solid in every respect. So my advice is to choose the one you like!"

In all these examples the nurse has offered a reason for his or her preferences and turned the final decision back to the client. If we want clients to take charge of their own healthcare, we can offer them our professional opinions yet make it clear that the final responsibility for a choice is theirs.

With your colleagues on the healthcare team, you might include your rationale in the following ways:

"Mrs. Jones is beginning to improve, so I think it would be a mistake for us to transfer her just now. Maybe Mrs. Hanes could be moved first so that Mrs. Jones would have an extra week of physical therapy. What do you think?"

"I think we should ask the instructor to go over the section on neuroanatomy one more time before the examination. It's worth 40%, and she spent only one lecture period on it. What do you think?"

"I think we should consider purchasing wireless laptop computers to enter data on the home health clients, since timely, proper documentation affects reimbursement. Do you think administration would agree?"

"We have nursing students from two different universities on this unit this month. Even though they are on different shifts, the patients have to answer the same questions over again and have commented about it. Do you see this as a problem?"

"I think we should have a first-year student representative on the faculty curriculum committee in addition to the second-year rep. We need a student there to get our perspective across to the faculty, don't you think?"

"Since you ask, Dr. Kenson, I have been Mr. Jones's nurse for the last week and a half, and I feel strongly that he could be discharged sooner than you are recommending. His condition is stabilized, and the home care nurses could see him daily for his injection and dressing change. He is very anxious to get back to his own surroundings and begin to take up his life again, especially to start a bit of writing on his home computer. What do you think?"

These examples demonstrate how to present your opinions assertively and still consider your colleagues' viewpoints. Giving your opinions does not mean co-ercing your colleagues into adopting your ideas. Providing a rationale for your point of view and inviting others' opinions makes the decision making a collaborative process.

The decision-making climate set by nurse executives and managers may influence the style of decision making used by staff nurses with their clients. The model of shared governance encourages nurses to participate in running the unit (Watson, 2002). Nurses may be organized as a council to oversee the clinical, administrative, research, and educational areas of nursing practice (Miller, 2002). Nurses who are committed to a mutual problem-solving approach with clients want the same kind of respect and collegiality in the work environment as in a participatory management structure. Nurses can influence how decisions are made by staying alert and assertively making and taking opportunities to express their opinions as another source of information for the workplace decision-making process. Become involved in setting the local, state, and national legislative agenda on issues related to healthcare, nursing, and advocacy for special client populations, such as the aging (Watson, 2002). At a time of change in a healthcare system, along with uncertainty comes opportunity. Nurses are positioned to become more involved in health policy and advocacy. Building skills in expressing opinions supports your role in the political arena to articulate issues you believe are important. Nurses who find this arena of nursing rewarding and exhilarating can pursue further education in advocacy and health policy (Stokowski et al, 2010).

Expressing your opinions is also assertive and responsible. It protects your right to have your point of view included in the decision-making process and respects others' rights to know what you are thinking. By including your views, you are ensuring that another piece of information is available to the decision makers.

How to Share Your Positive Regard for Others

You may notice a particular behavior of a client, family member, or colleague that, in your opinion, is noteworthy. Giving specific positive feedback is another form of expressing your opinions that can demonstrate your assertive communication style. Berent and Evans (1992) give examples of how to compliment and commend people for their actions:

> "You're always willing to help."
> "You're always open to new ideas."
> "I see improvement in . . . "
> "It took a lot of courage for you to . . . "

Contribute your opinion of shared good work:

> "We've worked hard on this."
> "We came up with some good ideas."

In work groups or other successful collaborations, humorous positive comments create energy and goodwill:

> "Are we a great team or what?"
> "We are so wonderful, I can hardly stand it."
> "We want a prize . . . we did so well."
> "Just call us terrific!"

Sharing positive opinions sets the stage for others to feel comfortable in loosening up a bit and sharing their ideas in a friendly, accepting environment. This promotes creativity and teamwork—a noninvasive, cost-effective tool! In a climate in which professional and personal change comes at an unprecedented rate, rewarding colleagues with praise or by other methods becomes important.

How to Master the Art of Not Expressing Your Opinions

Some of us do not need any help expressing our opinions, but rather need an awareness of knowing when not to share and the strength not to be right. When someone tells a story in which the details are not absolutely correct, consider whether the accuracy is crucial. You hear someone say it was "100 degrees" yesterday, but you heard on the weather report that there was "a high of 99 degrees." Is your usual response to correct the person? Consider the results. The correction is experienced as a put-down comment, which does not build relationships. This is a startling concept to some of us. Just give it some thought. Exercise 5 (near the end of this chapter) will help you explore this further.

> *The antidote to extraversion is measured words.*
>
> **WIT&** *Wisdom*

How to Empower Yourself by Expressing Opinions

At times in your career you may feel powerless in the face of decisions that are made without your input or with which you disagree. You can make a choice about when to share your disagreement even if you see no choice but to comply with the decision. For example, if a new policy is to be implemented that seems unreasonable to you, but not unsafe, you can say the following:

> I understand that this new policy is in place. I will comply with it, but I do want to voice my disagreement for the following reasons . . . I will try it this way and see how it goes, but I'll get back to you with any problems we encounter.

A teenage patient with asthma has chosen to smoke cigarettes. You might say the following:

> John, of course, your choice to smoke is your decision, but I want to express my concern for how this can affect your health. I can tell you more about how that can happen if you are willing to hear, but I can't in good conscience avoid opening up the discussion.

Sometimes just being able to voice your disagreement makes you feel more authentic and more assertive. Assertiveness is a matter of choice and is not necessary or appropriate in every situation. You may have a strong sense of fairness, but if another customer who is obviously belligerent and inebriated cuts in front of you in line at the grocery store, you would probably make a choice not to share your opinion about fairness. This does not mean you are nonassertive but that you have good judgment. You make decisions about what opinions to share, with whom, and when. Some of these decisions are based on unpleasant results from past experience. Try to remember that everyone has to learn some things the hard way. As you learn when to take appropriate risks to express your opinion and earn the respect of clients and colleagues, you may find that your input is requested because you are viewed as an authentic person who is willing to take a stand.

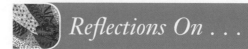

Reflections On . . .

Expressing Opinions

Consider what you read about expressing opinions. Think about your own experiences in healthcare and how expressing opinions makes a difference.

What? . . .
Write one thing you learned from this chapter.

So what? . . .
How will this affect your nursing practice?

Now what? . . .
How will you implement this new knowledge or skill?

Think about it . . .

Practicing Expressing Opinions

Exercise 1

Write about a time when you expressed your opinion and were glad you did. Write about a time when you did not share your opinion and regretted it. Reflect on what you learned from these experiences that can apply to your professional life.

Exercise 2

Over the next few days, note the way others express their opinions to you. Check whether they ask your permission and consider your particular situation, how tentative they are, and whether they provide a rationale. Your reactions to receiving advice from a variety of people can tell you a lot about how to express your opinions effectively.

As a class, compare and contrast your observations and conclusions about expressing opinions.

Exercise 3

Over the next few days, observe how you express your opinions to others in your day-to-day encounters. Assess the assertiveness of your approach. Congratulate yourself on your effectiveness and make note of where you need to improve.

Exercise 4

For 1 day, observe opportunities to express your positive opinions of others. Take the plunge and give one compliment that you would ordinarily not share. How did the person respond? Commit yourself to giving one compliment each day for a week and ask one colleague to try the experiment, too. Arrange for a specific time to sit down and share your experiences. This kind of positive energy can do wonders for the profession. Imagine if every nurse gave one compliment each day!

Exercise 5

Practice not sharing your opinion. Do you ever feel the need to correct someone whose facts in your opinion are not accurate? For 1 week, note when this happens. Ask yourself if it is important that you correct the person. If it is not a life-and-death matter, try resisting the impulse to be right. This may well be a stress-reducing activity for you and others the area of letting it go!

Exercise 6

What beliefs are important to you? Create a poem by completing a list, each line starting with "I believe . . . " Continue until you have exhausted your ideas. Keep this in your journal. Add to it with lessons learned and reread the list occasionally.

Exercise 7

Nurses have been criticized for not sharing their opinions on health-related issues (Morley, 2004). A well-written letter to an editor can often be an important way to make your opinions known. Identify an issue about which you have a strong opinion, in your nursing or personal life. Compose a letter to the editor of an appropriate publication expressing your opinion and thinking behind it. You may or may not submit it; that is up to you. Read your letter to one or two other appropriate people to generate discussion.

References

Berent IM, Evans RL: *The right words: the 350 best things to say to get along with people*, New York, 1992, Warner Books.

Jensen PS, Josephson AM, Frey J: Informed consent as a framework for treatment: ethical and therapeutic considerations, *Am J Psychother* 43(3):378, 1989.

Miller ED: Shared governance and performance improvement: a new opportunity to build trust in a restructured health care system, *Nurs Admin Q* 26(3):60, 2002.

Morley B: The world is LOUD, but nurses remain silent, *Aust Nurs J* 11(10):15, 2004.

Raica DA: Effect of action-oriented communication training on nurses' communication self-efficacy, *Medsurg Nursing* 18(6):343, November/December 2009.

Stokowski LA, Sansoucie DA, McDonald KQ, et al: Advocacy: it is want we do, *Adv Neonatal Care* 10(2):75, 2010.

Thomas CM, Bertram E, Johnson D: The SBAR communication technique: teaching nursing students professional communication skills, *Nurse Educ* 34(4):176, July/August 2009.

Watson DS: The perfect storm (president's message), *AORN J* 75(6):3, 2002.

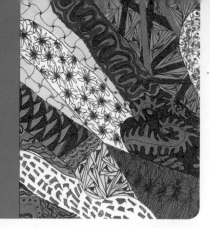

Chapter 15

Humor

Objectives

1. Define therapeutic humor
2. Distinguish between positive and negative humor
3. Identify three criteria for the appropriate use of humor in healthcare
4. Discuss the functions of humor in healthcare
5. Identify strategies to implement humor in healthcare
6. Discuss the use of a humor kit in healthcare
7. Identify three ways humor can be used to promote positive communication in healthcare
8. Discuss creative ways to add humor and play to relieve stress and build relationships
9. Discuss the use of play and humor to promote creativity
10. Identify possible health benefits of laughter
11. Participate in exercises to build skills in the appropriate uses of humor

Definition of Humor

The Association for Applied and Therapeutic Humor (AATH) defines therapeutic humor as "any intervention that promotes health and wellness by stimulating a playful discovery, expression or appreciation of the absurdity of or incongruity of life's situations. This intervention may enhance health or be used as a complementary treatment of illness to facilitate healing or coping whether physical, emotional, cognitive, or spiritual" (AATH, 2000). Humor is an important part of human behavior and everyday life, the ability to see the amusing side of a situation rather than being serious all the time, an exceptional way of perceiving life, and a perspective that frees us from conformity and puts us in touch with our authentic, spontaneous self (Kipplinger, 1987; Astedt-Kurki and Isola, 2001). You don't have to tell jokes or be a comedian to use humor successfully in nursing (Smith, 2000). Yet one nurse reports that as a nursing student she could improve a child's mood. "I would make goofy faces, sing silly songs and imitate popular characters . . . such as Barney" (Starr, 2009, p. 72AAA). Reflect on your own comfort with humor in the clinical setting as you read this chapter. As we begin to discuss humor, remember that the best advice is to follow the client's lead and to "dip a toe in the water" to see if humor fits the occasion (McGhee, 1998). The therapeutic effects of a study of nurse friendliness include mutuality, humor, fondness, and reciprocity in nursing interaction (Geanellos, 2005). Studies support the positive effects of the use of humor as a nursing intervention in cancer treatment and end-of-life settings to promote coping, hope, joy, and relaxation. Humor research in health caring situations involving aging, crisis intervention, and disaster demonstrates similar results (Adamle et al, 2008).

To be able to laugh at yourself in uncomfortable situations, in the face of life's incongruities, is essential to good mental health. Former Chrysler Chairman Lee Iacocca would often exchange jokes with members of the press and with stockholders. His humor put people at ease and built upon his image as a leader who had high self-esteem and control of situations (Green, 1994). Nurses can use positive humor with the same effect. "Humor is not only the telling of jokes to patients. It is the attitude, the relaxation and the smile that really make the difference" (Bakerman, 1998). One study showed that four times as much laughter was initiated by droll phrases as by formal jokes (Smith, 2000). "Just put on this air-conditioned patient gown! It's a one-size-fits-nobody." Remember to be yourself. Often it is the immediacy of a genuine, light response that makes the connection (Fonnesbeck, 1998).

To be able to laugh at a tough situation provides temporary relief from fear and worry. This changes the perception of a stressful event and adds a sense of control, the power to choose your own attitude or response. A nurse who has experienced the challenges of menopause, for example, may use her own humorous perspective to reframe or alter the view of the situation for her client. Hot flashes become "power surges." This can lead to a discussion of the positive side of the middle years.

Humor can also help nurses build relationships with clients and colleagues. After all, it is hard not to like a person who makes you laugh (McGhee, 1989). Analysis of observations of client–nurse interactions in a cancer treatment unit demonstrated the importance of social exchange, trust, and humor (Lotzar and Bottorff, 2001). A study of humor between nurse and client and among staff demonstrated that nurse–client humor helped both nurse and client to cope with unpleasant procedures. Humor among staff facilitated coping with the work environment (Astedt-Kurki and Isola, 2001). From observations and interviews in an intensive care unit and a palliative care unit, Canadian researchers concluded that humor promotes positive team relationships and adds a human dimension to support and care given to seriously ill clients and their families (Dean, 2008). Humor does the following (Green, 1994):

- Invites interaction
- Puts others at ease
- Wins affection
- Helps us cope with stress and fear

If you can laugh at your own shortcomings and learn from your mistakes, you are free to be creative. Being creative means taking the risk to fail. Nurse managers who can tolerate personal mistakes create a safe environment in which staff can dare to be innovative. Healthcare staff whose managers use humor effectively and appropriately are viewed as more effective and report higher job satisfaction (Cansler College, 2008).

Positive versus Negative Humor

Distinguishing between positive and negative humor is important. Positive humor, "constructive, empathic humor" (Fry and Salameh, 1987), is associated with love, hope, joy, creativity, or a gentle sense of playfulness. Its intent is to bring people closer together. Negative humor puts people on the defensive and makes them feel put down. It may be sarcastic, racist, sexist, or ageist, and it reinforces negative stereotypes about different cultures, age groups, or conditions. Negative humor isolates you and alienates people (Box 15-1).

> *A person without a sense of humor is like a wagon without springs—jolted by every pebble in the road.*
>
> **Henry Ward Beecher**
>
> **WIT&**Wisdom

Positive humor communicates that the human condition is shared, that we all have problems, and that no one is perfect. The highest form of humor is the ability to laugh at ourselves. Follow this adage: "Take your

Box 15-1	*Negative Humor Can Build Barriers between People*

Avoid the following:
- Racist humor
- Sexist humor
- Ageist humor
- Sarcasm
- Put-downs

work seriously, but yourself lightly." One nurse who volunteers as a clown in her hospice work relates an example of humor with an elderly man whose movements have slowed with his illness. The nurse and the client often joke about this because she admits to being slow in the mornings, too. The nurse gave her client a button that showed a turtle saying, "I may be slow, but I won't the race." The client loved the gift and wears it whenever the nurse visits. Positive humor adds to your relationships with clients, families, and colleagues by eliciting cooperation (Box 15-2).

Your response to another person's humor says something about who you are. To reinforce positive humor by laughing and sharing your own humorous perspective, but to refuse to laugh at or participate in demeaning humor by remaining quiet or gently commenting, "I don't think that's funny," is an assertive statement of your belief system. Although it may be difficult to make this type of response to demeaning humor, this is a responsible way to deal with such humor and does not encourage or reinforce put-down humor as does nervous laughter. Recognize, however, that humor serves to relieve tension, and negative humor may be a coping mechanism in tough situations. The medical humor, or gallows humor, that staff use to cope is appropriate when kept among staff because it permits sharing of frustration and promotes group cohesion (Simon, 1988).

Negative humor may serve to relieve tension for the sender of the communication, but it can demean others and undermine your credibility if shared inappropriately. When information about acquired immunodeficiency syndrome (AIDS) first became public, several radio stations aired macabre jokes about the illness. It was not uncommon to hear people repeat these jokes. People often make jokes about subjects that cause

anxiety, such as sexuality, relationships, and death. AIDS is one issue that touches all three.

National tragedies, such as the space shuttle disaster, can also be the source of jokes. Humor is often used as a catharsis to provide relief. In a study of such jokes, this humor was found to serve as an "antidote to personal tension and pain" and helped "neutralize the pain of a nation" (Green, 1994).

Humor is listed as an adaptive response to terminal illness by the End-of-Life Nursing Education Consortium curriculum (American Association of Colleges of Nursing, 2000). Joy Ufema, a well-known expert on death and dying, tells us that it is right to provide relief from the seriousness of being terminally ill but advises that you take your cue from the client. She writes of the courage of a woman with leukemia who agreed to be interviewed on *60 Minutes* while they were discussing funeral preparations; the client wondered if she should ask her friend, the church organist, to play. When the interviewer said she was sure that were their situations reversed, the client would do it for her friend if asked, the client retorted that she didn't think she would be asked, since she couldn't play the organ (Ufema, 2002).

Humor is highly individualized. People find different things funny. Pay attention to the subjects of your clients' jokes or humorous comments. This gives you a clue about their topics of concern. If a preoperative patient lightly says, "Well, I won't die from it," it is likely he would benefit from a little extra time to talk about these fears. Be alert for what seems like inappropriate humor in timing or subject. This is a clue that clients or colleagues may benefit from more serious discussion of the issue. Allow your clients the right to hostile or macabre humor but do not participate in it yourself. To listen without using off-putting body language shows your ability to allow for individual coping responses. To build on this negative humor may create problems. Consider a situation in which you are upset with a relative or close friend. You make negative comments or jokes to relieve tension. If a friend or spouse joins in, you may be offended. It's OK for me to joke about my mother, but not for you to!

In humor workshops held for clients who test positive for human immunodeficiency virus, participants suggest that nurses "allow us our own form of humor. We know it is black humor. Don't take offense at it and please, touch us more; don't act as if you can't wait to get out of the room." Although this may be seen as

---

Box 15-2	*Positive Humor Can Build Bridges between People*

- Laugh at yourself.
- Follow the patient's lead.
- Remark on humorous cards.
- Share cartoons.
- Share jokes.
- Use gentle banter: "Our gowns aren't skimpy; they're air-conditioned!"

negative humor by nurses, it is initiated by clients as a way of coping with anxiety. Coping styles vary. What people find funny varies. What is constant is your clients' need to feel that someone understands and accepts them wherever they are along their own journey of coping with illness.

If humor should become offensive, you can change the subject or tell your clients that you appreciate their need to use humor but that you are embarrassed by it.

> *Laughter is the most inexpensive and most effective wonder drug. Laughter is a universal medicine.*
>
> **Bertrand Russell**
>
> **WIT&** *Wisdom*

Criteria for the Appropriate Use of Humor

Have you heard the adage, "There is a time and place for everything"? Pay attention to timing, receptivity, and content (Leiber, 1986) in the use of intentional humor as an intervention.

Timing: When patients are admitted to an acute care setting such as the emergency department, they and their families want efficient, caring attention and treatment. Humor may be inappropriate unless initiated by patients or family members. You will be able to distinguish between banter among clients and family members to ease tension and the put-down humor or sarcasm that needs intervention. In chronic illness, humor may be a much-needed coping technique. One woman with arthritis refers to her condition as "Old Arthur."

Receptivity: Some people have been raised to believe that humor is frivolous; thus a humorous intervention would not be appreciated. If you use humor and it offends, apologize and explain that your intentions were to be helpful.

Content: Avoid sexist, racist, or sarcastic humor. Remember, just because someone makes light of an issue such as obesity does not give you permission to joke about these personal issues. Your efforts might be interpreted as ridicule.

Nurse–client relationships may provide occasions for humor that seems less amusing when it is retold and thus taken out of context. Trust your own judgment when relating a story. Observe a colleague whose sense of humor you admire. If you have an idea about how to use humor and question its appropriateness, check it out with a co-worker.

Functions of Humor in Healthcare

Robinson (1990), dubbed the fairy godmother of humor in nursing, examined the functions of humor used in the hospital setting by studying the jokes that were told. She found that humor serves both social and psychological functions.

Social functions include the following:

- *Coping with disruptive acts of hospital custom*. Consider the banter about "air-conditioned" hospital gowns.
- *Establishing relationships*. Clients who are disfigured may have a series of one-liners they use to break the ice when someone seems shocked by their appearance.
- *Coping with social conflict*. One nurse who has good rapport with a physician was surprised by his irritability one day. Realizing that he was having a bad day but was unaware of the effect of his behavior, she retorted, "Dr. Smith, did you have nails for breakfast this morning?" He laughed and apologized.
- *Promoting group solidarity*. Two teams of nurses with separate medication carts competed to dress a stuffed animal attached to their carts with a different costume for every holiday.

Psychological functions include the following:

- *Relief of tension*. One supervisor of a telemetry unit puts on oversized clown sunglasses and strolls down the hall when staff members are irritable.
- *Release of hostility and anger*. A Nerf basketball and hoop or a Koosh ball to toss in the staff lounge is helpful.
- *Denial of reality*. Humor in the operating room that would seem offensive elsewhere helps staff diffuse tension.
- *Coping with disability and death*. Individuals infected with human immunodeficiency virus practice their "death rattle" and laugh about it.

In a study analyzing the use of humor in healthcare among registered nurses in a graduate nursing program (Beck, 1997), five themes emerged about humor:

1. It helped nurses to manage difficult situations and difficult clients.
2. It helped build cohesiveness in nurse–client and nurse–colleague relationships.
3. It helped nurses intervene to address clients' anxiety, depression, and embarrassment.
4. It could be part of the routine or could be spontaneous.
5. It produced positive effects beyond the moment of humor.

A qualitative research study of personal health resources in elderly women demonstrated the use of humor, beauty, and cultural activities as strategies used to maintain physical health and mental well being. The interviews revealed these women had clear ideas about what helped them feel well even in the face of serious disease. Joking with others helped them cope with low-status jobs, pain, and marital difficulties. The researchers reported that study participants' lifelong experience as caregivers and homemakers provided special information about what can promote health, a wisdom that we can tap when supporting elders (Forssen, 2007).

Studies have shown that hospitalized children use humor, laughter, and play to deal with stressors that make them feel bad, nervous, or worried; to provide distraction from anxiety and pain; and to reduce fear of injury and chemotherapy, and they respond to clowning, jokes and riddles, puppets, games such as peek-a-boo for young children, music, storytelling, and stickers from staff (Dowling, 2002). Jill Sonke, a dancer-in-residence in the Arts in Medicine program at the University of Florida, Gainesville, uses the energy of dance and movement to raise a child's spirits. Helping a child create and fly paper airplanes in his room boosted his morale and his energy. Mary Lisa Kitakis, an artist-in-residence in the same program, brought T-shirts and paint for a child on a bone marrow transplant unit. The child would stand at the window waiting for her to come (Samuels and Lane, 1998). A nurse artist offered touch drawing (Koff-Chapin, 2002) to an 89-year-old hospice client, who exclaimed, "I am having FUN!" This occurred 1 week before she died. Play and humor bring us into the present moment (Burkhardt and Nagai-Jacobson, 2002). A review of the research literature on caring revealed that humor was a part of the emotional care of clients (Watson, 1993).

> . . . *[R]espectful humor used judiciously can buoy clients' spirits, bring spoonfuls of levity to a sea of seriousness, show humility that softens the stiff authoritarian semblance of control and increases clients confidence that their proverbial exposed underbellies are in safe hands.*
>
> **Craig (2009, p. 18)**
>
> **Wit&***Wisdom*

Nursing Practice Confirms the Research

Humor can be used in healthcare settings in simple interventions that serve these functions. A nurse in a veterans hospital, for example, says, "G.I. issue comes in two sizes, too big and too small; welcome back to the military!" Pediatric staff on one unit wear customized buttons with teddy bears in addition to formal name pins. A nurse in a heart center wears a button that says, "Speak slowly, I'm a natural blonde." This pin consistently breaks the ice with patients. Computer-generated certificates or banners can be used for clients to illustrate a shared funny experience, such as a "Best Dressed" certificate for clients with an elaborate cast. "Happy Birthday" banners can make a client feel more like a real person, not just a collection of symptoms.

When asked how they think humor works in healthcare, nurses reply as follows:

- Humor shows you care.
- Nurses are accepted better when they have a sense of humor.
- Humor shows you your clients' personalities with their defenses down.
- Humor reduces tension and helps you get on with work.
- Humor makes us equals, because we all laugh at the same things.

Clients initiate humor as an important means of self-expression. If humor has been a coping strategy throughout the client's life, then humor is likely to be even more important. Sometimes in the face of serious illness, humor may be the only personal attribute unchanged by disease and the one thing in the client's control. A study of oncology nurses' responses to client-initiated humor demonstrated the nurses were more likely to recognize and respond to spoken humor or inflection, pitch, or manner of speech than to nonverbal behavior (Adamle et al, 2008). When you recognize and respond to a client's humor you are demonstrating an understanding of the client's perception of the illness experience. Clients using humor expect a response from you even if it is not a humorous retort. Without an acknowledgment, the client may experience embarrassment, withdrawal, or humiliation. This can become a barrier to communication and affect the "physical and psychosocial function and informally damage the trust and confidence in nurses that patients need to subsist during illness" (Adamle et al, 2008, p. E7).

Clients initiate humor that shows creative coping skills. An 83-year-old woman in a rehabilitation unit of a nursing home, for example, takes great delight in wearing large, colorful earrings. She lives in southern Florida and wears her "resort" jewelry when she goes to physical therapy. Now her therapist has begun wearing wild earrings, and a nurse has gotten in on the act by presenting a pair of earrings to the client to fuel the competition. This same woman has also been given a pair of purple high-top basketball sneakers by her daughter. The client has been asked to wear shoes that help her navigate better in her wheelchair, since she has weakness on one side. At the nurse's encouragement, the daughter has glued jewels to the purple sneakers. Her mother is thrilled and calls people to her room to see them. This woman clearly has a rich sense of humor that she has passed on to her daughter. Walking down the hall, you can hear them laughing and talking. The physical therapist and nurse see the use of humor and playful attitude as positive coping strategies in this family and build upon them. This strengthens their working relationships and creates an environment in which the patient can talk about serious concerns with people who understand her.

To teach humor as a coping strategy, consider children's books. An especially useful book is *The Jester Has Lost His Jingle* (Saltzman, 1995). This book was written and illustrated by a young man who died of Hodgkin's disease at 23 years of age. His mother published the book and donates copies to children's hospitals.

A hospice client using the expressive arts for life review, meaning making, and legacy worked with the process of making collages for each of the five decades of his life. He was a social worker who worked with troubled youth. His dream was to be able to share lessons learned from this work. We worked with collage words to summarize concepts in several long articles he had been unable to get published. When we put these words together, they became poems. Below, as a tribute to him, is one of these poems that illustrates his values, which include laughter and whimsy. He died shortly after the completion of his legacy work.

On Dealing with Cancer
Simple solutions?
Be Thankful

Do you see emptiness
Or possibilities?
Making peace with the process . . .
Are you ready?

The moments you live for,
Uncertain,
Living the dream . . .
No kid was born bad

You're invited
to be delighted
Never give up your dream

Blessings
It's never too late
to learn
something new

Yes you can!
When opportunity knocks
Make sure you can hear it

Life is a ride
Dare to be extraordinary
Variety is the spice of life

Off the beaten track
Belly laughs
Shades of whimsy
Love in bloom

By Roger Skinner, MSW/LCSW, July 2009; used with permission and in hope of making a difference in your life

Humor Strategies

WIT&*Wisdom*

The word "silly" comes from the Greek word *selig*, meaning "blessed." Perhaps there is something sacred in being silly.

Try Gentle Banter

"A light touch may be the right touch" (Green, 1994). Humor provides comic relief from tension and worry. For example:

A client rushing onto a gynecology unit for an early morning admission was greeted by a nurse who said, "Congratulations! You win. You're the first one here." The client laughed and talked about how "wild" her morning had been trying to get there on time.

A client was wearing a large fabric protective shoe after foot surgery. One nurse said, "I hope you got that in some glamorous way . . . maybe skiing in Aspen?" The client laughed and shared her story.

A home health nurse reported working with an elderly couple while giving insulin injections to the wife. They had a running joke about how the client could make healthy food choices at the fast-food restaurant the couple went to each day. When the nurse would leave she would tell the wife, "No sausage biscuit today, OK?" They shared many good laughs over this. The nurse talked with pride about this couple's mobility well into their 80s. She used humor to try to teach, yet recognized that these trips to the restaurant were the highlight of this couple's days.

Let Humor Take the Lead

To Green (1994), letting humor take the lead is the "art of putting things lightly." Observe what is happening to your clients and see how you can add a light touch. Try using the "good news, bad news" approach.

The bad news is you have to leave your room for a test. The good news is we can have a fascinating conversation on the way.

Green offers some examples of putting things lightly:

The doctor says, "Well, Mr. Saunders, you'll be able to resume your normal activities soon, but you may not be able to play shortstop for the Detroit Tigers this season."

"This injection will make you feel like a kid again—getting your first bee sting."

Being able to laugh at yourself may provide some great material. Consider all those embarrassing moments that you can use to make a real connection with a client. A hospital chaplain relates the story of another chaplain new to the hospital who was shy about approaching clients for fear of disturbing them. One day, after trying to visit a client several times, the chaplain entered the room, tripped, grabbed onto the curtains to keep from falling, swung widely, and landed face down in the bed beside the client. The chaplain looked up and said, "This certainly is an icebreaker, isn't it?" The client laughed and was able to initiate a conversation about her own discomfort at being in the hospital and how hard it was for her to talk; this was the beginning of a very human relationship!

> *There is nothing left to say at this moment but to have a good laugh.*
> **Zen master**
>
> **WIT&** *Wisdom*

Look for the Positive

Take the initiative to encourage a positive attitude. Ask your client, "Do you have joy in your life?" (Smith, 2000). Ask, "What brings joy to your life?" or "What do you do for fun?" Ask your clients what is going well for them today. Share your own positive moments.

"I saw the first rose in my garden today."

"My grandson is visiting and watched me shave this morning. His father uses an electric razor, and my grandson asked, 'Grandpa, why do you put whipped cream on your face?'" (Green, 1994).

"There was a rainbow after the storm today."

"I saw a hot air balloon on my way to work this morning."

Encourage clients and staff to share their own stories. Listening for clues about your clients' interests suggests positive conversation ideas. Asking about children or grandchildren may be well received, too.

Be Creative

Each of us has different talents. Often we separate our personal selves from our professional selves. Consider people who love and raise animals. One director of a human resource department brought his eight Dalmatian puppies to work one day for a visit. Never has staff from that department been so united in their delight on any one subject! One home health agency was forced to require a family to contain its dog before a home visit, because the nurse had once been bitten and was afraid of dogs. The family sent the dog to obedience school and mailed the diploma to the agency. Grateful, the nurse delivered a bone as a graduation present for the dog.

Staff and volunteers who are clowns can share their talents by visiting pediatric or geriatric facilities. Staff who play musical instruments or sing can perform for other staff members on special occasions.

One hospital has a plant-filled atrium in its central hall. The maintenance staff in plant facilities keep a large rubber lizard among the plants and reposition him frequently. He gets a bow for special occasions. This little bit of humor provides visible relief for people who linger a moment to see something of beauty in a hospital.

To contribute to the morale of staff and clients, consider how you can use your own talents and ideas to add a little joy to your workplace (Box 15-3). Box 15-4 lists strategies cited by nurses for using humor, joy, and play to build positive communication.

Use Toys and Props

A humor kit in a colorful basket can be useful to add a light touch. A clown doll that laughs can be used when staff is tense. Wearing a clown nose adds a bit of comic relief.

Green (1994) shares the story of wearing funny glasses while visiting her father in the hospital. He loved them and used them to greet his physicians. Some hospitals have humor carts or humor rooms equipped with items to pass the time or get a good laugh. Table 15-1 gives suggestions for building your own humor kit.

Ways in Which Humor Promotes Positive Communication

Humor works in three ways:

1. *Prevention*: Using humor strategies before a crisis occurs in a work environment makes staff more willing to work together when tension is great. Have a baby picture contest for staff. Provide a

---

WIT&*Wisdom*

Laughter

A formed, formless
sound of joy.
The ripple
of a bubbling brook.
The sight of a child
at play.
A task done . . .
near perfectly.
A beautiful thought.
A new idea.
Laughter
is the clean freshness
of pine trees . . .
the ghostly echoes
Of invisible feet
touching
the quiet places
on the forest's floor.
Laughter
is a worldly life
accepted . . .
of an inner peace
given a quiet soul.

Copyright © Howard G. Kirkman. Used with permission.

Box 15-3 | *Get Creative*

- Celebrate holidays; decorate your unit or office. One intensive care unit staff hung handmade paper snowflakes from the ceiling at Christmas.
- Enlarge and post cartoons on the ceiling over examining tables or on walls in examining rooms.
- Use cartoons or funny clip art in client teaching materials or newsletters.
- Give stickers to adults and children after a procedure. The stickers given when people donate blood are popular.
- Blow up a glove and draw a funny face on it to make an instant balloon to cheer a child.
- Use crafts. One examining table has crocheted "booties" on the stirrups. Wear holiday accessories, a crocheted pumpkin pin, festive earrings.

Box 15-4   *Humor Strategies*

Following are ideas collected from nurses at various humor workshops:
- Put cartoons on bulletin boards.
- Collect cartoons in a photo album and share the book with patients as needed.
- Sing at holidays, for clients' birthdays, or whenever the mood strikes.
- Wear a funny hat on Halloween (full costume may be inappropriate).
- Share jokes.
- Use funny coffee mugs and give them as gifts.
- Provide a tiara for the birthday person at a staff party.
- Stage silly puppet shows.
- Use light banter (e.g., when strapping a client onto a stretcher, say, "Time to fasten your seat belt!").
- Use pet therapy.
- Keep Silly Putty or Koosh balls on hand for tension relief.
- Blow bubbles.
- Keep the television tuned to comedy shows.
- Play humorous audiotapes.
- Stage theme days for dress (e.g., Western Day).
- Wear a clown nose.
- Smile!
- Keep a positive attitude.

Table 15-1   *Building and Using Your Humor Kit*

SUPPLIES	USES
Magic wand	"ABRACADABRA . . . now you will have a better day." At a health fair with long lines, try "ABRACADABRA, you'll be finished soon!"
Whistles	Blow to start off an in-service or staff meeting to grab the attention of attendees and inspire creativity
Bubbles	Use to lighten up a tough time
Joke books	Lend to amuse a discouraged client
Koosh ball	Toss around to aid in brainstorming session or just to get a smile
Games such as cards, checkers, and chess	Offer these to clients to help pass the time
Clown nose	Carry for emergencies

These items can be used with patients and staff. Let your imagination, a bit of whimsy, and your good judgment be your guide!

candy jar labeled "Grump Beans" for a grumpy day. Get involved in a community project in which people can work together in an informal setting. Organize a community project for colleagues that could be done in conjunction with the traditional Christmas party.

2. *Perception*: Injecting humor into a situation changes the perception that the situation is so terrible that it cannot be handled. Keep a magic wand at the desk. When the pace is hectic, grab the wand and make a promise that the end of the day is in sight!

3. *Perspective*: Humor helps us to keep the big picture in view and not to take ourselves too seriously. Make light of your own idiosyncrasies. Get people to laugh with you (Riley, 2004a).

Consider that "humor endears the person who is engaged in it to others; such an individual can enjoy a sense of the outrageous as well as the sublime. The ability to play defuses anger, disarms grief. . . . Mirth often derives from a joint recognition of the ridiculousness of life" (Van Wormer and Boes, 1997, p. 87).

Comic Vision: Humor and Play and Creativity

Being able to keep your perspective, to play with problems, can lead to creative solutions. Pink (2005) delineates six skills or abilities to help us thrive in the changing work world, where he says we are moving from the Information Age to the Conceptual Age. Play, cultivating humor and valuing laughter, is one of these six skills. In the Conceptual Age, we will apply "R-directed," right brain thinking to "bring unconventional thought, emotional meaning, and aesthetic style to interactions, programs, and product design" (Carlson, 2005). Carlson suggests that nurses have already evolved to the Conceptual Age. Several other skill sets he delineates that inform this conclusion are empathy, caring, and imaging the world as it seems to another; story, understanding, communication, and self-knowledge; and meaning, spiritual fulfillment, beyond the material and financial (Carlson, 2005; Pink, 2005).

Pink (2005) writes that play is important in our work and personal lives, manifesting itself in games, humor, and joyfulness. Fifty percent of all Americans over 6 years of age play computer and video games and evidence supports that they enhance the right brain's ability to use pattern recognition in problem solving. The use of such gaming is found in the military and in healthcare. A game called GlucoBoy used with Nintendo's Game Boy can help children with diabetes monitor their glucose levels. Video games are being used to treat phobias and anxiety disorders with virtual reality technology.

Play is diversion. Consider the process of studying for an examination or writing a paper. Try building in a plan to take a playful break to clear your mind and make your study and writing more efficient. A student vowed to study "all weekend" for an anatomy test, but found that she wasted time with so much time allowed. When she scheduled a designated time for study with the reward of seeing a movie for a break, she found she returned to study with more efficiency.

Humor is a part of play and taps the right brain's ability to put situations in context, to see a big picture, and to explore new ways of looking at problems. Humor is a part of the emotional intelligence needed for a whole-mind worker. Humor can help clarify a situation in a team meeting. It can contribute to cohesion, decrease hostility, and improve morale. Brainstorming can often take a silly turn when off-the-wall ideas are introduced, but not censoring any ideas can promote creativity. Consider the 3M sticky notes we use for reminders and how they might have been invented.

> There is no question that a playfully light attitude is characteristic of creative individuals.
>
> **Mihalyi Csikszentmihalyi**
>
> WIT&*Wisdom*

Humor and play help develop your comic vision, the ability to bring perspective and not take oneself so seriously. See Box 15-5 for strategies to develop your comic vision.

Box 15-5	*Strategies to Develop Your Comic Vision*

1. Start with yourself. Laugh at yourself. Give yourself permission to be human. If you trip, laugh out loud.
2. Read the comics and political cartoons in newspapers as examples of comic vision. Look at local newspapers when you travel to get the community perspective and learn about regional humor.
3. Start an album with cartoons that track current work issues and encourage all team members to contribute.
4. Attend funny movies and comedy clubs. Rent classic comedy videos.
5. Listen to humorous CDs on the way to work to begin your day looking for humor.
6. Collect humorous one-liners that are "inside" jokes with your work team.
7. Laugh with others for what they do, at the incongruities in life in which we all share.
8. Pay attention to your own self-talk. Replace negative thoughts with positive ones. Focus on being someone others find pleasant company.
9. Ask yourself, "Does anyone look forward to seeing me walk down the hall toward them?"
10. Share your comic vision to make other people laugh. Laughter is CONTAGIOUS and adds much needed joy in all our lives.

The Healing Power of Laughter

Think about how good it feels to laugh. Consider a time when you just cannot stop laughing, perhaps, in a greeting card shop when one card after another evokes more laughter. Gelotology is the study of the physiology of laughter. Dr William Fry is known for his research in this field and acknowledges that there is evidence of the usefulness of laughter in wellness but that there is much work to be done (Bennet et al, 2003). These studies suggest that laughter may produce:

- Stimulation of the production of catecholamines and hormones that enhance feelings of well-being and pain tolerance
- Decrease in anxiety
- Increase in cardiac and respiratory rates
- Enhancement of metabolism

- Improvement of muscle tone
- Perception of the relief of stress and tension with increased relaxation, which may last up to 45 minutes following laughter
- Increased numbers of NK (natural killer) cells that fight viral infections of cell and some cancer cells
- Increased T cells (T lymphocytes) that fight infection
- Increased antibody IgA (immunoglobulin A) that fights upper respiratory infections
- Increased gamma interferon, which helps activate the immune system (Riley, 2004b)

Dr. Madan Kataria, a physician in Mumbai, India, created World Laughter Clubs and teaches exercises to create laughter that are practiced regularly by these groups. Over 2500 of these clubs exist internationally. Steve Wilson at http://www.worldlaughtertour.com certifies laughter trainers. Bayfront Medical Center, a trauma center in St. Petersburg, Florida, hosts facilitator training. Kataria's purpose with these clubs is to help people be more playful and more creative.

Consider different aspects of humor that are effective coping strategies, such as reframing negatives into positives, optimism, and hope. Research demonstrates that a belief in the benefits of laughter is sufficient for the body to experience positive benefits (Wilkins and Eisenbraun, 2009).

Humor in Healthcare Education

Humor can create a climate of trust in the classroom and can engage the learner in the process of learning. A smile and a sense of humor can help in client education. We can laugh at our own mistakes and help students and clients to address their own mistakes. A humorous name for a client in a case study on an examination might elicit a smile, a deep breath, and decrease of anxiety at test time. The addition of humor into mandatory training in a healthcare setting would be welcome (Box 15-6).

He Who Laughs, Lasts

The first step along the journey is to smile a little, then a little more, then laugh, then laugh a little more (Feeg, 2002). R. Dale Leichty (1987) delivered

Box 15-6	*Humor Goes to School*

- Design games to review medical terminology. "The Gastric Voyage" . . . burp . . . go back two spaces. Use a television game show format such as Jeopardy.
- In fire safety classes, distribute Fire Ball candy. Play songs with the word fire in them. Dress as a firefighter. In electrical safety training, try a tombstone with the words, "She was the ground."
- To limit negative comments, take a roll of pennies to class. Give each person two pennies. A student may make a negative comment but must pay 1 cent each time. When they have put their "2 cents' worth" in, they cannot complain again.
- When teaching a controversial topic, put a bull's-eye on your chest or wear a construction hard hat to break the ice.
- Begin the class with something funny so participants know it is safe to laugh.
- Make a list of quotes by funny people and add quotes frequently used by participants.
- Slip in unknown abbreviations. TSWNE is "this shift will never end." RP is a "real person."

Ideas compiled from the Carolina Society of Health Education and Training conference, Myrtle Beach, SC, March 26, 1998, conducted by the author.

an address, "Humor and the Surgeon," in which he concluded:

> Humor is an innate but fragile part of human life . . . and this scary world can sometimes erode it. To hold on to this gift of laughter, we must develop two faculties. The first is perspective, knowing that we exist somewhere between the tiniest and the infinite mysteries. Perspective is indeed the secret of philosophy. The second is a humorous outlook . . . that senses "the world is mad" . . . but also understands that human vanities and pretenses have made it that way. It tells us, from time to time at least, to stand back and smile or laugh at them.

Life must be lived as play.

Plato

WIT&*Wisdom*

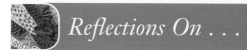

Reflections On . . .

Humor

Consider what you read about the use of humor and how you already use humor. Can you comfortably add humor to your skills for relating to clients and colleagues?

What? . . .

Write one thing you learned from this chapter.

So what? . . .

How will this affect your nursing practice?

Now what? . . .

How will you implement this new knowledge or skill?

Think about it . . .

Practicing Humor

Exercise 1

"An average 6-year-old child laughs 300 times each day" (How in the World, 1998). How often does a typical adult laugh?

What is your guess?

Answer: 15 to 1000 times per day (How in the World, 1998).

Discuss your ideas about these statistics.

Exercise 2

Write five things that make you laugh.

Exercise 3

In a small group, make a group list of 20 things to do just for real FUN! Now, contract to do one fun thing within 2 weeks from this day. Complete the following: I, promise to by (2 weeks from today) _____.

Exercise 4

Recall an incident in which you were the recipient of negative humor. Describe how you felt.

Exercise 5

Identify someone with a rich, positive sense of humor. Describe how you feel when you are with this person.

Exercise 6

For this exercise, work with a small group of students. Each student is to briefly interview a nurse who uses humor in a positive way in the clinical setting. Ask for examples of situations in which humor worked with a client. Compare the results of these interviews, compile a list of interventions, and share these with the class.

Exercise 7

Bring the comic strips from several newspapers to class. Share your favorites and discuss what is funny. Comment about why certain individual comics are funny and compare your favorite comic strips to see differences in humor styles.

Exercise 8

Read the following poem and discuss humor in coping with illness and disability:

Thorny Path to Sanity

Hospital walls
Enclosing hospital walls
that echo the sounds of the living
and the dying.
Whispering feet echoing
whispering thoughts and actions,
both covert and overt.
Within this sick prison
lie tales of the honorable,
And the dis-honorable.
Through this mysterious, noisy,
noiseless river of human sluff,
an observant, and absorbing mind
has swam and soaked up the good
and the bad . . .
and it has been a bountiful harvest
of both . . .
Never quite
wholly defeated
by the fears
the tears

Continued

the unholy size
and depth
of this smothering grave
that continually threatened to bury me.
Too dumb . . .
or too stubborn
to ever finally learn,
or admit,
that there was not
some tiny light
somewhere, somehow,
that would inject courage
and a kind of hopeless hope
into my living.
I somehow
developed a sense of humor
that enabled me . . . to survive.
Survive, that is
with some semblance
of sanity and
relatively leeched free
of bitterness.
Who can really say
that this is necessarily good . . .
or completely bad . . . ?

Copyright © Howard G. Kirkman. Used with permission.

Moments of Connection . . .
A Touch of Magic

A nurse received a magic wand at a workshop given by the author. She wrote to tell a story of its use. When visiting a friend who had just had a mastectomy, she took her several gifts, including the magic wand. The friend inquired about the use of the wand and the nurse replied it was so she would always have a nurse when necessary. About this time, the door to the room opened and in came a nurse asking if the client needed anything. The friends looked at each other and burst into laughter. Later, the door opened and another nurse entered asking if the client had called. Now they were true believers. As they talked, the friend was able to share her fears and joked that the surgeon had also taken a few nips and tucks for figure improvement. The wand had been an icebreaker, and laughing together had set the stage for comfort in sharing concerns.

From Riley JB, From the heart to the hands: keys to successful healthcaring connections, *Integrated Management and Publishing Systems*, Ellicott City, Md, 1999.

References

Adamle KN, Ludwick R, Zeller R, et al: Oncology nurses' responses to patient-initiated humor, *Cancer Nurs* 31(6):E1, 2008.

American Association of Colleges of Nursing and City of Hope National Medical Center: Module 6, Communication. In: *The-End-of-Life Nursing Education Consortium (ELNEC) faculty guide*, Duarte, Calif, 2000, The Medical Center.

Association for Applied and Therapeutic Humor: *Official definition of therapeutic humor* (website). http://www.aath.org/. Accessed January 29, 2011.

Astedt-Kurki P, Isola A: Humour between nurse and patient, and among staff: analysis of nurses' diaries, *J Adv Nurs* 35(3):452, 2001.

Bakerman H: Nursing humor: a perspective, *Therap Humor* 12(3):6, 1998.

Beck CT: Humor in nursing practice: a phenomenological study, *Int J Nurs Stud* 34(5):346, 1997.

Bennet MP, Zeller JM, Rosenberg L, et al: The effect of laughter on stress and natural killer cell activity, *Altern Therap Health Care* 9(2):38, 2003.

Burkhardt MA, Nagai-Jacobson MG: *Spirituality: living our connectedness*, Albany, 2002, Delmar/Thomson Learning.

Cansler College: *Laughter is the best medicine* (website). http://www.sciencedaily.com/releases/2008/01/080124200913.htm. Accessed June 2011.

Carlson K: A red hat and a new mind, *J Perianesth Nurs* 20(6):453, 2005.

Craig K: Hitch up your humor suspenders, case managers, *Prof Case Manage* 14(1):18, 2009.

Dean RAK, Major JE: From critical care to comfort care: the sustaining value of humour, *J Clin Nurs* 17(8):1088, 2008.

Dowling JS: Humor: a coping strategy for pediatric patients, *Pediatr Nurs* 28(2):123, 2002.

Feeg VD: Laugh a little—it might help, *Pediatr Nurs* 28(2):92, 2002.

Fonnesbeck BG: Are you kidding? *Nursing 98* 28(3):64, 1998.

Forssen AS: Humour, beauty, and culture as personal health resources: experiences of elderly Swedish women, *Scand J Public Health* 35(3):228, 2007.

Fry WF Jr, Salameh WA, editors: *Handbook of humor and psychotherapy: advances in the clinical use of humor*, Sarasota, Fla, 1987, Professional Resource Exchange.

Geanellos R: Sustaining well-being and enabling recovery: the therapeutic effect of nurse friendliness on clients and nursing environments, *Contemp Nurse* 19(1–2):242, 2005.

Green L: *Making sense of humor: how to add joy to your life*, Manchester, Conn, 1994, Knowledge, Ideas, and Trends.

How in the World, *USA Today*, July 29, 1998. B-1.

Kipplinger B: Humor in psychotherapy: a shift to a new perspective. In Fry WF Jr, Salameh WA, editors: *Handbook of humor and psychotherapy: advances in the clinical use of humor*, Sarasota, 1987, Professional Resource Exchange.

Koff-Chapin D: *The Center for Touch Drawings: resources for creative awakening, 2002* (website). http://www.TouchDrawing.com. Accessed October 25, 2002.

Leiber DB: Laughter and humor in critical care, *Dimens Crit Care* 5(3):162, 1986.

Leichty RD: Humor and the surgeon, *Arch Surg* 122(5):519, 1987.

Lotzar M, Bottorff JL: An observational study of the development of a nurse–patient relationship, *Clin Nurs Res* 10(3):275, 2001.

McGhee P: RX: laughter, *RN* 28(7):50, 1998.

McGhee PE: *Humor and children's development*, New York, 1989, Haworth Press.

Pink DH: *A whole new mind: moving from the information age to the conceptual age*, New York, 2005, Riverhead Books.

Riley JB: *Humor at work*, Ellenton, Fl, 2004, Constant Source Press.

Riley JB: Taking life lightly: humor, the great alternative. In Eliopoulos C, editor: *Invitation to holistic health: a guide to living a balanced life*, Sudbury, Mass, 2004, Jones and Bartlett Publishers.

Robinson VM: *Humor and the health professions*, Thorofare, NJ, 1990, Charles B. Slack.

Saltzman D: *The jester has lost his jingle*, Palos Verdes Estates, Calif, 1995, The Jester Co.

Samuels M, Lane MR: *Creative healing: how to heal yourself by tapping your hidden creativity*, San Francisco, 1998, Harper San Francisco.

Simon JM: Therapeutic humor: who's fooling who?, *J Psychosoc Nurs* 26(4):9, 1988.

Smith KL: Humor as a clinical skill: are you joking?, *Urol Nurs* 20(6):382, 2000.

Starr C: Lighten up!!, *Am J Nurs* 109(2):72AA, 2009.

Ufema J: Communication: lighten our souls (Insights on Death and Dying column), *Nursing* 32(4):28, 2002.

Van Wormer K, Boes M: Humor in the emergency room: a social work perspective, *Health Soc Work* 22(2):87, 1987.

Watson J: *Nursing: human science and human care: a theory of nursing*, Boston, 1993, Jones and Bartlett.

Wilkins J, Eisenbraun AJ: Humor theories and the physiological benefits of laughter, *Holist Nurs Pract* 23(6):349, 2009.

Resources on Therapeutic Humor

Association for Applied and Therapeutic Humor: Website at http://www.aath.org. Membership includes a newsletter and bibliographies.

The Humor Project at http://www.humorproject.com

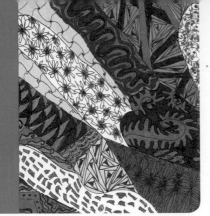

Chapter 16

Spirituality

Objectives

1. Discuss themes of spirituality
2. Examine the FICA (Faith and Belief: Importance, Community, and Address in Care) tool for taking a spiritual history
3. Discuss strategies to nurture the spirit
4. Identify nursing interventions to meet the spiritual needs of the client and family
5. Describe behaviors that the nurse can use to adopt a hopeful perspective and offer hope
6. Review a spiritual assessment tool for use in a clinical setting
7. Discuss the role of the nurse in helping the client find meaning in illness
8. Participate in exercises to build skills in meeting spiritual needs in health

Definition of Spirituality

Spirituality comes from a Latin word meaning "breath of life" (Brillhart, 2005, p. 31). The concept of spirituality is elusive because it is "heart" language not "head" language and is hard to put into words (Carson and Koenig, 2008). Donnelly and Cook (1989) reflect that "to be spiritual is to be connected—to the inner self, to others, or to a transcendent being or energy." Spirituality in practice is "to demonstrate a unique capacity for love, joy, caring, compassion, and for finding meaning in life's difficult experience." Nurses' spiritual interventions "reflect the human traits of caring, love, honesty, wisdom, and imagination . . . a belief in a higher power, higher existence, or a guiding spirit . . . something outside the self and beyond the individual nurse or patient" (Dossey, 1998b, p. 47). Spirituality includes "unconditional love, trust, forgiveness, hope, and imagination . . . a sense of awe and wonder regarding life" (Brillhart, 2005, p. 31). In a study measuring the attributes of caring relationships created by nurse practitioners, spiritual expression proved to be a significant factor (Thomas et al, 2004). The use of a spiritually based complementary group intervention with U.S. combat veterans experiencing symptoms of posttraumatic stress disorder (PTSD) from the wars in Iraq and Afghanistan showed promising results (Bormann et al, 2008).

> Spirituality is good science . . . Over 250 studies now show that religious practice—the specific religion doesn't seem to matter—is correlated with greater health and increased longevity . . . some say that clinicians have no business taking on the role of spiritual guide . . . but we are not being asked to become spiritual counselors. We're being asked to integrate a holistic approach and extend love, compassion, and empathy . . . the bedrock upon which nursing has always rested. (Dossey, 1998a, p. 37)

Harold Koenig, MD, at Duke University's Center for the Study of Religion/Spirituality and Health, reports on the results of over 70 data-based, peer-reviewed published papers. Findings show that people who attend religious services on a regular basis have better health outcomes, have stronger immune systems, have lower stress, and recover from hip fractures and open-heart surgeries more quickly than do less religious people. Elders with religious faith seem to be better protected from cardiovascular disease and cancer (Koenig, 1999). Spirituality has been shown to be an important variable in quality of life in persons living with human immunodeficiency virus infection (Tuck et al, 2001). In a study of persons with spinal cord injury, life satisfaction increased as spirituality increased (Brillhart, 2005). Exploring meaning in life and prayer has been associated with increased psychological well-being in breast cancer survivors (Meraviglia, 2006). Spirituality has been part of the vision of nursing since the time of Florence Nightingale (Calabria and Macrae, 1994). From his continued review of the literature and research, Koenig concludes: "Addressing spiritual issues in clinical practice can bring back life into our profession and, for many of our patients, can help them regain their lives by finding hope, meaning, and healing" (2007, p. 232). The goal of practicing spiritually sensitive care is to support clients in the search for meaning and solace without injecting our own opinions or values (Lackey, 2009).

Erickson and colleagues (1983) believe that human beings are holistic with multiple interacting subsystems. "Permeating all subsystems are the inherent bases . . . which include the genetic and spiritual drive" (p. 44). Our "spiritual drive starts before our biophysical existence, continues through our lifetime, and culminates during transformation. It is always present, and pervades our subsystems even though we may not be consciously aware of it. It inspires us to search for our Life Purpose" (Erickson, 2006, p. 8). As nurses, every interaction we share with our clients allows us to nurture and facilitate the client's spiritual essence and drive. Through this sharing of experiences, moments, and events the nurse and client journey together to gain a better understanding of and to work toward their Life Purpose or Reason for Being (Erickson, 2006, p. 8).

In this chapter, we will explore the concept of spirituality, a notion that may be feared or ignored by healthcare professionals, perhaps because it reminds us of the fallibility of science in healing (Donnelly and Cook, 1989). It is this spiritual connection that is the essence of being present with clients in moments of tragedy where the seeds of personal triumph are planted. This discussion is not based on religious denomination but on the spiritual path to finding personal meaning and to helping the patient and family find meaning in illness and suffering (Travelbee, 1970). This chapter helps you recognize opportunities to introduce clients and families to the idea that we learn lessons from life's difficulties and that we find meaning in life by sharing these life lessons as part of our legacy.

Themes of Spirituality

Nagai-Jacobson and Burkhardt (1989) review general themes that emerge in the literature that broaden the concept of spirituality. They found that spirituality has the following characteristics:

- It is a broader concept than religion.
- It involves a personal quest for meaning and purpose in life.
- It relates to the inner essence of a person.
- It is a sense of harmonious interconnectedness with self, others, nature, and an Ultimate Other.
- It is the integrating factor of the human person.

Discussions of spirituality in nursing suggest that interactions between nurses and their clients involve the spirituality of both and that this relationship can transform them all in the search for a meaning in life. The nature of such client–nurse relationships is sacred. It is a walk on holy ground as two people meet at what Newman (1989) calls choice points presented by health crises. These choice points or events are "opportunities to experience more fully the reality of the patterns of our lives." These are times when former ways of coping and relating to life no longer work. When a person is confronted with disability, new ways of existing, of behaving, and of finding meaning are necessary. A woman whose husband was experiencing the deterioration of Alzheimer's disease, for example, found her own health affected by the strain of being a caregiver. Unable to drive or visit with friends, she befriended a wild, stray cat who was reluctant to make physical contact. Over time, the mother cat brought her kittens to the woman. Feeding these kittens and playing with them gave this woman's life a purpose and some joy in the midst of the suffering she was sharing with her husband. "God sent me this cat," she said. "We needed each other." She slowed down and stayed focused in the present.

A qualitative research study of opportunities for enhanced spirituality in well adults revealed six themes: connectedness, relationships with "self, others, nature, the universe, or a higher power"; beliefs, such as a belief in God or in good versus bad; inner motivating factors, guides for behavior and attitude; divine providence, belief in a higher power; understanding the Mystery, looking for meaning and purpose in life; and walking through, using our inner resources on life's journey (Cavendish et al, 2000). The researchers concluded that nurses need to be more aware of the significance of life events in clients' lives to make accurate nursing diagnoses and to intervene in meaningful ways. Support of clients' coping strategies, inner resources, and beliefs, and an understanding of spirituality that allows nurses to foster even small changes in the spiritual aspect of their clients' lives, can have a significant impact (Cavendish et al, 2000).

FICA—Taking a Spiritual History

A documented spiritual history is mandated by The Joint Commission (TJC) for clients who are admitted for care in an acute care hospital or nursing home and those seen through a home health agency (Koenig, 2007). Beginning this conversation opens a dialogue about spiritual issues and gives the client permission to talk about spirituality with you (Koenig, 2007).

The acronym FICA stands for Faith and Belief: Importance, Community, and Address in Care, a tool developed by Christina M. Puchalski, MD, founder and director of the George Washington Institute for Spirituality and Health (Box 16-1). This brief tool is a good way to begin to incorporate spiritual assessment in your work. A more detailed assessment can be found later in this chapter (see Box 16-7).

Before beginning this history taking, it is helpful to explain why you are asking these questions. Clients may find the conversation anxiety producing because they expect it might mean that they are facing a terminal diagnosis. Simply say the questions you will ask are to be more sensitive to any spiritual needs a client may have.

The Essence of the Spiritual History

A single question concerning spiritual history can be, "Do you have any spiritual needs or concerns related to your health?" Sometimes the initiation of even this

---

Box 16-1   *FICA—Taking a Spiritual History*

F—FAITH AND BELIEF

"Do you consider yourself spiritual or religious?" or "Do you have spiritual beliefs that help you cope with stress?" If the patient responds "No," the nurse might ask, "What gives your life meaning?" Sometimes patients give answers such as family, career, or nature.

I—IMPORTANCE

"What importance does your faith or belief have in your life? Have your beliefs influenced how you take care of yourself in this illness/situation? What role do your beliefs play in regaining your health?"

C—COMMUNITY

"Are you part of a spiritual or religious or faith community? Is this of support to you, and if so, how? Is there a group of people you really love or who are important to you?" Communities such as churches, temples, and mosques or a group of like-minded friends can serve as strong support systems for some clients.

A—ADDRESS IN CARE

"How would you like me, your nurse, to address these issues in your healthcare?"

Copyright © Christina M. Puchalski, MD, founder and director of the George Washington Institute for Spirituality and Health.

---

short history is met with the response that the client has no interest in religion or spirituality and does not use these for coping with illness. At this point, you can take a different tack and ask about other ways the client is coping—what gives meaning and purpose in the face of illness, what social supports are useful, and what cultural beliefs may influence the treatment of illness. This gets at the essence of the spiritual history (Koenig, 2007, pp. 44–45).

Knowing that in times of crisis clients may feel at a loss for coping strategies, ask if the client has ever been in a similar situation and, if so, what was helpful then—what has been a source of strength for you and who have you talked to in the past that has been helpful to you? Such questions may stimulate problem solving about what might be helpful at this time.

The Nurse as a Spiritual Person and Caregiver

Life is a journey. Peck (1998) suggests that we must appreciate the fact that life is complex. This means to "abandon the urge to simplify everything, to look for easy answers, and to begin to think multi-dimensionally, to stay in the mystery and paradoxes of life." Those who would simplify nursing practice would teach students how to do "things"—treatments, techniques, procedures. How easy it would be if the quality of nursing care could be quantified by how accurately or quickly procedures could be performed. Consider that "the essence of nursing is not doing . . . but being open to whatever arises in the interaction with the client. It is being fully present with an unconditional acceptance of the client's experience" (Newman, 1989). Perhaps we can think of life not as a series of problems to be solved but rather as a mystery to unravel.

To facilitate your clients' growth and coping, you must be open to your own life experiences, continue on your own journey to make sense of life, and nurture your own spirit. Your own unmet needs can get in the way of being able to be fully present with your clients and their families.

Spiritual Care Begins with the Nurse

To be a nurse is to be given a sacred trust. Clients and families come to us fearfully in their darkest hours, in the face of their own mortality, or, at the time of childbirth, in the face of the wonder of creation. Burkhardt and Nagai-Jacobson (1994) speak of a "reawakening spirit in nursing practice." To have the ability to stay connected to the experience of another, you must pay attention to nurturing your own spirit. Moore (1998) speaks of living artfully as a necessity for the care of the soul or spirit. To do so, he suggests the following:

- Pause—the opposite of being busy—stop, reflect, savor the moment, experience wonder at the things around you, be still.
- Take time for self, people, relationships, and things— living creatures, too! To take time for relationships, even difficult ones, deepens our understanding and appreciation.
- Be mindful of, or pay attention to, what is happening all around you so that you recognize the need to stop and focus on this moment rather than thinking about the past or the future.

But how can you slow down, considering the demands of nursing? Other chapters in this volume address methods such as relaxation techniques and meditation. Practicing these techniques helps you to be in touch with your own spirit and helps you to be centered. The process of centering helps you focus on this moment. Remember the value of rest, of time to do nothing, and of playful leisure time. Focusing on the moment can mean slowing down to really enjoy the taste and texture and smells of the food you eat, taking time to stroke the fur of a cat or dog, listening to the sound of birds singing, enjoying music rather than using it for background noise, stroking the hair of a child, listening to another person without offering an opinion, hugging a friend, and listening to laughter and joining in. In a series of community classes for cancer patients and their families, one man said that cancer had changed his focus from "working for a living to the art of living." These simple suggestions are mindful activities. They are what clients tell us they do to stay connected to life in tough times. For them, these are the things that make life worthwhile. Nurses reported spiritual renewal practicing mindfulness and other spiritual self-care processes such as meditation, time in nature, yoga, and music in retreats as part of a study to support nurses' spirituality (Bay et al, 2010). Perhaps such activities can replenish your energy to do your life's work.

Communication is more than verbal and nonverbal behavior. The ability to stay present in the moment requires conscious effort, which is sometimes a struggle. When you feel overwhelmed, take time to return to being still and paying attention to the gifts of the senses. When you are frightened, remember the lyrics, "when you are troubled and cannot sleep. Just count your blessings instead of sheep." Emmons (2007) discusses results of gratitude research. Study participants who kept a weekly gratitude journal exercised with more regularity, had fewer physical complaints, felt better about their lives, and were more optimistic than the control group who kept journals about neutral events. Participants who kept a daily gratitude journal were more likely to offer emotional support to someone else. People who are grateful are more likely to believe in an interconnectedness of all life and demonstrate a commitment to others. Consider starting your own gratitude journal, writing a few words each day about the things for which you are grateful or just spend a few moments before you go to sleep to say thank you for the things for which you are grateful or for the people and things in your life that you appreciate.

Reflect on this mnemonic for fear when you are afraid and in spiritual distress. FEAR is:

F—Forgetting
E—that Everything
A—is All
R—Right

Offering simple strategies that work for you may be useful for your clients.

Meeting the Spiritual Needs of the Client

Spiritual care is not separate from all other aspects of nursing care. In Watson's conceptual model of nursing, spirituality is central. "The human spirit is regarded as the most powerful force in human existence and the source behind striving for self-transcendence through spiritual evolutions and the achievement of inner harmony. Nurses practicing within this framework promote harmony of body, mind, and spirit, regardless of the external health problem, age, or life circumstance of the person" (Touchy, 2001).

Caring in nursing requires intention, relationship, and actions (Touchy, 2001). Spiritual care is how you do what you do. It is an attitude, an openness, to the shared experience of the human condition. When you assist a patient with morning care, when you offer a bedpan or a urinal, when you take a temperature, when you bathe a person who has soiled himself—these ordinary tasks, when done mindfully, provide spiritual care. In a book on spiritual fulfillment in everyday life, Fields and colleagues (1984) talk about performing simple daily tasks as a way to get in touch with the natural cycles of life and death.

When searching for meaning, a client may have a need to explore spiritual and psychological issues and to talk about religious feelings or the lack of them. The client is not asking for advice or opinions but a time to talk about feelings and to express doubts, fears, and anguish. Even clients with strong religious beliefs may need encouragement in crisis. You can support a client with religious beliefs by encouraging prayer or meditation (Narayanasamy, 2004). Consider the role of spirituality, religion, and culture in healthcare beliefs. Participants in a study of spiritual practices in the self-management of diabetes in African Americans used prayer, reading the Bible, listening to Christian radio and television programs, church attendance, and

testimonies from people with diabetes (Casarez et al, 2010). Perhaps a selection of scripture, a morning prayer, or a testimony of success about the use of spiritual practices in making better food choices is a "nudge" to make better food choices or take a walk that day, ways to get us to think before we choose (Donnelly, 2010; Thaler and Sustein, 2008). Clients can be very vulnerable and not comfortable sharing sensitive information such as their belief system. It is important to respect the individual's freedom of choice about a personal belief system and not to try to persuade or encourage a patient to adopt your personal point of view (Buswell et al, 2006).

Spiritual needs may be greater during times of illness and a separation from routine comforting spiritual or religious practices can be a source of stress. The spiritual history and spiritual assessment may provide information that helps in mutual problem solving to find ways to meet these needs (Delgado, 2007).

Being Fully Present

The daily routine of nurses is not routine to clients. One reason it takes courage to be fully present with clients is that to be present is to understand their fear and pain. Words and procedures you will come to see as commonplace strike fear in the hearts of company presidents who find themselves in a setting they cannot control. Do not be fooled by clients who seem to be calm and confident. Assume that your clients and their families see you as a lifeline, and work from there.

"Spiritual care begins with presence. . . . In essence, the presence of love we bring to any situation is the basic way we integrate spirituality into care" (Burkhardt and Nagai-Jacobson, 2002). Presence is "a conscious act of being fully present—body, mind, emotions, and spirit—to another person" (McKivergin and Daubenmire, 1994). It is about how we do the things we do, who we are, and how we are with one another. Each moment is new. Each moment is different. In the chapter on empathy, you read about the highest level of empathy, in which you recognize the other's humanity and personhood regardless of the illness, its circumstance, or its stigma. You understand that we are all connected. Consider for a moment: can you view all of your work as sacred and feel that you are standing on holy ground day by day? (O'Brien, 1999). In the accompanying Moments of Connection, one nurse is fully present with a novice nurse and her client, sharing her own convictions. She responded "as whole being to whole being, using all of her . . . resources of body, mind, emotions, and spirit" (McKivergin and Daubenmire, 1994). This response was brief. Spiritual care does not take extra time. It is a part of all you do.

Offering Prayer

In a national study of more than 2000 Americans, about 75% of those responding report they pray to prevent illness and 22% report they pray to alleviate a medical condition with a high degree of perceived helpfulness (McCaffrey, 2004). Prayer "is an intimate conversation between us and God"; it is "an expression of spirit that is a fundamental way of connection with our inner self and the Sacred Source" (Burkhardt and Nagai-Jacobson, 2002); it is "an expression of the spirit . . . a deep human instinct that flows from the core of one's being where the longing for and awareness of one's connectedness with the source of life are blended . . . [and] represents a longed for communion or communication with God or the Absolute" (Dossey and Keegan, 2008). Prayer as a nursing intervention—praying with a client, praying aloud in the presence of a client, offering time of silence for prayer, fostering a supportive environment for prayer, or praying in your own quiet time—is based on an assessment of the spiritual needs of a client. Praying at the end of a time with a client or praying prematurely may be seen as dismissive, a way to escape after the content of an interaction has been emotional, of cutting off conversation (Bayfront Medical Center, 2002). Consider the use of prayer in the middle of a visit, which allows time for the client to respond emotionally to the prayer if appropriate. See the thoughts on prayer listed in Box 16-2.

Moments of Connection . . .
Where Can I Begin?

"The foundation began in my first year of nursing, at age 21, when an experienced nurse noticed my confusion and helplessness in dealing with a dying patient one evening. I didn't ask for help; I never did. The patient had no family present, so it really was up to me. This nurse took me into the room and said, 'Hello. We're with you. You are not alone.' She was speaking to the patient and to me. It was years before I finally believed what she said. By the grace of God, I know that we are never alone, and I can share this belief now with conviction."

Box 16-2	*Thoughts on Prayer*

Consider . . .
- Not everyone is receptive to or believes in prayer.
- Prayer traditions vary.
- Clients may offer cues that they are open to prayer by verbal references or the presence of inspirational or religious reading material or religious objects.
- Prayer may help the client with feelings of isolation.
- It is appropriate to ask the client if he or she would like a prayer and for what.
- Prayer can express what the clients would pray if they were able.
- Prayer may be a brief, simple statement of the client's hopes, fears, and needs and God's ability to be with the client in difficult times.
- Prayer for the greatest good for all involved is an inclusive prayer.
- Prayer allows for "intimacy without exposure."

Modified from *Pastoral care volunteer training manual: the use of prayer* St. Petersburg, FL, 2002, Bayfront Medical Center (handout).

Being Silent

Being still, being comfortable with silence, understanding that it is acceptable not to have answers—or even words—may come naturally to the introvert, a person who thinks to talk. For the extravert, a person who talks to think, such a realization may be growth. One therapist who is an extreme extravert said that the only way he could still his mind and his mouth was to learn to meditate. Yes, it is acceptable and even therapeutic to be quiet, just to be, not to do all the time. Thirty years ago, a nursing instructor said, "If you don't know what to say, just be quiet and stay there. Try saying, 'I don't have any words to help, but I will stay with you a while.'" These words are still good counsel.

A psychologist, when talking about her experience as a patient, said, "I want the nurse to understand that I am not myself when I am ill. I'm not the person I present to the outside world. I appreciate your understanding this and not judging me or my behavior. I don't want you to try to fix my problems. All I want is for you to acknowledge my pain, even by just a kind look when you stop in to check on me."

Silence means acceptance. There are no expectations that clients or nurses must have all the answers. There is no right thing to say or perfect nursing care plan to write that can make things all better for clients. Part of the challenge for all nurses is to live with this realization.

WIT&*Wisdom*

Don't just say something!
Sit there.

Using "Oh . . . ?," "Hmm . . . ," and "Really?"

Although asking questions may seem to be a good way to encourage a distressed person to say more, questions may be experienced as attacks, intrusions, or demands (Bogia, 1985). Rabbinical pastor and chaplain Kate Fagan, in a hospital training class for pastoral volunteers, recommends the use of encouraging or questioning sounds or body language as cues that encourage the client to continue talking. Try "Oh . . . ?" when you sense that the client has more to say and then be quiet. It is not always easy to wait, but it is essential. You can also say "Hmm . . . " or ask "Really?" again, followed by silence. These strategies may elicit further conversation more effectively than more involved verbal responses, but they need to be used with discernment and not overused.

Other strategies are useful when a client is in crisis. Try an observation about the physical facts of a situation. When a client is crying, saying "There arc tcars in your eyes" encourages elaboration because you have acknowledged the tears. Use an "I" statement, such as "I wonder if you have some ideas about that?" when a client presents a scenario that seems puzzling to him or her. The "seems-to-me" approach is useful; for example, "You seem to be upset." Avoid the overused question "How does that make you feel?" which may lead clients to believe you are trying to analyze them (Bogia, 1985). Remember that humor can be an element of spiritual coping as clients try to gain perspective and make meaning, and our humor can foster deeper, more trusting relationships with clients (Johnson, 2002).

Recognizing Opportunities for Moments of Connection

Martin Buber (1958) distinguishes between two types of relationships, the I–It and the I–Thou. The I–It relationship can be experienced as nurses do the work of patient care. Teaching and caring can become routine and, although excellent in form, may lack substance or a real connection with the patient. The I–It is the world of "experiencing and using . . . a typical subject–object relationship." The I–Thou relationship can be experienced only with the whole being. The I–Thou is "characterized by mutuality, directness, presentness, intensity" (Friedman, 1966). "The It is the eternal chrysalis, the Thou, the eternal butterfly" (Buber, 1958).

Just as the world of the nurse provides the potential for a genuine relationship with the patient, the I–It can become the I–Thou in special moments of connection to the patient or to a family member in the potential crisis situation of surgery and illness.

A nurse's personal or family experience with surgery and/or illness can contribute to a deeper understanding of patient and family needs. Nursing is a sacred trust in which the patient and family agree to give up conventional constraints on behavior in exchange for acceptance of their personal response to the traumatic experience of surgery. The nurse's ability to stay connected to the pain of the human condition is one ingredient that can create I–Thou relationships. These moments of connection, however brief, sustain the patient and family throughout the crisis and provide the meaning the nurse so badly needs to revitalize in the nursing practice.

Tapping Resources

So that spiritual care can be provided to clients from a variety of traditions, it is helpful to take the initiative to learn about available resources. As part of a spiritual assessment, you can find out about clergy with whom the client is acquainted who may be contacted with the client's permission. Find out if your organization has access to a pastoral care department for referral, and find out what faith traditions are represented. Take responsibility for learning about rituals, sacred texts, devotional articles, prayer, and sacred music from different traditions (O'Brien, 1999). Martin recommends three strategies for enhancing spiritual well-being in nursing homes: offer religious activities in the facility;

with permission, inform the local church of choice about the admission; and offer opportunities for the expression of clients' faith. Martin writes, "Residents of extended-care facilities must give up a great deal of their former lives and possessions when they embark on this new chapter. Connection with the sacred should not be among the losses" (Martin, 2004, p. 16).

Family members with online access sought and received spiritual comfort using an Internet-based pancreatic cancer chat room through Johns Hopkins Hospital (Nolan et al, 2006). If you find ways to combine personal interest and skills with computers with your nursing career, you might design a website as a resource to assist clients and families in receiving information and support.

Nearing Death

As clients near death, nurses work as part of a team to provide spiritual care. When is the right time? Nurses learn to trust their intuition about the right time to talk about the client's concerns. Nurses offer nurturing touch, silent presence, a prayer, or, if the client prefers, a chance to speak to a member of the clergy. Remember that some clients may be able to attend all or part of a religious service held in your facility. Encourage family to provide sacred music that has offered comfort to the client in the past. Some clients like to listen to recordings of sermons or sacred texts. Nurses create a climate for hope to grow and flourish (Box 16-3). The nurse can ask clients to consider special messages or special mementos for which they want to make arrangements (Piemme, 1998).

Helping in Life Review and Life Repair

Clients near death may find peace by engaging in life review and repair. You can suggest reflection through journal writing. Life review raises issues of forgiveness. There may be a need for forgiveness or acceptance of self. Recent research distinguishes between "decisional forgiveness," a behavioral intention to forgive, and "emotional forgiveness," a shift from negative, unforgiving emotions to positive other-oriented emotions. Emotional forgiveness was found to have more positive effects on health and well-being (Matters of Note, 2008). Nurses in hospice and palliative care may build open and deep relationships with clients. For nurses in such a position, the following question might assist the process of life review: "If you had your life to live over

---

Box 16-3 | *Notes on Hope*

Hope is trust and confidence. Hope is patient. Hope brings enthusiasm and adds animation. Hope is a fuel to keep us going, a tonic to energize, a driving force to move us forward, daily bread to feed the soul. Hope is in contrast to expectation, which takes us from the present to a focus on the future; this can bring disappointment when things do not go as we planned (Brussat and Brussat, 1998). "Hope is the belief . . . that one can have a life in the midst of trauma and suffering. Hope that you will be able to cope with the suffering, hope that something good will come from it, hope for remission—if not a cure, hope for an extension of time, hope for the future welfare of your family, hope to keep your dignity, hope for life after life" (Hampton, 1998).

To *bring hope* you must have hope. To keep a hopeful countenance, learn to forgive yourself for your mistakes so you can take the risk of opportunities of the future; learn to leave room for the future, love yourself, laugh and keep a sense of humor, trust in God, celebrate your imagination, cherish your dreams, create visions, set goals. In the face of difficulties, remember: within every problem there is a lesson. Embrace the lesson and release the problem. To face the uncertainty of life, consider this notion: I am uncertain about the future, but I am certain it will be positive.

To *instill hope* you show it in your face; in your kind, positive words; in your ability to truly face someone—to look into the eyes; in your presence rather than avoidance; in your presence in the face of suffering; in your openness to hear hopeless words; in your offered prayer. Encourage clients to display cards and have family bring photographs or art from children or grandchildren. Suggest the family provide favorite music. Comment on flowers as reminders of connection in the client's life.

---

again, what would you like to be different?" (Kemp, 2001). It may be helpful to ask the client if there is unfinished business in life that they might now be able to address. One hospice client replied that she did not believe she had ever told her daughter how truly proud she was of her. The nurse helped her determine a good time to do this and supported the client's resolve to do it, even though talk of feelings did not come easy. After the talk, the client seemed to experience more peace. Rabbi Zalman Schachter-Shalomi, founder of the Spiritual Eldering Institute, offers an in-depth process in his work and in the book *From Age-ing to Sage-ing* (1995).

The accompanying Moments of Connection help illustrate the different forms communication may take as nurses support clients and families in these intimate times.

Moments of Connection . . .
Having the Courage to Share a Prayer
"A patient who had been on the acute pain service three previous times during the same admission was received in the postanesthesia care unit (PACU) after an exploration of the abdomen and was in a great deal of pain as I started her patient-controlled analgesia (PCA). I told her I would stay with her until the pain was controlled. For the next 2 hours I gave her multiple boluses, but her pain was not relieved satisfactorily. During this time I patted her forehead and moistened her lips. When I asked her what else I could do for her, she asked if I would pray with her. We were still in the PACU, and I was aware that several other nurses were rolling their eyes. We said the Lord's Prayer. She soon relaxed and appeared more comfortable."

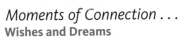

Moments of Connection . . .
Wishes and Dreams
"It was springtime, and she was a young leukemia patient who would probably not leave the hospital before a 'celestial discharge.' We had chatted for days about her wishes and dreams. She had never gone to a circus, seen a bluebird, or been to Disneyland. Several nurses got together. Mickey Mouse appeared in her room. I came as a clown with my 'trick' dog, bringing a video of the circus. A pet shop owner brought in two blue birds to spend the afternoon. She was laughing and crying. She said she didn't know nurses did all these things. I asked her if she was happy and content. She replied, 'The only thing I haven't seen is God, and I'll see Him soon, but I know I've seen the angels.'"

Moments of Connection . . .
I Clearly Felt Her Presence
"I was working as a hospice nurse with a very independent client who always wanted to be in control, up in the chair each day. As her pain increased and my visits became more frequent, I took on more of a nurturing role. I am also a massage therapist, and when she became bedridden, I would frequently give her a massage. She asked to purchase a gift certificate for a massage for her sister. On the day she passed, I went into her room where her body lay, cold and still. I thanked her for the opportunity to be her friend and nurse. I clearly felt her presence and love. A month later, her sister came for a massage after having been very distraught over her loss. It was a marvelous experience for both of us. She still returns monthly for a massage, and each time we remember her sister and her gift."

Finding Meaning

By understanding that meaning can come from suffering, you can be alert to times when clients or family members want to share what they have learned. Clients may give you clues that they want to talk further. Here are some things your clients might say and possible interventions to help them share their understanding of what has happened:

> *Client 1:* "So much has happened in such a short time. I never knew I could handle so many things."
> *Nurse:* "You've been thinking about all the things you've been through. Tell me about it."
> *Client 2:* "Having AIDS makes me value life more."
> *Nurse:* "Can you share how you see life now?"
> *Client 3:* "When you lose a child, your other children become all the more precious."
> *Nurse:* "How do you think things will change between you and your children?"

Hannaford and Popkin (1992) report things that people have learned from loss, as listed in Box 16-4. Their book *Windows* is used as a text for a grief class that is taught to caregivers who may support clients and families during loss. They suggest questions and statements that may "encourage the griever as he turns loss into meaningful experience." Box 16-5 lists questions and statements that might be helpful, and Box 16-6 lists comments that might be harmful.

Box 16-4	*Possible Meanings of Illness and Suffering*

I have learned . . .

- That I can love.
- That loving hurts.
- That I can survive.
- That healing occurs.
- That I have grown.
- That I can forgive.
- That I can forgive myself.
- That you taught me much.
- That I can be a receiver.
- That change is a necessary part of life.
- That I am grateful for the many things you gave me.
- That I wouldn't miss you if you hadn't been so important to me.
- That I cannot control everything.
- That I can care.
- That I can become involved.
- That I need a significant other.
- That I can reevaluate myself.
- That a new page of my life is being written.
- That I will have to change.
- That I can start again.
- That I am wiser.
- That I have discovered a new level of courage.
- That I am more open.
- That I can make new contacts on my own.
- That I can ask for support.
- That I am stronger, more independent, more joyful, happier.
- That I have choices.
- That I am really never alone.
- The value and importance of the present.
- To fill my days in new ways.
- To appreciate this disruption in my life as motivation to grow.
- To enjoy aloneness.
- To appreciate life more.

Reprinted from Hannaford M, Popkin, M: *Windows: healing and helping through loss,* Atlanta, GA, 1992, Active Parenting, pp. 77–78.

Box 16-5	*Questions or Statements That May Help*

As you look at this experience, is it possible that you have found new meaning in relationships that you were not aware of before?

- Have you considered your growth during this time, the changes in you that this loss seems to have brought?
- How has the experience changed your life?
- How has it influenced your life purpose and belief system?
- What positive action have you taken or might you take as a result of this lesson?
- You seem to have learned that there are a lot of things over which we have no control.
- You have gained a lot of self-confidence in your ability to handle a crisis.
- You seem to feel that with all the loss, you are gaining a kind of independence that you never knew you could enjoy.
- I like to hear you laugh; it seems that you are more able to express your feelings since your recent experience.

Reprinted from Hannaford M, Popkin M: *Windows: healing and helping through loss,* Atlanta, GA, 1992, Active Parenting, pp. 129–130.

Finding God in the Busyness

How do you as a nurse find God for yourself with the pace you keep? Hanrahan, a writer, anthropologist, and painter, speaks of "finding God in the busyness."

She writes about the great longing for stillness and silence and the assumption that it is necessary to go "on retreat" to find God. She suggests that quiet and withdrawal are not necessary for spiritual health and that to be busy does not have to mean a disconnection from God. Hanrahan works with indigenous people in Canada, people who have always seen God everywhere and in everything. "I saw God in the face of an Elder in the Yukon and heard in the prayers we said to open our meetings. I met God in the bubbly Turkish man who drove me to the airport . . . and in the Mexican professor–taxi driver, a refugee from the institutional Revolutionary Party's long, hard rule, a man empty of bitterness" (Hanrahan, 2006). She felt God as her head hit the pillow in a hotel on a business trip. Her advice speaks to slowing down for a moment of gratitude or connection.

Remember that there is often nobody better placed or better qualified to provide spiritual care than the nurse (Kemp, 2001). Consider that sometimes nurturing the sacred in your own life is the best approach.

Box 16-6   *Comments That May Do More Harm Than Good*

- As you look at this, you have no doubt learned never to do it again.
- Life's lessons are hard, and you have certainly made this one into a hard one.
- When you make mistakes, you always have to pay.
- If you had kept in touch, you wouldn't feel so bad.
- You'll learn from this one to be kind from now on.
- I do hope you've learned your lesson.
- Everything will be all right.

Reprinted from Hannaford M, Popkin M: *Windows: healing and helping through loss*, Atlanta, GA, 1992, Active Parenting, pp. 129–130.

We come full circle. Spiritual care begins and ends with the caregiver. You nurture your own spirit, thus becoming open to your clients' experiences in a genuine, holistic way. Your experience with your clients nourishes your spirit and offers renewal. "Presence becomes a gift to ourselves and others in the shared moment of the present and enhances the fullness of our being, filling our cups to overflowing" (McKivergin and Daubenmire, 1994). A number of retired nurses have continued their commitment to spirituality through becoming parish nurses.

 Reflections On . . .

Spirituality

Consider what you read about spirituality. How do you see your own spirituality? What spirituality interventions are you already using? Answer the following questions.

What? . . .
Write one thing you learned from this chapter.

So what? . . .
How will this affect your nursing practice?

Now what? . . .
How will you implement this new knowledge or skill?

Think about it . . .

Practicing Spirituality

Exercise 1
Visit www.journalofsacredwork.typepad.com. This is a site of ecumenical daily devotionals and inspiring narratives for strength and support for professional and lay caregivers for loving care for self and others (Jackson, 2010).

Exercise 2
Answer these questions for yourself, which are a sample of those used in a 2-day course taught to nurses on the subject of presence (McKivergin and Daubenmire, 1994).

- What are the characteristics or qualities of presence?
- What does it mean to be fully present to another?
- How can I become more aware of opportunities to be present to others?

Exercise 3
Keep a journal for a day.

1. Choose a clinical day and be aware of how you can live artfully in an ordinary day, not just on vacation.
2. Pay attention to your senses. Record pleasurable moments.
3. Consciously take time to pause and reflect on your thoughts, feelings, and actions. Record these.
4. Take at least 15 minutes in the day for yourself. Surely you can take that time even if you must study for a test. In fact, that is a great time to do this to build your energy and stimulate your creativity.
5. Be mindful of your clients' experiences and pay special attention to understanding their perspective. Consider ways in which these experiences relate to any of your own and how they may have affected your life. Record these thoughts.

Exercise 4

Ask yourself this important question: "How do I experience the sacred?" People have a variety of ways of nourishing the spirit (Burkhardt and Nagai-Jacobson, 1994). Share your answers with at least three other students or peers. If you don't understand the question or can't think of an answer, discuss that instead.

It will stimulate your thinking.

Exercise 5

Use this poem to begin a discussion of nature as a source of spiritual connection.

Take a Quiet Walk for Me

Walk slowly
    by the quiet path
And look at the trees
    and the sky
    by day and night . . .
Remembering the good times
    on the lakeshore,
    in the woods
Near the meadows
    and the black softness
    of the friendly hollows . . .

Copyright © Howard G. Kirkman. Used with permission.

Exercise 6

Examine the Spiritual Assessment Tool (Box 16-7). This tool has been published in a number of sources and includes different ways of looking at the concept of spirituality. Read and reflect on the tool, and put a check by the questions you would be comfortable asking a client. Share your responses with several other students. Talk about how you can use this tool or parts of it in your current clinical setting. File this tool for future use.

Exercise 7

Examine Box 16-1 on the FICA tool. This simple acronym, FICA, can easily be memorized. Remember that throughout your career, anything you memorize is yours forever. Commit this tool to memory and use it with a client, another nurse, or student, whichever is appropriate for your role. Share your response with another nurse or student and reflect on the application of this tool to your clinical setting or preferred specialty.

Exercise 8

Visit http://www.hmassoc.org to learn about health ministries. Parish nursing is a specialty area in which nurses create an atmosphere of trust in a faith community, parish, or church that allows parishioners to bring up health concerns they might not otherwise address (Brooks et al, 2005).

Exercise 9

Think of someone still living toward whom you feel great gratitude that you have never expressed. Spend 10 minutes writing that person a gratitude letter and then pair up with someone here, and each of you read your letter to the other. The final step is that you pay a personal visit to that person sometime in the near future and read that letter aloud (Yalom, 2009, p. 135).

Exercise 10

The Blessing of the Hands is a nondenominational ceremony or ritual with the intent to renew and honor nurses. It is often conducted at Nurse Week celebrations. It could also be incorporated into celebrations in a school of nursing. Research this tradition online and discuss with other students and staff interest in conducting such a ceremony in a clinical setting or school of nursing celebration (Wolpert, 2010).

Box 16-7   *Spiritual Assessment Tool*

The following reflective questions may assist you in assessing, evaluating, and increasing your awareness of spirituality in yourself and others.

MEANING AND PURPOSE

These questions assess a person's ability to seek meaning and fulfillment in life, manifest hope, and accept ambiguity and uncertainty.
- What gives your life meaning?
- Do you have a sense of purpose in life?
- Does your illness interfere with your life goals?
- Why do you want to get well?
- How hopeful are you about obtaining a better degree of health?
- Do you feel that you have a responsibility in maintaining your health?
- Will you be able to make changes in your life to maintain your health?
- Are you motivated to get well?
- What is the most important or powerful thing in your life?

INNER STRENGTHS

These questions assess a person's ability to manifest joy and recognize strengths, choices, goals, and faith.
- What brings you joy and peace in your life?
- What can you do to feel alive and full of spirit?
- What traits do you like about yourself?
- What are your personal strengths?
- What choices are available to you to enhance your healing?
- What life goals have you set for yourself?
- Do you think that stress in any way caused your illness?
- How aware were you of your body before you became sick?
- What do you believe in?
- Is faith important in your life?
- How has your illness influenced your faith?
- Does faith play a role in recognizing your health?

INTERCONNECTIONS

These questions assess a person's positive self-concept, self-esteem, and sense of self; sense of belonging in the world with others; capacity to pursue personal interests; and ability to demonstrate love of self and self-forgiveness.

- How do you feel about yourself right now?
- How do you feel when you have a true sense of yourself?
- Do you pursue things of personal interest?
- What do you do to show love for yourself?
- Can you forgive yourself?
- What do you do to heal your spirit?

These questions assess a person's ability to connect in life-giving ways with family, friends, and social groups and to engage in the forgiveness of others.
- Who are the significant people in your life?
- Do you have friends or family in town who are available to help you?
- Who are the people to whom you are closest?
- Do you belong to any groups?
- Can you ask people for help when you need it?
- Can you share your feelings with others?
- What are some of the most loving things that others have done for you?
- What are the loving things that you do for other people?
- Are you able to forgive others?

These questions assess a person's capacity for finding meaning in worship or religious activities, and a connectedness with a divinity.
- Is worship important to you?
- What do you consider the most significant act of worship in your life?
- Do you participate in any religious activities?
- Do you believe in God or a higher power?
- Do you think that prayer is powerful?
- Have you ever tried to empty your mind of all thoughts to see what the experience might be?
- Do you use relaxation or imagery skills?
- Do you meditate?
- Do you pray?
- What is your prayer?
- How are your prayers answered?
- Do you have a sense of belonging in this world?

These questions assess a person's ability to experience a sense of connection with life and nature, an awareness of the effects of the environment on life and well-being, and a capacity or concern for the health of the environment.
- Do you ever feel a connection with the world or universe?

Box 16-7	*Spiritual Assessment Tool—cont'd*

- How does your environment have an impact on your state of well-being?
- What are your environmental stressors at work and at home?
- What strategies reduce your environmental stressors?
- Do you have any concerns for the state of your immediate environment?
- Are you involved with environmental issues such as recycling environmental

resources at home, at work, or in your community?
- Are you concerned about the survival of the planet?

From Dossey BM: Holistic modalities and healing moments, *Am J Nurs* 98 (6)44 (1998). Sources: Burkhardt MA: Spirituality: an analysis of the concept, *Holistic Nurs Pract* 3(3)69, (1989); Dossey BM, Keegan L, editors: *Holistic nursing: a handbook for practice*, ed. 2, Gaithersburg, Md, 1995, Aspen Publishers.

References

Bay PS, Ivy SS, Terry CL: The effect of spiritual retreat on nurses' spirituality, *Holist Nurs Pract* 24(3):125, May/June 2010.

Bayfront Medical Center: *Pastoral care volunteer training manual: the use of prayer* (handout), St Petersburg, Fla, 2002, Bayfront Medical Center.

Bogia BP: Responding to questions in pastoral care, *J Pastoral Care* 13(4):357, 1985.

Bormann JE, Thorp S, Wetherell JL, et al: A spiritually based group intervention for combat veterans with posttraumatic stress disorder, *J Holist Nurs* 26(2):109, June 2008.

Brillhart B: A study of spirituality and life satisfaction among persons with spinal cord injury, *Rehabil Nurs* 30(1):31, 2005.

Brooks D, Henry J, Leblanc H, et al: Incorporating spirituality into practice, *Can Nurse* 101(6):22, 2005.

Brussat F, Brussat MA: *Spiritual literacy: reading the sacred in everyday life*, New York, 1998, Touchstone Books.

Buber M: *I and thou*, New York, 1958, Charles Scribner's Sons.

Burkhardt MA, Nagai-Jacobson MG: Reawakening spirit in nursing practice, *J Holist Nurs* 12(1):8, 1994.

Burkhardt MA, Nagai-Jacobson MG: *Spirituality: living our connectedness*, Albany, NY, 2002, Delmar/Thomson Learning.

Buswell J, Clegg A, Grout G, et al: Ask the experts: spirituality in care [gerontological care and practice], *Nurs Older People* 18(1):14, 2006.

Calabria MD, Macrae JA, editors: *Suggestions for thought by Florence Nightingale: selections and commentaries* (a volume in the Studies in Health, Illness, and Caregiving series), Philadelphia, 1994, University of Pennsylvania Press.

Carson VB, Koenig HG: *Spiritual dimensions of nursing practice*, West Conshohocken, PA, 2008, Templeton Foundation Press.

Casarez RLP, Engebretson JC, Ostwald SK: Spiritual practices in self-management of diabetes in African Americans, *Holist Nurs Pract* 24(4):227, July/Aug 2010.

Cavendish R, Luise BK, Horne K, et al: Opportunities for enhanced spirituality relevant to well adults, *Nurs Diagn* 11(4): 151, 2000.

Delgado C: Meeting clients' spiritual needs, *Nurs Clin North Am* 42(2):279, 2007.

Donnelly GF: Health choices and heightened awareness: the art of the nudge!, *Holistic Nurs Pract* 24(4):179, July/Aug 2010.

Donnelly GF, Cook DC: From the editors, *Holist Nurs Pract* 3(3):vi, 1989.

Dossey B: Body-mind-spirit: attending to holistic care, *Am J Nurs* 98(8):35, 1998a.

Dossey B: Holistic modalities and healing moments, *Am J Nurs* 98(6):44, 1998b.

Dossey BM, Keegan L: *Holistic nursing: a handbook for practice*, Sudbury, MA, 2008, Jones & Bartlett Publishers.

Emmons RA: *Thanks: How the new science of gratitude can make you happier*, Boston, 2007, Houghton Mifflin Co.

Erickson H, editor: *Modeling and role-modeling: a view from the clients' world*, Cedar Park, TX, 2006, Unicorns Unlimited.

Erickson H, Tomlin E, Swain MA: *Modeling and role-modeling: a theory and paradigm for nursing*, Englewood Cliffs, N.J., 1983, Prentice-Hall. (Second–ninth printing, Cedar Park, Tex, 1988–2009, EST Co, Tenth printing, Cedar Park, Tex, 2010, Unicorns Unlimited.)

Fields R, Taylor P, Weyler R, et al: *Chop wood, carry water: a guide to finding spiritual fulfillment in everyday life*, Los Angeles, 1984, JP Tarcher.

Friedman MS: *The life of dialogue*, New York, 1966, Harper & Row.

Hampton C: Hope and healing after traumatic illness (paper presented to the Case Management Society of America, Georgia chapter, September 26, 1998).

Hannaford M, Popkin M: *Windows: healing and helping through loss*, Atlanta, Ga, 1992, Active Parenting.

Hanrahan M: *Finding God in the busyness*, The Social Edge: A Monthly Social Justice and Faith Website (website). http://www.thesocialedge.com/columns/maurahanrahan/index.shtml. Accessed June 19, 2006.

Jackson C: Using loving relationships to transform health care: a practical approach, *Holist Nurs Pract* 24(4):181, July/Aug 2010.

Johnson P: The use of humor and its influences on spirituality and coping in breast cancer survivors, *Oncol Nurs Forum* 29(4):691, 2002.

Kemp C: Spiritual care interventions. In Ferrell B, Coyle N, editors: *Textbook of palliative care*, New York, 2001, Oxford University Press.

Kidd SM: *The mermaid chair*, New York, 2005, Penguin Books.

Koenig HG: *The healing power of faith: science explores medicine's last great frontier*, New York, 1999, Simon & Schuster.

Koenig HG: *Spirituality in patient care: why, how, when, and what*, West Conshohocken, PA, 2007, Templeton Press.

Lackey SA: Opening the door to spiritually sensitive care, *Nursing* 39(4):46, April 2009.

Martin I: Nurturing that old-time religion, *Vibrant Life* 20(5):14, 2004.

Matters of Note: new forgiveness research looks at its effect on others, *Explore* 4(1):1, January/February 2008.

McCaffrey A: Prayer for health concerns: Results of a national survey on prevalence and patterns of use, *Arch Intern Med* 164(8):858, 2004.

McKivergin MJ, Daubenmire MJ: The healing process of presence, *J Holist Nurs* 21(1):65, 1994.

Meraviglia M: Effects of spirituality in breast cancer survivors, *Oncol Nurs Forum* 33(1):E1, 2006.

Moore T: *Care of the soul*, New York, 1998, Harper Collins.

Nagai-Jacobson MG, Burkhardt MA: Spirituality: cornerstone of holistic nursing practice, *Holist Nurs Pract* 3(3):18, 1989.

Narayanasamy A: The puzzle of spirituality for nursing: a guide to practical assessment, *Br J Nurs* 13(19):1140, 2004.

Newman MA: The spirit of nursing, *Holist Nurs Pract* 3(3):1, 1989.

Nolan MT, Hodgin MB, Olsen SJ, et al: Spiritual issues of family members in a pancreatic cancer chat room, *Oncol Nurs Forum* 33(2):239, 2006.

O'Brien ME: *Spirituality in nursing: standing on holy ground*, Sudbury, Mass, 1999, Jones & Bartlett.

Peck MS: *Further along the road less traveled: the unending journey toward spiritual growth*, New York, 1998, Touchstone Books.

Piemme JA: Discussing end-of-life decisions, *Innovations in Breast Cancer Care* 4(1):31, 1998.

Schachter-Shalomi Z: *From age-ing to sage-ing: a profound new vision of growing older*, New York, 1995, Warner Books. (The work of Sage-ing is facilitated by the Sage-ing Guild, at http://www.sage-ingguild.org).

Thaler RH, Sustein CR: *Nudge: improving decisions about health, wealth and happiness*, London, 2008, Penguin Books.

Thomas JD, Finch LP, Schoenhofer SO, Green A: The caring relationships created by nurse practitioners and the ones nursed: implications for practice, *Top Adv Pract Nurs* 4(4), 2004.

Touchy TA: Nurturing hope and spirituality in the nursing home, *Holist Nurs Pract* 15(4):45, 2001.

Travelbee J: *Interventions in psychiatric nursing*, Philadelphia, 1970, F.A. Davis.

Tuck I, McCain NL, Elswick RK Jr: Spirituality and psychosocial well-being in HIV+ adults, *J Adv Nurs* 33(6):776, 2001.

Wolpert NS: Blessing of the hands, *Nurs Manage* 41(5):29, May 2010.

Yalom ID: *Staring at the sun: overcoming the terror of death*, San Francisco, 2009, Jossey-Bass.

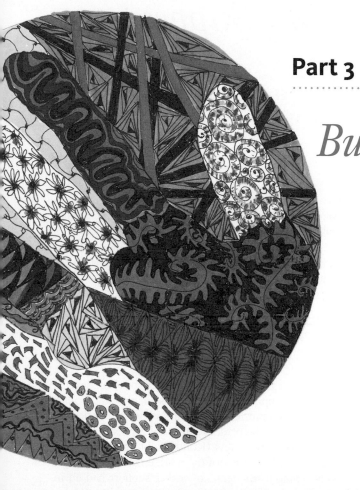

Part 3

Building Confidence

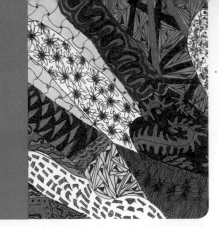

Chapter 17

Requesting Support

As a student nurse, and later as a nurse, you will have many occasions on which you will need support to do your work. This chapter provides you with guidelines for making your requests for support in a way that will bring the greatest likelihood of success. You will learn how to be specific about your needs for support and how to plan an assertive strategy. The exercises will give you the opportunity to practice assertive ways to request support.

Objectives

1. Discuss the relationship between social support and health
2. Complete a support system assessment
3. Distinguish between assertive, nonassertive, and aggressive requests for support
4. Practice making requests for support in selected exercises

Recognizing the Importance of Social Support for Health and Work Life

Research on the relationship between social support and health has important implications for nursing practice today. The literature suggests that a positive relationship exists between the presence of social support and health and coping with illness (Komblith et al, 2001; Adams et al, 2000). In a study of the work environment of secondary school teachers, co-worker support had an inverse relationship to anxiety and depression (Mahan et al, 2010). Employers are looking at ways to support nurses in order to reduce stress and promote recruitment and retention. The American Nurses Credentialing Center (2010) defines criteria for the selection of healthcare organizations that demonstrate sustained excellence in nursing care in the Magnet Recognition Program, by supporting nurses in professional practice. Nurse administrators are challenged to take the leadership role in creating work environments that support nurses by asking nurses how they want to be supported, being sensitive to nurses' stress, and understanding the emotional risks nurses face at work (Ingala and Hill, 2001; Kerfoot, 2001). Leaders are encouraged to demonstrate their own compassion and to recognize the economic benefits of institutional compassion in times of trauma. For example, Mayor Rudolph Giuliani's public display of grief strengthened people's resolve to rebuild and restore confidence in New York after the bombing of the World Trade Center on September 11, 2001 (Dutton et al, 2002).

Determining the Support You Need at Work or School

In the broadest sense of the word, support is anything that helps you work more effectively and feel better about how you are functioning. This general notion of support is vague and does not help you specifically articulate what you need or guide you in getting it. Conceptualizing support as being cognitive, affective, and physical can help you assess your needs and secure the support you require to work effectively as a nurse.

Cognitive support helps you think intelligently about your job, decide how to approach problems, and discover the how and why of doing things a certain way, and it also provides some criteria for doing your work. One method of providing nurses with cognitive support is through mentors. In a study using a mentorship model, newly graduated nurses who were mentored demonstrated a higher level of competency as evaluated by their head nurses than they did in two evaluations prior to the mentorship (Komaratat and Oumtanee, 2009). From mentors, nurses receive career advice, intellectual stimulation, and role modeling. New nurses receive needed support to promote retention, and experienced nurses are challenged to advance their knowledge base, sharpen consultative skills, and initiate needed change. Peer mentoring is another potential solution for support. At a university in southern Ontario, senior nursing students became role models and resources for other students in relationships that were mutually beneficial (Dennison, 2010). See "Looking for a Mentor" later in this chapter.

Affective support is acknowledgment for the work you do and a feeling of nurturance. Nurse managers need continued support and confirmation of their important role in today's world, in which nursing practices are changing, clients' conditions are more acute, and recruitment and retention are challenging issues (Sala, 2002). Respect, honor, and recognition of employees by the acknowledgment of positive performance are needed frequently, not only during an annual review. Expressing gratitude and appreciation can create feelings of goodwill and nurturance among nurses, which is a form of job gratification that makes them feel better about their workplaces, clients, and colleagues (Doherty, 2002). Mentoring can also provide affective support. In a study of a mentorship program initiated when the nurse turnover rate increased to 31%, nurses working in inpatient units, surgery, and emergency rooms who participated in a 1-year pilot program had a 0% turnover rate. Three years after the program continued and was expanded to other departments, the hospital staff turnover rate decreased to 10.3% (Fox, 2010).

Callahan (1990) believes that burnout occurs when nurses realize that no matter how developed their talents are, they receive no recognition. She urges hospitals to initiate a system of positive incident reports that can be posted on the unit's bulletin board and then be included in the staff nurses' personnel files. A commendation for work well done might look as follows: "I'd like to commend Sheila Jersey, RN, for the empathy she showed the client in room 1039 on the night of 10/12/98. Her words cut through his pain and delirium, grounding him in reality and allowing him to rest without further medication. She has a special ability to say just what the client needs to hear."

Physical support is being provided with the staff, materials, and processes needed to get work done. Staffing requirements, an essential aspect of physical support, are discussed in the abundance of articles on retention. In this era, the belief is that the provision of adequate cognitive and affective support will attract nurses. The requirements for supplies, equipment, and environmental conveniences have likely been met in most nursing workplaces through technology, computerization, and adherence to stringent occupational hazard and safety regulations.

As nurses, we need to be assertive about securing the support necessary to function comfortably and confidently at work. The clearer we are about the support we need to do our jobs, the more likely we are to secure it. We devote a lot of energy to attempting to improve the health status of our clients. Getting the support we need to do our work can help us maintain our own health and enhance how we feel about both our work and our co-workers.

Conceptualizing cognitive, affective, and physical components of support provides you with an organizing framework for your individual support assessment. The first step in your systematic approach is to determine whether you are satisfied with the quality and quantity of each facet of support. Quality refers to the nature or characteristics of the support; quantity refers to the amount of support.

Look at the checklist in Box 17-1, grab a pencil, and indicate the pluses and minuses in your support system.

After you have completed this checklist, take note of those areas in which you do have the support you need at work or school. It is easy to take for granted the support we do have, and noticing the benefits makes us more appreciative.

Next, look at those areas in which the support you would like is not available. Answer the following questions about those instances in which you are not satisfied with the quantity or quality of the support you receive:

- What exactly dissatisfies me about the quantity or quality of the support?
- If I had a choice, how would I change things to ensure that I receive the support I need?

Be as specific as possible in answering these questions. The clearer and more detailed you can be about the gaps in your support system at work or school, the greater are your chances of rectifying the situation. By answering these questions, you indicate your desired outcome.

Requesting the Support You Need at Work or School

The first step is to identify your needs for support. The next step is to decide if you wish to pursue the acquisition of this support. Can you manage without it, or would the presence of that support really enhance your working situation? Once you have decided to try to obtain the support, your next step is to design your strategy. You need to answer the following questions:

- Who is the best person to ask for this support?
- What is the best way to seek this support?
- How can I present my case in a way that increases the probability of securing the support I want at work or school?

Let us take an example from each domain—cognitive, affective, and physical—and demonstrate effective and ineffective methods of seeking support.

Making a Request for Cognitive Support

You are a student nurse in a small college. Although the school has several computers with access to databases, you and most of your classmates have your own

computers and would prefer to work in your dormitory rooms. You could work more efficiently if there were telephone lines in each room so that modems could be used. In the area of cognitive support, you need better access to information. Knowing that several other colleges have recently decided to equip rooms with telephone jacks, you decide to approach the dean of your school of nursing with your request.

After making an appointment with the dean, you begin to prepare your strategy. In the 20 minutes you have been allotted, you must make the dean aware of the problem and how it is affecting the students' ability to access recent information. You want to urge the dean to explore your recommendation so that you and your colleagues will have the support you need.

You obtain information on comparably sized schools in your region and learn that these schools have completed or begun the process of providing in-room telephone access. Next, you survey your classmates to see how many have computers or would get them if they had the facilities to use modems, and how many have used modems in the past. You also obtain specific information from your colleagues about how often they have been delayed in their work by having to wait for computer access in the library.

Armed with this information, you next prepare yourself for the interview with the dean. You envision yourself looking relaxed and calm. In your mind's eye you see yourself presenting your arguments in a clear, straightforward, assertive manner. You notice how the dean is paying attention to what you are saying and taking notes. You visualize the dean agreeing with your concerns and promising to explore the feasibility of installing the necessary equipment.

Here is an example of how your interview with the dean might go if you were assertive:

Assertive Approach

Assertive you: "Thank you for seeing me, Dr. Thomas. I want to talk to you about the library resources and the students' concerns about their ability to do timely literature reviews by computer."

Dr. Thomas: "Oh? Is that the case? Can you tell me any more about the situation?"

Assertive you: "Yes, I can. Although our library has excellent computer access to information, there are too few terminals to allow us to get our work done in a timely way. Most of us have our own computers or would bring computers if we had

Box 17-1 *Credits and Debits in Your Support System*

For each cognitive, affective, or physical support item, ask yourself the following:
- Am I satisfied with the quality of support I get to do my job?
- Am I satisfied with the quantity of support I get to do my job?

| | SATISFIED WITH: | | | |
| | QUALITY | | QUANTITY | |
	YES	NO	YES	NO

COGNITIVE SUPPORT

1. Inspiration: You work with people whose knowledge and skill levels show how you can improve your nursing care.
2. Information: Resources (books, procedural manuals, memoranda, online information) are available to provide clear information or instruction about relevant nursing procedures.
3. Advice: Colleagues offer expertise and show a willingness to help guide and/or direct you.
4. Challenge: Colleagues intellectually stimulate you by encouraging you to examine, question, and critique your nursing care.
5. Direction: Colleagues exhibit or freely share their philosophies and beliefs about nursing in a way that is helpful to you.

AFFECTIVE SUPPORT

6. Empathy: Colleagues show interest in you and listen to you, and you feel respected and understood.
7. Recognition: Colleagues acknowledge the knowledge and skills you possess, and you are able to make independent decisions and use your talents properly.
8. Praise: Colleagues express admiration for your work and compliment you or show attention and genuine interest in your nursing.
9. Reassurance: Forgiveness for imperfections of omission or commission is offered with acceptance and encouragement for you to continue to do your best nursing.
10. Concern: Colleagues show warm, caring interest in you as a person, and you have a sense that they look forward to working with you; they are concerned for your welfare as a person (not just as a nurse or student).
11. Feedback: Honest, forthright evaluation of your work is offered or is available to you when you ask for it; constructive criticism is given in a straightforward, clear manner and is worded in such a way that you can accept it.
12. Cooperation: Colleagues share ideas with you; there is little greedy competitiveness, and nurses enjoy working together to improve client care.
13. Enthusiasm: Nurses and others are motivated, and the atmosphere is lively; creative ideas to improve nursing care are encouraged.

PHYSICAL SUPPORT

14. Adequate personnel: Staff with essential knowledge and skills is available to carry out the necessary nursing functions.
15. Sharing: When circumstances dictate, colleagues share the workload and help each other; rarely do colleagues avoid helping or refuse to pitch in and lend a hand.
16. Supplies: Sufficient nursing or administrative supplies are consistently available to allow you to smoothly carry out your work.
17. Equipment: Equipment on your unit is efficient, in working order, and is easily accessible.
18. Environment: The physical design and decor of your working environment allow you to work without inconvenience, hassles, or unpleasant distractions.

Adapted from Smith SP: Need support at work? Think CAPs, *Can Nurse* 81(8):40, 1984.

phone access in our dorm rooms. I have checked with other schools of comparable size in this region and can show you their progress on this issue. I have surveyed the student body and have responses that indicate how many students are affected by the problem. I have made a copy of the information I have compiled that you may keep [hands dean a well-organized information packet]. We are excited about the quality of education we are getting here, and the complexity of the assignments makes them challenging. We believe we could work more efficiently if we could use modems in our rooms, especially since, as you can see by the survey, most of us have been accustomed to doing our research in this manner."

Dr. Thomas: "I can't argue with your facts. You have certainly done your homework. Your suggestion sounds like a good solution to the situation. I certainly want our students to have access to the most current information. I assure you that I will bring the matter up at the next faculty meeting. We have been talking about this, and your concern and initiative on behalf of the students to get the support you need are impressive. We have a faculty meeting this week. I'll share your data and get back to you in 1 week. Thank you for bringing this important matter to my attention."

Your assertive approach has brought the students' concerns to the dean's attention. By thanking Dr. Thomas for seeing you, you showed your respect for her busy schedule. You reinforced your awareness by getting right to the point of your visit. Your acknowledgment of the assets of your school library indicated to the dean that you were appreciative of the positive resources available and were not just complaining. You clearly outlined the situation, indicating why it is a problem, and respectfully offered a possible solution. Your research and approach to the dean helped you present your needs and provided data to increase the possibility that the cognitive support requested could be provided.

In contrast to this assertive approach, you could have used a nonassertive or aggressive approach with the dean. Let us examine the consequences of both of these less effective approaches.

Nonassertive Approach

When we act nonassertively in any situation, we come across as being unsure, undecided, and without confidence. These nonassertive qualities give others the message that we do not expect to receive what we are seeking. Messages of uncertainty work against us by putting doubts about our requests in the minds of potential providers. Here is an example of a nonassertive approach:

Nonassertive you: "I appreciate your seeing me, Dr. Thomas. It's about the computer problem. Uh, did you know that we have trouble getting the information we need?"

Dr. Thomas: "What's this about a computer problem? What problem?"

Nonassertive you: "Well, I'm not the only one who has had to wait to use the computer to get the information I need for my assignments. It's quite a problem you see . . . I mean, it takes a lot of time to get this information."

Dr. Thomas: "Yes, I know. Library research is very time consuming. Is there a problem with the computers?"

Nonassertive you: "Well, no. You see, that's just the problem. There aren't enough computers. We have some in our rooms. What I mean to say is, I think we need to be able to use modems in our rooms."

Dr. Thomas: "Well, how big a problem is this?"

Nonassertive you: "Well, last week I had to wait a long time for access to a computer in the library. Others are complaining, too."

Dr. Thomas: "If you want my assistance, I need to know more about how many students are affected by this problem, to see if any action is necessary. I'll be happy to look into this matter when you provide me with the information to do so."

When we are nonassertive, we are asking to have our requests for support ignored. In this example you were not armed with the information you needed to convince Dr. Thomas of the importance of the problem. Your content was not delivered in an objective, forthright manner. Because of your style, delivery, and preparation, being nonassertive lost your case.

Let's look at an aggressive approach.

Aggressive Approach

When we are aggressive, we go after what we want in a way that is upsetting, disrespectful, or threatening to others. When we attack other people in our endeavors to get what we want, we create bad feelings that take considerable energy and time to overcome.

Here is an example of an aggressive approach:

Aggressive you: "Thanks for seeing me, Dr. Thomas. You've just got to do something about this computer situation. I'm fed up with having to go to the university library to get the stuff I need to complete the assignments required for this program when I could use my modem if I had a telephone in my room. It's got to change. It's unfair to students when they can't get the latest information. How would you like to hand in assignments based on half-baked ideas?"

Dr. Thomas: "I can see you are upset about this, and it sounds quite important. When you have calmed down and can talk to me rationally about the problem, I'll be glad to meet with you."

Being aggressive did not get you what you were seeking. But it did create an unpleasant relationship between you and your dean. Now there are two problems. When we are aggressive, we are often out of control and do not present our arguments in a logical, clear way. A rational, well-planned, assertive approach is more likely to secure the needed support and maintain a good relationship with the person whose help we are seeking.

Making a Request for Affective Support

You are a senior nursing student. You have noticed that as each academic quarter begins your colleagues are becoming more and more competitive about grades. When grades are posted, students converge on the posting and hover around, checking out how each student did. Some students are very upset or depressed for days if they receive anything less than a B+.

There is less sharing of articles, ideas, and material that would help colleagues do well on assignments. Students are starting to hoard materials, hoping that another person will not do well if the material is not easily accessible. Trying to get the academic edge is the name of the game, and it has resulted in bickering, unfriendliness, and backbiting. You are aware of the loss of cooperation among your colleagues. This situation leaves you feeling isolated and bereft, and you sense it makes others feel that way too.

You decide to try to rectify or reverse the situation. After giving the matter some thought, you decide that the best strategy is to get your closest colleagues together and raise your concerns. Having the whole group present would provide more influence than trying to reach each person individually. You decide to invite your group over for coffee, with the plan to bring up your agenda.

In preparation, you think through how you will approach the topic. You decide to allow some time for chitchat and for everyone to get reacquainted. You plan to have coffee and snacks to break the ice and get everyone mixing. You decide that the best way to broach the subject is to begin with your feelings of loss. You don't want the discussion to disintegrate into a gripe session, so you come up with several suggestions that the group could consider.

In addition to planning the content, you spend time preparing yourself emotionally for the meeting with your fellow students. You envision yourself and your colleagues looking relaxed. You imagine that when you raise the issue of lack of cooperative support, your classmates will look interested and agree with your assessment of the situation. In your mind's eye, others look eager to return to more cooperative ways of relating to each other, and there are even suggestions from the group members.

When you are prepared, you carry out your plan. The following is what an assertive approach to your request for support might be like.

Assertive Approach

After your colleagues have enjoyed getting reacquainted, you bring up your issue in the following way:

Assertive you: "I'm really enjoying seeing all of you again. It's like old times. Something I've noticed as we get further along in the program is that we are becoming more obsessed with grades. It's really bothering me that we don't share ideas and materials the way we used to. It's as if we are all operating in isolation—each student for herself. It's too cutthroat for me. I'd like to propose that we restart our weekly study group so that we can share our ideas and knowledge as well as our books and articles. I think we could really help each other, and it would make us feel more like we were in this thing together instead of in competition. What do you think?"

Colleague: "I think it's a great idea. I've been feeling lonely for our shared times, but I guess I just assumed you guys were so 'nose to the grindstone' that you didn't need our group support. I'd love to start meeting again."

Another colleague: "I think it would be a good idea to make a list of what projects on which we are working and circulate it. Then when we find articles on someone's topic, we could let them know. It wouldn't take any more time, and it would really help us all out."

Another colleague: "I'm house-sitting for my brother, and he has a huge dining room table that we could use for our meetings."

Your assertive strategy worked. By putting effort into setting the scene and allowing the opportunity for people to realize how much they had missed each other, you furthered your cause immensely. By expressing your feelings, you avoided blaming anyone. Including a suggestion got the ball rolling and gave others a chance to present their ideas. It is likely that your strategy has set things in motion for securing the cooperative support you were after.

Consider how things might have gone if you had chosen a nonassertive approach.

Nonassertive Approach

When we are nonassertive, at some level we are conveying the feeling that we do not have much faith in ourselves or our ideas. If we are not able to convey that we believe strongly in what we are saying, it is highly unlikely that we will convince anyone else. Being nonassertive involves little advance preparation and little visualization of positive outcomes. When we are nonassertive, we look unsure and sound hesitant.

Here is what your strategy might have been like if you had taken a nonassertive approach.

You invite your colleagues over for coffee, and sooner or later the conversation rolls around to school and grades. Soon everyone is comparing how they are doing on their assignments, and an uncomfortable atmosphere of competition surfaces. You attempt to intervene as follows:

Nonassertive you: "Uh, this is the kind of thing I find so disappointing . . . I mean, all we ever talk about anymore is grades and who's got an A."

Colleague: "Well, it's only natural. That's what we're here for. Grades are the most important things in our lives as students."

Nonassertive you: "Well, they are important, I agree. But so is feeling good and sharing things with friends."

Colleague: "Yes, but when we get good grades that's the thing that makes us feel good these days."

Nonassertive you: "Well, I was wondering if we could help each other out more, like we used to do. Don't you ever long to get our study group together?"

Colleague: "Those days were fun. Now, though, we hardly take any of the same subjects. I'm afraid it would take more time and energy than I've got to get us together and make it time well spent."

Nonassertion got you nowhere except feeling more discouraged about the situation. By not presenting a positive, concrete solution to your complaints, you missed an opportunity to influence your colleagues' outlook on the situation. You avoided emphasizing the benefits of sharing, and consequently your colleagues swayed the argument to the negative aspects of meeting. Not only did you fail to obtain cooperation, but you are likely feeling disappointed in your lack of assertiveness.

Consider how the scene might change if you were aggressive.

Aggressive Approach

Although we may get what we want when we are aggressive, we lose out on the good feelings between ourselves and the other person. Sometimes the bad feelings generated by aggressiveness take extensive time to repair.

Here is one possible scenario if you were to use an aggressive approach:

Aggressive you: "Come on, you guys, stop talking about school and grades. I've had enough of it. You've got your heads buried so deeply in the books that you can't even take time to have fun. I remember when you used to be a fun group to be with. Now I get the feeling that if anyone does well, it's like stealing points from someone else. When are you going to wake up and realize that those little numbers on your papers aren't nearly as important as having some contact as people?"

Colleague: "Well, you may not care about grades, but I do. I might want to go to graduate school some day, and my grades have to be good. You don't even take that into consideration."

Another colleague: "If you can't even see how important school is to some of us, then there's no point in getting together. I think we're on different wavelengths."

By being aggressive, you have further ostracized yourself from your colleagues. Your demonstration of insensitivity about the value your friends put on school has cost you their cooperation. By not seeing things through their eyes, you have lost your connection to a valuable source of support.

Making a Request for Physical Support

You are a nurse working on a surgical unit in a general hospital. About 6 months ago, the head nurse asked all nursing personnel to complete a health history on newly admitted clients. Part of this history involves asking personal questions about, for example, drug use, religious beliefs, and sleeping habits. Any information that might be important for the nursing staff to know about clients who will be undergoing anesthesia is included. There is no place to interview clients in private on your unit, and you have felt uncomfortable asking clients some of these questions within the hearing range of other clients and staff. To complete these initial histories, you need the physical support of adequate private space.

You have identified what dissatisfies you about the lack of private space; now you need to decide how you would like to see things changed. You know there is absolutely no possibility of getting a room designated for interviewing alone because of budget cutbacks. What would be satisfactory is a room that could be booked in advance for a private interview with clients and used for other purposes as well. There is a room on the unit that is designated for Dr. Gait, the physician in charge of the unit. She makes rounds each morning and occasionally uses her room then, but at other times it is not used by anyone. You decide to attempt to secure access to Dr. Gait's office for the purpose of completing the initial histories on clients. It is important to have the privacy, and you are certain that you can complete the histories more accurately if you have it.

Having decided to seek support, the next step is to determine how to go about acquiring it. The interpersonal style you use to make your request will greatly influence the outcome. A meek or indirect approach leaves you open to being misunderstood or ignored. An aggressive or overly confrontational presentation will put others on the defensive and likely result in rejection. A balance of speaking up for your rights for support without hurting others is what the situation requires.

You already know that the other nurses on the unit agree that a private room is necessary. The lines of communication on the unit dictate that you should make your request to the head nurse. You decide that she needs some advance notice about the issue, and you approach her with a request for a meeting time to discuss the issue. Your request for a meeting is simple, straightforward, and clear:

Assertive you: "Ms. Peters, I would like to make an appointment with you to discuss the need for some private space in which to conduct our initial histories. I'm on duty for the next 3 days. Do you have about 15 or 20 minutes during that time when I can discuss this matter with you?"

Once the meeting has been arranged, you need to plan your strategy. You have asked for about 15 minutes during which time you must convince Ms. Peters of the importance of having a private place to interview clients. You prepare for the meeting by itemizing all the reasons you and your colleagues have concerning the need for privacy. You are well aware that you will have more success in getting your request granted if you can present a reasonable solution, so you itemize the reasons for using Dr. Gait's office.

Having secured your facts, you now ready for your encounter with Ms. Peters. You prepare by visualizing yourself talking to her in a relaxed, confident manner. In your mind's eye, you envision her listening to you intently, nodding her head in agreement with the points you are making. You imagine yourself successfully countering any arguments she has against the use of Dr. Gait's office. All in all, your mental rehearsal of the meeting is successful, which increases your confidence.

Here is an example of how your meeting with your head nurse, Ms. Peters, might go if you were assertive.

Assertive Approach

Assertive you: "Thank you for setting aside the time to meet with me, Ms. Peters. As you know, I wish to discuss the need for some private space to complete the initial health histories on our clients. I've talked to the other nurses, and we all agree that the histories provide some important information about our clients that increases their safety in undergoing anesthesia. Also, it gives us a chance to relax the clients and put them at ease. However, there is one major problem we have encountered. There is no designated space for us to talk to our clients, so we end up interviewing them in the corridor, or their rooms, or in the sunroom; in all these locations what they say can be overheard by other clients and staff. We are concerned that some clients may hold back information about themselves that might be important because of the lack of confidentiality. We would like to have a room in which we could take newly admitted clients and interview them in private. A little checking shows that Dr. Gait rarely uses her office in the afternoons. The other nurses and I suggest that Dr. Gait's office might be a place we could use. What do you think of this idea?"

Ms. Peters: "I can see your point about the privacy. As you know, I'm interested in having the histories completed, so I would like to push for a room if the privacy will mean that the histories will be more accurate. In the past Dr. Gait has wanted her office off-limits to nurses because she has done her dictating and teaching to her residents in there. But from what you are saying, she doesn't use the office for those purposes anymore. I will talk to her about making her office available to our nursing staff in the afternoons. Thank you for your interest and your suggestions."

Your assertive strategy worked. By stating that you and your colleagues supported the history taking, you avoided putting your head nurse on the defensive and you invited her to listen. Your reasons for needing a private room were sound on two counts: client safety and client respect. Your astute inclusion of the data about the vacancy of Dr. Gait's office added credibility to your suggestion. You ended your suggestion by respectfully asking for the head nurse's opinion. Your delivery was forthright. Never once did you beat around the bush or sound hesitant. You did not even have to rush because you had already made an appointment with your head nurse.

Here are some examples of ineffective ways to make the same request for a private room.

Nonassertive Approach

When we are nonassertive, we do not give full credit to our needs. We act shy or make light of factors that are really important to us. When we avoid expressing ourselves clearly and forthrightly, we waive control over our legitimate rights. Being nonassertive invites others to walk all over us.

In this situation, a nonassertive nurse would not likely book time with her manager but probably would hope that she could catch the head nurse's attention without advance notice. Nonassertive nurses would not likely plan an effective strategy in advance and would not envision themselves being successful. Verbally nonassertive approaches are limp and unclear,

and do not convey confidence or conviction. Here is an example of nonassertion:

Nonassertive you: "Uh, Ms. Peters, do you have a few minutes?"

Ms. Peters has no idea what you want to talk to her about, nor how long it will take. If she is a typically busy head nurse, she will probably have other things planned for that moment.

Ms. Peters: "I can see you briefly. What is it about?"
Nonassertive you: "Well, it's about those histories you want us to take from the new clients. I think it's rather hard . . . I mean, sometimes there are so many people around. It's hard to talk to the clients when there's no privacy, do you know what I mean? Something's really got to be done, I think."

It is possible that this approach may put Ms. Peters on the defensive. By not finishing your sentence you have given the impression that completing the histories is difficult. You have provided no rationale for the idea that privacy is essential. By not clearly explaining your points, you are ensuring that Ms. Peters will not understand and consequently will not be sympathetic to your cause.

Ms. Peters: "Well, I realize that it might be difficult to do the histories, but it's essential that the information be collected. Client safety in the operating room depends on this information."
Nonassertive you: "Uh, yes . . . it is important. It's just that, you know, it's hard to talk to the clients when there are other people around. Isn't there a quiet place we could go to? How about Dr. Gait's office?"
Ms. Peters: "Well, you know that she needs her office to be available to her. You can always use a quiet corner of the sunroom, or even ask the other clients to leave the room if you want to have a private interview."
Nonassertive you: "Yeah . . . I guess so. I haven't tried that yet. Maybe that'll work . . . I hate to ask a client to leave . . . but I'll give it a try."

You have lost your case. By not being clear about what you wanted and not defending your suggestion, you have permitted your manager to overlook your suggestion and to force you to continue taking histories the way you have been doing. Had you better prepared your defense and your speech, you might have secured the support you were requesting.

Aggressive Approach

When we behave aggressively, we forget to give due respect to the other person's rights. We become so intent on getting what we want that we tend to bulldoze the other person. Here is an example of an aggressive approach to trying to secure a private place for interviewing:

> *Aggressive you:* "Ms. Peters, I need to see you as soon as possible about the initial histories. When can you see me? Today?"

This rush on Ms. Peters does not give her much breathing space. You have indicated there is urgency about your need to see her that is out of proportion to the truth. In no way have you respected her own timetable or any agenda she may wish to complete. She is probably already on the defensive.

When you get to see Ms. Peters, you begin as follows:

> *Aggressive you:* "You've got to do something about getting us a quiet place to do these initial histories you want done on all the clients. It's impossible to do them when everyone can hear what you are saying. How would you like to spill your guts about your sex life or pills you take when every client and staff member around can hear? If you don't get us a quiet place, then they just won't be done right. Why can't we use Dr. Gait's office? We nurses don't have any private space, and this one doctor has a whole office to herself, even when she's not around."
>
> *Ms. Peters:* "It's not up to you to dictate how the office space will be assigned on the unit. When you've learned proper etiquette and protocol, I'd be glad to discuss this issue with you. In the meantime, do the best you can. That'll be all for today."

You have made your dissatisfaction very clear. In the process of doing so, however, you have put your manager on the defensive and created a rift between you. There are now two problems to be solved: the lack of privacy and the discord between the two of you. When you attack other people, they are likely to divert energy to their injured feelings instead of attending to the issue for which you are fighting. Using an aggressive approach diminishes the chances that you will secure the physical support you were hoping to get.

Planning an Assertive Strategy for Making Requests

The preceding examples illustrate the importance of planning and implementing an assertive strategy for seeking cognitive, affective, or physical support. If it is important for you to have the support you have identified, then it is important to invest the time and energy to secure it. As a nurse, you spend considerable energy trying to meet your clients' needs for support. If you can secure the support you need at work or school, then it is more likely that you will have the energy to extend support to your clients and colleagues. Nurses who keep on giving without adequate cognitive, affective, or physical support are draining their own reserves. We spend a lot of time trying to get our clients to take care of their health; securing the support we need as nurses provides them with an example to follow.

Just because you use an assertive approach does not mean that you will get the support you seek. Sometimes support is not forthcoming, no matter what strategy is used. On occasion your colleagues may not have the interest or skills to support you. Other times there may not be the money or time to provide you with the support you are seeking. At those times you must decide whether you can continue to work in the system without the support. If you cannot secure the support you need from others at work or school, you may be able to get some support from friends or family to see you through. Only you can decide whether the support is adequate. Because you are the seeker and receiver, it is your perception of the support that is important.

Providing Support at Work and School

The CAPS (Cognitive, Affective, Physical Support) framework is helpful for articulating exactly what support you need at work and school. It can also be a guideline to help you determine your colleagues' need for support. Support is a nebulous concept; breaking it down into cognitive, affective, and physical components helps you to decipher your colleagues' needs for support. One way to obtain support is to offer it to others. In so doing, a bond is built between you that encourages both parties to give and take. Contributing to the effort to build a solid support system at work and school will add to your feelings of confidence and competence. It is worth the effort to learn the assertive way to make requests for the support you need.

Looking for a Mentor

Murray looks to Greek mythology for the definition of a mentor as "loyal friend and advisor of Odysseus and teacher of his son, Telemachus" (1999, p. 1). In business, a mentor takes a mentee, the one mentored, "under his wing" to help him or her advance. Murray (1999) further describes a mentor in nursing as one who represents excellence in knowledge, skill, and competence. She adds that affective components necessary for a mentor are warmth, acceptance, friendliness, empathy, compassion, patience, a willingness to learn from many sources, including the mentee, generosity, and a willingness to share what one knows and rejoice when another excels and surpasses. McMahon (2005) describes her first 6 months as a new nurse as a difficult time during which she felt she had to prove herself in a hostile environment without support. Yet, when she confided in a nurse from another unit whose leadership skills she admired, she found herself in her first mentoring situation. She had expressed her thoughts and feelings and opened the door to get just the support she needed to grow into her new role. How did she do this? She identified her problem, assessed who was a safe person to whom she could ventilate, expressed her thoughts and feelings, and built a rapport with someone who was able to mentor her.

What roles does a mentor fulfill? Servodidio (2006) identifies the roles as counselor, coach, role model, advocate, and energizer. Mentors have a positive outlook, they are loyal and nurturing, they enjoy nursing, and they have superior communications skills. As a new nurse consider trying to find a mentor through professional associations, networking at organization events, and explore online mentoring (McMahon, 2005). Consider, too, what qualities you have and can develop that would make you a good mentor as you develop your professional career. Look for "teachable moments" that you can use to teach others (Servodidio, 2006). As you move and grow in comfort with your knowledge and skills, consider how you can offer support to new graduates or nurses new to your work setting.

Remembering That We're All in This Together

The changing healthcare climate makes the ability to ask for and give support an imperative. The healthcare industry and other industries are responding to economic concerns by decreasing staff, by reassigning the work of staff whose positions are not filled when vacated, and by cross training. Charlie Brown's friend Linus clings to his tattered blanket to help face change. Koerner (1994) sees Linus's strategy as similar to that of nurses who expect job security by competently performing all the tasks they have always done. She suggests that only by "re-scripting our roles and relationships can true transformation occur to create a care delivery system that is relevant to the changing needs of the twenty-first century society." Like the anthropologist Bateson (2010), she sees us needing to rely on the skills of improvisation and adds the skill of imagination. She suggests that role relationships are not predetermined but must be renegotiated. This involves the ability to be aware of the needs of others and of ourselves, to be able to give and seek the support necessary to cope with the ambiguity of change. Imagination helps us to see new ways of working together to respond to change. We must come to see that security lies not in the job itself but in our own demonstration of innovation and flexibility (Koerner, 1994). The ability to know what we need and how to ask for support is increasingly important to move beyond our fears and face the challenge of change.

Ulrich and Ulrich (2010) in their book *The Why of Work* challenge us to look for meaning in our work, to look for opportunities to use our talents to pursue our aspirations, and to work synergistically with others with creativity, resilience, hope, and resourcefulness in a work environment in which we can all thrive. To be able to do this you must identify what you need to enable you to do your best work and seek the support needed. Look for ways to incorporate skills you want to grow at work and interests you have that might add value in the work setting, thus making it more likely colleagues will support you. Perhaps you have organization skills or computer skills that might be useful in problem solving. This process, called "job crafting," may help you and others embellish the work with individual gifts and talents (Wrzesniewski et al, 2010). Remember, we are all in this together.

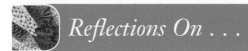

Reflections On . . .

Requesting Support

Consider what you read about the importance of support. Can you identify your own need for support? How can you get what you need? Answer the following questions.

What? . . .

Write one thing you learned from this chapter.

So what? . . .

How will this affect your nursing practice?

Now what? . . .

How will you implement this new knowledge or skill?

Think about it . . .

Practicing Requesting Support

Exercise 1

For this exercise, work in groups of three. One person requests support from another in your group. The third person gives feedback on how assertively the requester sought support. When you are the requester, choose one of the cognitive, affective, or physical supports that you would like to secure. Explain to the person role-playing the provider of this support some details of his or her role (the provider is a teacher, a colleague, etc.).

When you are clear about your roles, act out a scene in which you request support. After you have completed your request, seek feedback from the person providing the support and the feedback giver on how assertive you were in making your request.

What have you learned about your ability to be assertive in requesting support? Where do you excel in being assertive? What suggestions do you have for improving your ability to be assertive?

Switch roles so that each person has the opportunity to role-play the requester, the provider, and the feedback giver.

After you have done this exercise in your small group, join your colleagues in the rest of the class and compare what you have learned about requesting support.

Exercise 2

Being aware of the environment includes an awareness of your own limitations as well as knowledge concerning the capacity of those around you. Effective teams "watch each other's backs." Mutual support is an important teamwork behavior and requires knowing our own limitations in delivering safe care and maintaining a watchful eye across the team. Write a reflective case study at the end of your clinical experience according to the following:

- Identify instances in which you felt you needed assistance in completing care assigned to you.
- Which team member did you ask to assist you?
- What influenced your decision to ask this person?
- How can you use improved self-awareness to recognize your limitations to stay within a safety zone but also continue to expand your learning?
- What is your response when you notice another team member needs assistance?
- How does the concept of mutual support influence a culture of safety?

QSEN Competencies: Teamwork and Collaboration; Safety

Exercise 3

Consider your personal support system. Make a list of people, relatives, and friends from whom you might be able to ask for support. Write a journal entry about strengths and weaknesses in your personal support system. Identify what support you might need and what support you might be able to offer others. If you have difficulty asking others for help consider a quote from a cancer patient in an I Can Cope cancer support program. "When you refuse to ask others to help, you deny them the pleasure you get when you are able to help another."

Exercise 4

Search www.google.com or your favorite search engine to learn about possibilities for online mentors. Explore articles such sites offer that further describe the role of mentor and nurse who is mentored.

Moments of Connection...
The Loss of a Cat, a Friend, a Companion
A nurse was finding it hard to concentrate at work and was often moved to tears. "I was just on overload. My husband had just asked for a divorce. I was worried about being a single parent and how I would survive financially. It was just so overwhelming. Then we had to have our cat put to sleep because of massive cancer. I knew only one person would really understand: the oncology supervisor. She responded right away when I told her about the cat. She's an animal lover, too. I made an appointment to see her on my lunch break. She listened and really knew my grief was just compounded. It's like losing a child. She didn't make fun of me. She is so special."

WIT&*Wisdom*

Why Not?

Marion was a hospice client whose speech was limited after having had a stroke. One thing she could clearly say was, "Why not?" She would say it with a different voice inflection depending on what she was trying to communicate. It became almost a life philosophy. Take a risk . . . ask for what you want and need . . . allow others to have an opportunity to help you . . . your might just be surprised . . . "Why not?"

References

Adams MH, Bowden AG, Humphrey DS, et al: Social support and health promotion lifestyles of rural women, *J Rural Nurs Health Care* 1(1), 2000. Available from http://www.rno.org/journal/index.php/online-journal/article/viewFile/65/64.

American Nurses Credentialing Center (website). www.nursingworld.org/ancc. Accessed December 10, 2010.

Bateson MC: *Composing a further life: the age of active wisdom*, New York, 2010, Knopf.

Callahan M: Applauding the artistry of nursing, *Nursing* 20(10):63, 1990.

Dennison S: Peer Mentoring: Untapped potential, *J Nurs Educ* 49(6):340, 2010.

Doherty R: Tune up your employee retention efforts, *Healthcare Rev* 15(6):11, 2002.

Dutton JE, Frost PJ, Worline MC, et al: Leading in times of trauma, *Harv Bus Rev* 80(1):55, 2002.

Fox KC: Mentor program boosts new nurses' satisfaction and lowers turnover rate, *J Contin Educ Nurs* 41(7):311, 2010.

Ingala J, Hill K: Building two-way streets, *Nurs Manage* 32(5):34, 2001.

Kerfoot K: The leader as retention specialist, *Urol Nurs* 21(4):298, 2001.

Koerner J: Drawing on the art of nursing practice, *J Prof Nurs* 10(2):68, 1994.

Komaratat S, Oumtanee A: Using a mentorship model to prepare newly graduated nurses for competency, *J Contin Educ Nurs* 40(10):475, 2009.

Komblith AB, Herndon JE II, Zuckerman E, et al: Cancer and Leukemia Group B: Social support as a buffer to the psychological impact of stressful life events in women with breast cancer, *Cancer* 91(2):443, 2001.

Mahan PL, Mahan MP, Park N, et al: Work environment stressors, social support, anxiety, and depression among secondary school teachers, *AAOHN J* 58(5):197, 2010.

McMahon L: Mentoring: a means of healing new nurses, *Holist Nurs Pract* 19(5):195, 2005.

Murray R: What does it mean to be a mentor? Presentation at the Fall Faculty Senate Assembly November 16, 1999, upon receiving the Saint Louis University 1999 Burlington Northern Faculty Excellence in Teach Award (website). http://www.slu.edu/organizations/fs/resources/Murray.html. Accessed June 19, 2006.

Sala RD: A message from one of our sponsors, St Joseph Hospital uses creative ways to retain nursing staff, *Healthcare Rev* 15(4):23, 2002.

Servodidio C: Oncology nurses of today mentor the cancer caregivers of tomorrow, *ONS News* 21(2):1, 2006.

Ulrich D, Ulrich W: *The why of work*, New York, 2010, McGraw Hill.

Wrzesniewski A, Berg JM, Dutton JE: Turn the job you have into the job you want, *Harv Bus Rev* 88(6):127, June 2010.

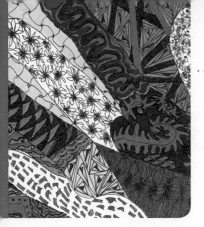

Chapter 18

Overcoming Evaluation Anxiety

> *The enemy of the good is the better.*
>
> **Unknown**

Objectives

1. Define evaluation anxiety
2. Describe characteristics of evaluation anxiety
3. Identify strategies to handle job performance appraisals assertively
4. Discuss techniques to decrease test anxiety
5. Identify benefits of criticism
6. Identify assertive strategies to handle difficult situations in student performance evaluations
7. Participate in exercises to overcome evaluation anxiety

Defining Evaluation Anxiety

Pause for a moment and take a deep breath. Reflect on the old saying, "To err is human." Yes, it applies to all of us. We know this and yet we still think we have to be perfect. In our competitive culture we idolize excellence in personal performance, products, and services. Advertisements about "better" or "improved" products bombard us from billboards, radio, and TV. We spend years in an educational system that makes judgments about our physical and psychological abilities through a variety of examinations and elaborate grading systems. Emphasis on standardized achievement testing in American school systems has increased with the passage in 2001 of House Resolution 1, the No Child Left Behind Act, and has made for high stakes in test taking. Making mistakes is the antithesis of our cultural standard for excellence. Because of our preoccupation with perfection, it is difficult to believe that making mistakes is a normal part of human endeavor. We face these unrealistic expectations whenever we are in a situation in which our knowledge, skills, and behavior must be evaluated. In this chapter you will learn how to approach evaluations, test taking, and criticism in more positive ways so you can learn from them. These approaches will help you as a student and throughout your career as a nurse.

Evaluation anxiety occurs when we are upset about having our performance judged and are intimidated by the evaluation process. We cannot directly control others' responses to our work, and overvaluing the responses of others creates a kind of anxiety that interferes with performing at our best. One form of evaluation anxiety is test anxiety, which has negative effects on academic performance (Bowie, 2010; Black et al, 2008). For nursing students, test anxiety can be evident in both written examinations and evaluations of clinical proficiency. Instead of focusing on relevant parts of a task, students with high test anxiety worry about how they are performing and how well others are doing and ruminate about alternatives (Meichenbaum, 1972). High test anxiety is associated with intrusion of irrelevant thoughts such as preoccupation with feelings of inadequacy, anticipation of punishment, and loss of status and esteem.

Accompanying these cognitive aspects of test anxiety are emotionality, the autonomic arousal aspect of anxiety, and a variety of physical symptoms including increased heart rate, increased muscular tension, gastrointestinal changes, changes in breathing, and dietary and sleep pattern disturbances (Meichenbaum, 1972). These physiological symptoms are distressing and must be alleviated just as much as negative thought processes. Learning to relax and decrease unpleasant symptoms helps diminish their negative effects.

One of the most significant and recurring problems experienced by health professionals is a fear of making a mistake and being evaluated negatively. Clinicians in practice have revealed fears about committing errors in diagnosis or treatment. Nursing students and nurses, too, fear making mistakes.

Examples of other nursing situations that engender anxiety in students are the initial clinical experience on a unit, nursing procedures, hospital equipment, patient simulators, evaluation by faculty, observation by instructors, tardiness, and conversations with physicians (Kaplan and Ura, 2010; Moscaritolo, 2010).

The two major factors underlying our evaluation anxiety as nurses are concern for client safety and concern for our own security.

WIT&*Wisdom*

No Knowing, No Growing
It's safe to perform
Your tasks, do your duty.
Look inside yourself
And see only beauty.
Have you the courage
To ask for inspection?
Can you face hearing
You're less than perfection?
Have you learned yet
We're better for knowing?
To take bad with good,
A chance to keep growing.

Concern for Client Safety

Nursing involves caring for the health of fellow human beings. Health is a precious commodity, which makes the stakes high if a nursing error negatively impacts our clients' health or pushes them into illness. This responsibility underlies our anxiety about making an error in our nursing practice.

Concern for Our Own Security

Clients are becoming more knowledgeable and critical about healthcare and its cost. No longer content to passively submit to treatment, consumers of healthcare are demanding to know the rationale for regimens and to have access to a second opinion. In extreme cases clients are suing physicians and other healthcare professionals, including nurses, for ineffective healthcare. This potential threat from clients represents a powerful source of disapproval, with implications for career advancement and public embarrassment. The loss of your job and financial assets could also result from unsafe care. Today, nurses are aware of their accountability for the nursing care provided and their vulnerability to investigations of these actions through the legal process.

Evaluation anxiety is an unpleasant, ever-lurking phenomenon that threatens nurses and other health professionals. As nurses, we are committed to making a positive difference for our clients, yet today's work environments are loaded with potential deterrents to this goal: inadequate staffing, the more acute health conditions of clients, technological complexity, information overload, and the uncertainty of healthcare reform. In its mildest form, evaluation anxiety can detract from enjoyment in the workplace; when strong, it can be overwhelming and interfere with our ability to perform competently as nurses.

As nursing students, or as practicing registered nurses, we need to develop ways to minimize evaluation anxiety so that we can confidently handle clinical or written examinations, job performance appraisals, and everyday criticisms—all naturally recurring events in the professional life of nurses.

Characteristics of Evaluation Anxiety

People who suffer from evaluation anxiety exhibit ways of thinking that make them feel uneasy and interfere with their ability to perform in adaptive ways. Those experiencing evaluation anxiety have been reported in the literature to have the following characteristics (Dweck and Wortman, 1982; Wine, 1982):

- *Self-focus versus task focus.* Some people spend more time thinking about their performance than they do completing the actual task. Attention to their performance detracts from the necessary attention needed to do the task adequately. Self-focused thoughts are negative and self-devaluing, and they lead to self-doubt. Not only does a focus on self versus task detract from task performance, but the focus on negative aspects of one's performance engenders feelings of anxiety.
- *Self-blame.* Some people with evaluation anxiety tend to blame themselves for their poor performance more than they blame circumstances or other external factors.
- *Worry and concern about evaluation.* People with high evaluation anxiety tend to place great emphasis on how they are doing in comparison to others and how the examiner is evaluating them.

Those with low evaluation anxiety react to performance evaluation with an external, situational, task-oriented focus. For those with high evaluation anxiety, failure signifies a lack of ability. Those with low evaluation anxiety generate thoughts about the task or situation that encourage solutions or completion of the task, whereas those with high evaluation anxiety give up and see themselves as the main reason for failure.

High-anxiety individuals do not fully explore options such as trying different strategies or looking for an external causative factor, which leaves them with feelings of failure and uneasiness. Mistakes are interpreted as failures, not as stepping stones in the process of discovering the best solution. People with high performance anxiety tend to attribute success to factors other than their own ability, yet they readily assume that failure is their own doing. This view leads to feelings of pressure in every new achievement situation (Dweck and Wortman, 1982; Wine, 1982). Consider, too, the effect of past negative experiences on the evaluation process. Students and nurses with previous work experience who have had a traumatic incident in performance appraisal may have so much anxiety that the process is highly emotionally charged (Marquis and Huston, 1998). It is useful to spend some time reflecting on your fears and worries to determine how realistic they are.

In our culture it is easy to berate ourselves when we make a mistake. In addition to our self-chastisement we sometimes invent disapproval or exaggerate the disapproval of others. How we internally evaluate ourselves can be constructive or destructive.

Examples of constructive and destructive thoughts in relation to being evaluated are given in Table 18-1.

Gaining Control over Your Evaluation Anxiety

Knight (2011), on the management faculty in the graduate program at the University of Pennsylvania, observes that students who are afraid of evaluation are

Table 18-1 *Constructive and Destructive Self-Thoughts*

CONSTRUCTIVE THOUGHTS	DESTRUCTIVE THOUGHTS
"I'm doing a good job. I can't do everything I'd like to do for my clients today because we're short-staffed, but I'll make sure I do the most important things."	"I've got to do everything for my clients or I'll feel like a failure." "If I don't do everything just perfectly, I'll be letting down my clients and the rest of the team."
"I've done the important things I can for the clients on the unit. Now I'll prepare a concise report for the evening staff."	"How can I possibly explain to the evening staff that I didn't get everything done on the day shift? They'll think I'm incompetent and disorganized."
"One thing I didn't make arrangements for was an extra load of linen for the evening staff. Now that I know you have to put your order in before 1 PM, I won't forget in the future."	"They're going to crucify me for not arranging an extra load of linen. They'll be mad at me for days for that mistake."
I can go home knowing I did the best I could today. It was very busy and we were short-staffed this evening but we gave our clients the best care we could under the circumstances."	"What a day! All I can think about is what still needs to be done. I'll be miserable mulling over how I could have done things better."

rendered incapable of engaging with a topic of learning and seeing it from multiple perspectives due to their fear of being wrong.

Because evaluation anxiety affects cognitive, affective, and psychomotor dimensions, a multifaceted approach is needed to help overcome it.

- You can use positive self-talk (see Chapter 22) to overcome your self-defeating internal dialogue. Making sure that your inner voice is reassuring comforts you in your day-to-day activities and during those times when you are having an examination or a performance appraisal.
- Relaxation (see Chapter 20) helps you focus on the task and act more efficiently. You feel more at ease and overcome the negative physiological effects of evaluation anxiety when you relax.
- Imagery (see Chapter 21) helps you picture yourself performing in a way that makes you feel good about yourself. Your positive visualizations keep you focused on performing your best and engender positive feelings that overpower the uneasiness generated by your anxiety.
- Learning how to make use of feedback from others (see Chapter 19) helps you prepare yourself for situations in which your performance is evaluated. Practice sessions with helpful colleagues can boost your confidence.

In addition to these four approaches, avoiding errors requires thinking before acting. Using the nursing process on a consistent basis helps to ensure that your nursing actions are safe, ethical, and helpful.

Handling Job Performance Appraisals Assertively

At many points in our nursing careers we receive both formal and informal evaluations of our performance. For us, the purpose of these evaluations is to learn what we are doing well (so that we can continue to do it) and where we need to improve our work performance. For the employer, evaluations serve as a check on whether employees are fulfilling the expectations of the work contract.

Evaluations are helpful to both parties and should occur regularly. As the employee, you can take an assertive approach to evaluations, which will help ease your anxiety. The following sections describe several assertive steps you can take to prepare for an evaluation. The example given is for a nurse employed in service.

As a student nurse, apply the same preparatory procedures for evaluations at your school of nursing. It is helpful early in your course or clinical experience to carefully read the guidelines for successful completion and clarify anything you do not understand. Review clinical competencies, procedures, and behaviors expected for this clinical rotation. Keep your own documentation of the completion of specific requirements in a clinical rotation and bring this to an evaluation meeting. Pay attention to the details of assignments on course syllabi.

Before Your Evaluation

1. Find out the schedule for evaluations in your agency. Many agencies offer an evaluation for new employees after 3 to 6 months of probationary employment and yearly thereafter.
2. Find out in advance the criteria by which your employer will be evaluating you. Having this information gives you the chance to make notes about how you think you have met the standards expected of someone in your position.
3. If your employer does not have a set of standard criteria for evaluation, suggest that one be developed soon. Request that your job description or the standards of nursing care prepared by your professional nursing association be used as the reference for determining your performance level.
4. Review what you and your colleagues in similar nursing positions actually do in the workplace. Compare this time and task allotment with what your job description outlines. At your evaluation, point out any discrepancies to your employer. If job descriptions are not updated, you may find that a significant part of your daily work is not being acknowledged.
5. Prepare your own evaluation of your work performance before meeting with your employer. Go to your appointment armed with specific examples of how you have met the requirements of your job description. Be aware of where you need to improve and what support you will need from your head nurse to make the necessary changes.
6. Develop goals toward which you would like to work. Be as clear, realistic, and specific as possible in the preparation of these work objectives so that you can articulate them clearly in your performance evaluation.
7. If the date at which your evaluation should have occurred passes, request an evaluation from your

employer. Evaluations protect you by providing guidelines for maintaining or changing your professional behavior. You need feedback to know if your nursing care is within the legal and qualitative expectations of your agency.

8. Prepare mentally for your evaluation interview by ensuring that your self-talk is encouraging and visualize yourself looking and feeling calm and confident during your interview.

During Your Evaluation

1. Inform your employer that you wish to discuss your goals at some time during the interview.

2. Allow your employer uninterrupted time to comment about your work.

3. Ask for clarification of any points that are not understandable. Request evidence of your employer's points so that comments are backed up with examples. These illustrations clarify the kind of behavior your employer expects.

4. Your employer may have suggestions about ways in which you can improve your performance. Agree only to those changes that are realistic given your time and potential and the support available in the workplace.

5. Share your performance goals with your employer and ask for support for the achievement of your career plans. Ask your employer for a list of goals toward which you should be working.

6. Do not sign your evaluation until you are fully satisfied that it is an accurate and fair assessment of how you do your job.

7. Thank your employer for the supervision and the feedback you receive.

8. Come to an agreement about the date for your next evaluation.

After Your Evaluation

1. Take time to reflect on how you handled the evaluation. Praise yourself for the ways you handled yourself assertively. Make note of things you would like to do differently in your next evaluation interview.

2. Follow up on the goals you and your employer set. Take time to develop your strategy to achieve your objectives and set intermediate and final deadlines. Think about people and resources you can tap to help develop your talents.

3. Keep a diary of your work performance in preparation for your next performance evaluation.

Consider the maxim to "underpromise and overdeliver." If you are asked when you can finish a project, overestimate the time it will take. When you deliver the results prior to the agreed upon date, you distinguish yourself. Avoid the temptation to give a date earlier than is reasonable in order to look good at the moment. Nurses following this practice should not feel anxious at job appraisal time.

Moments of Connection . . .
Beyond the Call of Duty

"A young woman with a newborn child and very poor support systems was angry at the world because of chronic pain from a neck and back injury. She would refuse treatment and medications, yet was angry that we wouldn't do anything to stop her pain. It was hard to continue to interact with her, knowing that she would be critical of everything we did. After a period of months of contact with her, just listening to her, not becoming offended by her attacks, and understanding what she was experiencing, she now relies on me as her support. In a crisis she will call. I calm her and help her think through the situation. Although this is beyond the normal attention given to a client, it is a special connection that can assist her to build her problem-solving skills, cope, and receive the care she needs, by simply offering caring and understanding."

Assessing the Validity and Reliability of an Employer's Appraisal System

The performance appraisal process should provide nurses with an evaluative component that rates their nursing behavior against established criteria and a career developmental component that seeks to improve their nursing performance through self-learning and growth (Flanagan, 1995). Many appraisal systems that fail to provide the necessary input or feedback to enhance employee performance do so for some, or all, of the following reasons (Flanagan, 1995):

- *The appraisal process is conducted by upper management rather than by the nurse employee's immediate supervisor.* Performance appraisal is best handled at the management level closest to the nurse, by supervisors who have firsthand knowledge of the work performance.

- *A single appraisal tool is used to evaluate all employees.* A nurse's job description should form the basis of any performance evaluation, anchoring the appraisal with a pertinent and appropriate focus.
- *Evaluation and assessment focus on personal traits rather than work behavior.* Using the nurse's job description as a reference focuses on observable, measurable behaviors.
- *Behaviors that are the subject of evaluation or assessment fail to reflect the major substance of a specific job.* A job description enumerates precise job content, including nursing duties, nursing activities to be performed, nursing responsibilities, and results expected by the nurse's employer.
- *The weighting of traits and behaviors does not reflect their significance in the performance of a specific job.* Ideally, a nurse and a supervisor develop the job description in concert so that both parties have a clear understanding of the job expectations at the outset.
- *Criteria for identifying an acceptable level of performance are vague, which leave them open to varying interpretations.* Tasks included in a nurse's job description should be specific and comprehensive and stated in action verbs, which minimizes the likelihood that the nurse will be evaluated on insignificant job behavior or personal traits. Acceptable levels of nurse performance must be clearly defined. If rating scales are used, the meaning of each rating should be open to a single interpretation.
- *Little or no informal feedback is given on job performance, and formal evaluation occurs infrequently.* The appraisal system should allow for sufficient interaction throughout the process. Job performance appraisal should entail systematic assessment and evaluation throughout the designated period. Feedback (employment counseling or coaching) should be ongoing and should include recommendations for improvement. The more frequent the evaluation of job performance, the more likely nurses are to view the evaluation as guidance and thus find the appraisal less stressful.

If you do your part to ensure that your job performance appraisals are objective, fair, and frequent, you will do much to minimize your own evaluation anxiety.

Coping with the Anxiety of Written Examinations

Taking examinations is part of student life. Even as a registered nurse, you may find yourself preparing for an examination as part of a continuing education course or degree program. Your grade symbolizes the level of achievement you have attained at a given point. Many examinations offer only one chance to demonstrate your knowledge or skill, so you may feel anxious about performing well at the time of the examination. The following sections describe some assertive steps you can take to make you feel better prepared and less anxious about examinations.

Before Your Examination

1. Find out all you can about what content (or skill) will be tested on the examination. This knowledge helps you narrow down the material to study.
2. Review the objectives for the course and focus on content that directly relates to these objectives.
3. Find out the format of the examination (whether it is multiple choice or essay). This information determines your study approach.
4. If you need guidance on how to study, consult your teachers, the counseling center, or a study guide.
5. Consider forming or joining a study group. Effective study groups can make preparation for examinations fun and fruitful.
6. Make a realistic timetable of study preparations for the examination and stick to it. Keeping pace with your schedule helps you integrate the material you are studying. If you are rushed, prioritize what is important to learn and cover it first.
7. Find out where the examination is being held and familiarize yourself with the room. Choose a seat where you will be comfortable. Be sure you know the exact hour of the examination.
8. Make sure you have all the necessary tools to help you in the examination, such as a calculator with a spare battery, sharpened pencils, a watch, tissues, and your good luck charm!
9. Mentally prepare before the examination by visualizing yourself in the examination room looking calm and smiling as you read the questions because you know the answers. As you study for the examination, be sure that your self-talk is positive. Tell yourself that you are learning and that you are covering the material in a sensible way. Encourage yourself and do not allow self-defeating thoughts about failure or mistakes to take over your internal dialogue.
10. Put yourself through a dry run of the examination. If it is a written test, obtain examinations from previous years and complete them in the specified

time limits. If there are no old examinations, make up your own questions and answer them in a simulated examination situation. If you are being examined on your nursing technique, perform the procedure in front of your colleagues. Have them evaluate you using the criteria that your instructor will use.

11. Plan a postexamination reward. This treat will give you something to look forward to and will prevent you from dwelling on the examination after it is over.

During Your Examination

1. Decide in advance what time you will be arriving at the place of the examination. If you are a person who likes to talk with colleagues before the examination, arrive early. If preexamination cramming with colleagues raises your anxiety level, time your arrival accordingly.
2. Take time to calm down before even looking at the examination. Sit calmly and do deep breathing.
3. Maintain this focused calm throughout the examination. If you are thinking about passing or failing, instead of staying focused on the examination questions, your concentration will slip. Just as athletes don't perform their best when they are thinking about winning the gold medal or breaking a record during an event, neither do you perform your best if you are thinking about anything other than the best response to the question in front of you. Thinking about anything else creates anxiety and interferes with your concentration on the questions.
4. If you are distracted by an external interference that can be stopped (such as noise from other candidates or the proctors, or uncomfortable conditions in the room), be assertive and ask the proctor to handle the situation. If nothing can be done about the external distractions, then tell yourself to refocus, giving all your attention to the question at hand.
5. Read over the entire examination before answering any questions. This way you know what is expected of you and you can pace yourself throughout the allotted time.
6. Before answering any question, be sure you understand what is expected so that your answers will be at the appropriate level. If you merely describe an issue when you are expected to critique it, then you will not get full credit.
7. Tackle questions to which you know the answers first. This strategy boosts your confidence.

8. Decide how much time to spend on any one question (usually determined by the number of points allotted) and stick to your timetable so that you are not rushed at the end.
9. If you finish before the allotted time, read over your answers before submitting them. This review ensures that you have answered all the questions. In addition, you may think of some points to add.

After Your Examination

1. Decide whether you wish to join your colleagues for a "postmortem." Sometimes going over an examination only increases your anxiety.
2. Follow through with your plan for celebration after the examination. Doing something fun helps clear your mind and relax you after all the hard work you did.
3. After you get your results, check to see where you did well and where you need to improve. Find out whether you need to study the content more or whether you need experience in interpreting the questions. This information will help you prepare for future examinations.

> *The person who never makes a mistake probably isn't doing anything.*
>
> **Rita Emmett**
>
> **WIT&**_Wisdom_

Dealing with Criticism

Many people feel anxious about receiving criticism. Here are some perceptions on criticism that shed a more positive light on the issue.

- Think about criticism as a gift instead of bad news. Criticism offers you the chance to reevaluate your performance. People who take time to criticize you are often interested in you or the job you are doing.
- Seek more information from the person who is criticizing you. Use negative inquiry, an assertiveness technique. Ask for specific facts about the particular behavior for which you are being criticized. This information helps you determine the validity of the criticism.
- You are not obliged to agree with all criticism you receive. Take time to review the criticism, extract

what fits your self-assessment, and discard what does not fit.

- If you receive criticism you have heard before, take note of it. There is likely some truth to criticism you hear repeatedly.
- Reply to unjust or aggressive criticism; do not let it pass without speaking up. You will feel better about yourself if you confront or correct the person who is unfairly criticizing you. Some people deliver destructive criticism to make themselves feel more powerful or superior. You do not have to accept the criticism. You can assert yourself.
- Reply with civility. Incivility or rude or discourteous behavior violates the desired climate of mutual respect (Clark et al, 2009; Feldman, 2001).
- Realize that criticism does not mean there is something wrong with you. You may be accurately criticized for doing something ineffectively or incorrectly, but that in no way means you are a bad or stupid person.

Assertively Handling Difficult Situations in Nursing Student Performance Evaluations

Some situations increase our evaluation anxiety. We need to prepare ourselves for uncomfortable situations such as those in which an evaluator is aggressive, we are given an evaluation without time to prepare, or serious allegations are made without evidence. Several examples of difficult evaluation situations follow, with suggestions for handling them assertively.

Harshly Delivered Criticism

Your clinical instructor tells you that your charting is fine and your treatments are carried out superbly, and she compliments you on your effective sterile technique. She also points out that your organization is poor. She notes that your rooms look disheveled and cluttered. "How can you or your clients find things you need in that confusion? Half the time your beds aren't made until after noon, and the room is a mess. This is a disgrace to the nursing profession."

You know that these comments are legitimate, even though they are delivered in an aggressive way. You tend to be disorganized and messy at home as well. Here is an assertive reply to this evaluation:

Assertive response: "Thank you for the feedback on my nursing skills. I don't know what to do about my organization. It's a bad habit I've had for years, even

before I came into nursing. I always admire nurses who can do things well and keep their work space uncluttered at the same time. I don't know where to begin. Can you give me some suggestions about how I can improve?"

This reply acknowledges both the compliments and the criticisms from your instructor. Your openness to improve your organization is demonstrated by your request for help. If you really want to improve, you will follow through with some of the suggestions your instructor provides.

WIT& *Wisdom*

The Secret to Success
Would you like to wow them
With your high self-esteem?
Want to hear a secret,
An instructor's dream?
Be willing to listen
To others' critique.
Your strengths and weaknesses,
What makes you unique.
If you knew all there was
To know when you came
Why come here at all?
Stay home, stay the same.
So be open to listen
And, yes, really hear.
Take a look at yourself
There's nothing to fear.
Don't be defensive.
Ask how you can change.
Old approaches for new
You soon can exchange.

Copyright © 1995 Julia W. Balzer Riley.

Unexpected Aggressive Criticism

You have been assigned to a telemetry unit in a general hospital for the past 7 weeks. It is your last week on the unit, so you decide to stop at the head nurse's office to thank her for the help she has given you during your practicum.

Without having requested it, the head nurse gives you this piece of advice: "I'm glad you enjoyed your time with us. Here's some advice I'd like to give you before you leave us: improve your charting. It's a mess to read. I spent 10 minutes trying to decipher one of your notes the other day. You'll never make a good nurse if you can't communicate to the rest of the world what you have done."

Assertive response: "I am aware that my charting is too long and difficult to read. Miss Jameson, my clinical instructor, has also pointed out my need to improve. Do you have any suggestions to help me learn how to improve my charting?"

This reply acknowledges the feedback from your head nurse. Although her feedback is aggressive, you maintained an assertive stance in your response. Your request for guidance invites her to contribute to your development in a more positive way.

Allegations without Evidence

Your clinical instructor is giving you your final evaluation on your performance on the obstetrical unit where you have been working for the past 3 weeks. She has made several negative comments about your handling of the babies and your interactions with the new mothers. However, she has given no examples to support her comments and she has never observed you directly. You believe that your performance is acceptable and that it meets the standards set out in the procedural manual. You reply in the following way:

Assertive response: "My own assessment of my handling of the babies and my interactions with the mothers is that I treat them both with respect and care. I would appreciate your providing me with more concrete evidence of any rough handling, since this charge has serious implications for my career. I have worked closely with Ms. Green in the nursery and Mrs. Nuthers on the unit. Both these staff nurses could provide you with a thorough assessment of my performance. I would like to have a joint meeting with you and these nurses to discuss my performance. I will not sign this evaluation form until this meeting has taken place."

This assertive response lets your instructor know that you intend to protect your reputation. You have made a reasonable request for another evaluation. Your straightforward manner, which is neither insulting nor disrespectful to your instructor, increases the likelihood of having another evaluation.

Moving from Reactive to Proactive Behavior

The ability to seek out opportunities for evaluation sets you apart as a person who has vision, who wants to improve rather than hide in hopes that no one will notice your mistakes. Consider beginning the process of reflective journal writing after each clinical day to gain insight into your actions, reactions, biases, and values. Lasater and Nielsen (2009) conducted research on a model for reflective journal writing as a student assignment with faculty input. You can use this process on your own as a proactive strategy, including entries such as a description of the situation, your previous experience, what you noticed, how you interpreted your observations, how you responded and set goals for the client's care, your reflection on the effectiveness of the interventions, and lessons learned. Covey (2004) suggests that "being proactive" is the first of seven habits of highly effective people. According to Covey, being proactive means that "we are responsible for our own lives." Proactive people "do not blame circumstances . . . for their behavior." For a student nurse, a proactive behavior is being prepared for a clinical assignment and open to questions and dialogue about the client's care. The reactive person blames other people and specific situations for problems. To be evaluated can be experienced as criticism and can evoke a natural tendency to look for excuses. As your skills improve and your confidence increases, you should find yourself moving from being reactive to being proactive, seeking out evaluation. You give your permission for others to give you feedback. You take responsibility for corrective action without having your feelings hurt.

They cannot take away our self-respect if we do not give it to them.

Mahatma Gandhi

WIT& *Wisdom*

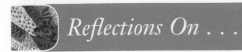

Reflections On . . .

Overcoming Evaluation Anxiety

Consider what you read about evaluation anxiety. In what areas do you experience evaluation anxiety? Answer the following questions.

What? . . .
Write one thing you learned from this chapter.

So what? . . .
How will this affect your nursing practice?

Now what? . . .
How will you implement this new knowledge or skill?

Think about it . . .

Practicing Overcoming Evaluation Anxiety

Exercise 1
Create a collage depicting yourself as you want to be, confident and accomplished. To do this collect several magazines that appeal to you, a background (use a piece of colored art paper, mat board, or even cardboard), scissors, and a glue stick or white glue. Set a goal of creating a full picture of you being your best self professionally and personally. Without a lot of thought, select images and words or phrases that appeal to you. Create a collage by gluing these to the background. When you finish, take a few minutes to write your thoughts and feelings about your expressive art. Set the collage in a place where you will see it frequently and hold these images.

Exercise 2
Dr. Barbara Bunch (1994), a nurse and psychologist, recommends the following technique to minimize arousal due to stress, a preventive strategy that you can practice throughout the day when you feel stressed. She believes the technique has a cumulative effect and will decrease the effects of stress in difficult situations such as evaluations.

1. Smile!
2. Take two abdominal breaths.

3. Drop your jaw.
4. Drop your shoulders.

Go ahead and laugh! You may look silly, but try this for several days and share your results with another student or colleague.

Exercise 3
Your colleague in the school of nursing has an important physiology test coming up in 2 days. Over coffee in the cafeteria she says the following:

Nervous Nina: "I'm terrified about this examination. Everyone says Dr. Capitell is such a hard grader. I did OK on the first test but the stuff we've covered since then is a lot more complicated. I can't fail because it will put my course selection out of sequence. I've put so much time into studying this stuff that I'd better pass. I'll be glad when it's over."

How would you intervene to help minimize your friend's evaluation anxiety? Prepare your suggested strategy, then work with classmates in groups of four to compare your suggestions.

Exercise 4
You are a staff nurse working in the operating room of a general hospital. A student doing her clinical practicum in the operating room is talking to you at coffee break. This is what she says:

Anxious Anita: "Tomorrow's going to be awful! I've got to scrub for Dr. Shark, and I've seen how he yells at students if they don't do exactly what he wants. And to top it off, my clinical instructor chooses tomorrow to evaluate me! I'll be a wreck by 4 o'clock tomorrow."

How would you help this student nurse cope with her evaluation anxiety? Prepare your own response and then work in groups of four to compare and share strategies.

Exercise 5
How can nurses follow the advice to jobholders to "underpromise and overdeliver"? Compare your views with those of your classmates.

Exercise 6

Read the following words of wisdom and write a journal entry discussing how you can apply them to your life.

- A hundred cartloads of anxiety will not pay an ounce of debt (Italian proverb).
- FEAR stands for Forgetting that Everything is All Right.
- I have found that for the most part most of what I worry about never happens.
- Feel the fear and do it anyway (Susan Jeffers).
- I think I can . . . I think I can . . . I think I can . . . (*The Little Engine That Could*).
- Courage is fear holding on a minute longer (George S. Patton).

References

Black SJ, Everhart DE, Durham TW, et al: The effects of anxiety on affective learning and serial position recall, *Int J Neurosci* 118:1269, 2008.

Bowie BH: Clinical performance expectations: using the "you–attitude" communication approach, *Nurse Educ* 35(2):66, March/April 2010.

Bunch B: Handling anxiety disorders (Lecture delivered at Baptist Medical Center), Jacksonville, FL, August 1994.

Clark CM, Farnsworth J, Landrum RE: Development and description of incivility in nursing education, *J Theory Constr Test* 13(1):7, Spring/Summer 2009.

Covey SR: *The seven habits of highly effective people*, New York, 2004, Free Press.

Dweck CS, Wortman CB: Learned helplessness, anxiety and achievement motivation. In Krohne HW, Laux L, editors: *Achievement, stress, and anxiety*, Washington, D.C., 1982, Hemisphere Publishing.

Feldman L: Classroom civility is another of our classroom responsibilities, *College Teaching* 49(4):137, 2001.

Flanagan L: *What you need to know about today's workplace: a survival guide for nurses*, Washington, D.C., 1995, American Nurses Association.

Kaplan B, Ura D: Use of multiple patient simulators to enhance prioritizing delegating skills for senior students, *J Nurs Educ* 49(7):371, 2010.

Knight A: *Andrew Knight* (in the Office of Graduate Studies) (Website). http://www.upenn.edu/grad/pennprize/2006/knight.html. Accessed March 3, 2011.

Lasater K, Nielsen A: Reflective journaling for clinical judgment development and evaluation, *J Nurs Educ* 48(1):40, January 2009.

Marquis BL, Huston CJ: *Management decision making for nurses: 124 case studies*, Philadelphia, 1998, Lippincott–Raven Publishers.

Meichenbaum DH: Cognitive modification of test anxious college students, *J Consult Clin Psychol* 39(3):370, 1972.

Moscaritolo LM: Interventional strategies to decrease nursing student anxiety in the clinical learning environment, *J Nurs Educ* 48(1):17, 2010.

Wine JD: Evaluation anxiety: a cognitive-attentional construct. In Krohne HW, Laux L, editors: *Achievement, stress, and anxiety*, Washington, D.C., 1982, Hemisphere Publishing.

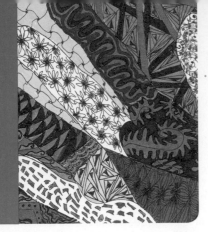

Chapter 19

Feedback

Objectives

1. Discuss the importance of feedback in communication
2. Identify strategies for giving feedback
3. Discuss steps for receiving feedback to promote self-growth
4. Practice seeking, giving, and receiving feedback in selected exercises

Why Feedback Is Important

Feedback is defined as the "transmission of evaluative or corrective information to an action, event, or process" (Merriam-Webster Online Dictionary, 2010). Discussions about how to give feedback distinguish between positive and negative feedback, and either one can be regarded as a gift. Consider the two parts of the word—"feed" and "back." In one sense of the word, "feed" implies to nourish, even to comfort, or to meet another's needs. "Back" in this context is the return of something to another. When these two notions are combined, feedback means the returning of nourishment to another person. In this sense, feedback is something positive—a gift for the other person. The gift that is given is one person's thoughts and feelings about another person's behavior. When you take a positive approach to giving or receiving feedback, this creates a comfort zone for others, "turns negative feedback into productive dialogue . . . fosters a learning environment . . . and turns criticism into pure gold" (Gallagher, 2009, p. 152). Cultivate positive people in your life by giving specific praise about colleagues, especially in front of people important to them (Anderson, 2002). This chapter invites you to use the technique of reframing, that is, seeing or describing a situation from a different perspective.

Feedback helps us see our behavior from another's perspective. This reflection indicates how someone else is reacting to our communication. This picture helps us decide whether to continue acting in the same way or to change. Viewed in this way, feedback is a springboard for self-growth. Feeling happy with ourselves is one of the most joyous experiences in life. This contentment is an acknowledgment of what we like about ourselves, and it solidifies our self-concept. Contemplating a change in our way of behaving is really envisioning a new self-concept. Feedback has the potential for expanding our development as human beings. To be most effective, feedback on our progress toward goals must be frequent and specific (Eisenberg and Goodall, 2001). Consider the nursing process as an example of a feedback mechanism. Assessment, planning, and intervention can change based on feedback from the client in the evaluation phases and on additional information obtained in continuing assessment. Improving care based on feedback has been a part of nursing since the days of Florence Nightingale. Continuous quality improvement, which is really just data-driven problem solving, examines processes in the delivery of care to improve service and depends on regular feedback for excellence. Three hundred and sixty–degree feedback, or multisource performance approval data, is used as a staff development tool because feedback is drawn from peers and subordinates to supplement direct observation by the manager (Watkins and Leigh, 2009).

Giving feedback differs from giving advice. Giving feedback is merely a reflection of how another person's behavior has affected us, not advice about how a person should change. After receiving our feedback, clients or colleagues may wish to make changes in their behavior. One thing we may be asked is, "What do you think I should do to change?" Often we have advice to give, but a note of caution is in order.

To avoid hurting the feelings of others and to ensure that we are being respectful, options we may offer should be made as suggestions for the other person's consideration. We can never know what changes will be comfortable or suitable for another person, because each of us must decide what suits our personal style and priorities. Our suggestions will be more readily received if they are offered tentatively, as in the following:

"Something I've tried is this."
    "Perhaps adding this change will help you."
    "When I was trying to change in the same way, my sister-in-law suggested I do this. . . . It worked for me, and maybe it will work for you."

These examples allow the receiver the final option of accepting or rejecting your advice.

For feedback to be integrated, it must be delivered in a way that is receivable, and the receiver must be open to considering the feedback. The following sections discuss some steps you can take to increase the probability that your feedback will be accepted.

How to Give Feedback

First, check your reason for wanting to give feedback. What is motivating you to give feedback? What do you hope to accomplish by delivering feedback? Any reasons based on the belief that your feedback will benefit the other person by increasing the opportunities for self-growth are in agreement with the intention of feedback. There are many reasons for giving feedback that are unacceptable in a caring, therapeutic relationship. Feeling irritable and wanting to lash out at another as a way of obtaining revenge, wanting to display your superior knowledge to discredit another, or wanting to rigidly control the behavior of clients or colleagues because of intolerance are not good reasons for giving feedback.

Gain Permission to Give Feedback

The next step is to gain permission from your client or colleague to give feedback so the individual will be more open to your input (Ambrose and Moscinski, 2002). Permission may be requested verbally by simply asking if the other person would like the feedback. Or the request can be made through nonverbal checking.

The following example includes verbal and nonverbal ways of obtaining permission to give feedback.

You have been teaching a new father to bathe his newborn, and he has given a return demonstration.

> I noticed how securely you have been holding your baby daughter—I'm sure it makes her feel safe and secure. It looks like she's enjoying the bath you are giving her and especially how you are talking to her. I'd like to point out one suggestion for improvement.

Here you pause and look at the father, who nods his approval for you to continue.

> When you allow your daughter's umbilical cord to get wet, it increases the chance that she'll get an infection. I've got some suggestions, if you'd like to hear them, for how you could keep her cord dry.

Again, you make eye contact with the father and do not proceed until he conveys his interest in hearing your suggestions.

> Some ways to keep the cord dry are to fill the tub with less water and hold her at about a 45-degree angle. Also, you can squeeze out the washcloth so that water doesn't accidentally drip on her cord.

Be Specific

Giving feedback to clients or colleagues is not your chance to bombard them with everything about their behavior that you like or dislike. To give your feedback impact, you must focus on specific, observable behavior. The following situation between two nurses illustrates how to be specific when giving feedback.

You are on the evening shift and are still relatively new to the procedures on the unit. Before the night shift comes on, you always have last-minute charting to do and tying together of loose ends for your report. For the past four nights, one of the night nurses has come on duty 30 minutes early and tried to engage you in a social conversation. Your hints that you don't have time to talk at that moment have been ignored, and she has persisted in bending your ear about her date or how she slept that day. You approach her with the following:

> Rhonda, I'd like to talk to you about how your coming on early and talking to me is affecting me.

At this point you wait until she's agreeable to discuss the issue and proceed as follows:

> I'd love to talk with you, but when you try to capture my attention at the end of my shift it agitates me because I'm trying to tie up so many loose ends and get things in order for the night shift. I find myself getting so tense that I can't pay enough attention to what you are trying to tell me, and I don't get my work completed the way I'd like to. Do you understand what I'm saying?

Here you must pause and give Rhonda a chance to respond. You might proceed as follows:

> I've got a suggestion that will allow me to get my last-minute work done and still give us a chance to visit before I leave. Want to hear it?

Restricting your feedback to observable behavior prevents you from blurting out something cruel such as "Can't you wait till your shift starts to talk my ear off?" or "I can't stand you bugging me like this!" Being specific helps you keep feedback realistic and acceptable.

Convey Your Perspective

When you give feedback, you must remind yourself that you are reporting your view of things. Nothing is innately or objectively right or wrong about your perspective; it is simply how you see the world. Because every relationship you have with colleagues and clients has significance and influence for both parties, however, your reactions are important to others.

When looking in the mirror after getting your hair cut in a new style, you might smile with approval, blush with embarrassment, or feel reluctant to pay for such an outrageous coiffure! The hairdresser might glow with pleasure at your sophisticated new image, and your friends may look ambivalent about the new you. Any of these reactions is legitimate, and none is better than the other. Each reaction is feedback based on the viewer's frame of reference. When you are giving feedback you need to keep in mind that as important as your views are, the receiver may not agree with your perspective.

To ensure that you give feedback respectfully, you can couch your comments with phrases such as these:

> "As I see it . . . "
> "I felt happy (sad) when you clapped (did not applaud)."
> "From my perspective . . . "
> "The way I see things is . . . "

Using the first person to convey your thoughts and feelings prevents you from accusing or labeling another person's behavior.

Because I am responsible for customer service training in a hospital setting, it is my job to give feedback when I observe poor customer service. When I am in the role of client, I am in a good position to assess the quality of service. When I give feedback, I share my perspective of someone who has "been there." When I went to the laboratory to have my blood drawn, a woman came into the room, did not identify herself, and was wearing no name tag. When I asked her about it, I learned she was a student. A staff member came in to help, and I learned that students were not routinely given name pins. I shared this information with the manager and indicated how uncomfortable it made me as a patient not to know who was working with me. She agreed and arranged to provide the students with name tags. It is not always easy to give feedback if it requires correction, but it may help others. In this case, we were able to upgrade the image of the staff as professionals.

Use This Formula to Give Assertive Feedback

In difficult situations in which you need to tell others how their behavior is affecting you and request a behavior change, the following formula, often used in assertiveness training, is helpful (Carr-Ruffino, 2001):

1. When you . . . (describe the behavior without judging it)
2. The effects are . . . (describe concretely how it affects your life in a practical sense)
3. I feel . . . (describe your feelings without blaming; the "I" statement implies ownership of your own feelings)
4. I prefer . . . (describe what response or change you would like or, if possible, give the other person a chance to come up with a solution)
   For example:
1. "When you speak in a loud voice when I am trying to listen to someone on the telephone . . . "
2. "I cannot hear, and I must ask the caller to repeat the message."
3. "I feel embarrassed that the patient might think the unit is in chaos."
4. "How can we handle this?" Or: "I would prefer you to speak more softly or finish the conversation away from the telephone."

Let's try this with the name pin issue:

When you don't wear a name pin, I can't call you by name and I don't know who to ask for if I need to talk with you later. I don't feel as if I'm in a setting in which people are professional, and I can't even be sure you work here. Were you given a name tag? No? In that case, I'd like to check into this because I think wearing name tags might make other patients feel more comfortable, too. Would that be all right with you?

Invite Comments from the Receiver

Because the feedback you give is from your perspective, it is important to keep in mind how others might feel when receiving your comments. One way to do this is to check out their reactions by using phrases such as "What do you think about my comments to you?" or "Could you tell me your reaction to what I've just told you?" Giving feedback requires consideration. You never know how others will respond to your feedback, and you must allow them to express their reactions. People need time to grasp what you are saying, mull it over, ask for more information, and express their feelings and thoughts about what you have said.

Be Genuine

It warrants saying that those who give feedback should be honest when expressing their views. If you do not mean it, do not say it! When you are sincere in giving feedback, you build trust. If you are verbalizing something positive but the frown on your face indicates displeasure, then the receiver of your feedback gets a mixed message. It is important to keep your verbal and nonverbal behavior congruent.

Check Out How Your Feedback Is Being Received

If you can honestly say that the feedback was given in the best interest of the receiver, if you gained permission before proceeding with your feedback, and if you were specific in your comments and gave them tentatively, then you know that you have given feedback in a caring way.

In addition to your self-assessment, you can also pick up clues from your clients or colleagues about whether your way of giving feedback is acceptable. If they indicate that they understand what you are saying and verbally and nonverbally indicate that they would like you to continue, then you know that your manner of giving feedback is respectful. If they become embarrassed or angry, or move away from you, they may be indicating that they are not yet ready to receive any feedback from you, or at least not in the dose you are administering. When you receive clues that your clients or colleagues are becoming defensive about your comments, it is important to pause and check with them on how to proceed. You might stop altogether or choose gentler and more receivable words.

How to Receive Feedback

Feedback is an opportunity for self-growth; therefore, knowing how to get the most out of the experience is worthwhile. Clearly, giving feedback requires risking another person's feelings and the relationship you have. Knowing about that risk has implications for how you can act when one of your clients or colleagues takes a chance on giving you feedback.

Get Focused

It is important to be focused when receiving feedback. This means not thinking or worrying about some other issue but attending to the feedback and listening respectfully. Remember that feedback can help you develop your clinical and interpersonal skills, build your self-confidence and self-esteem, and motivate you to continue to learn more about yourself (Clynes and Raftery, 2008).

Arrange to Have Enough Time to Receive the Feedback

Being unrushed when feedback is being given is also important. If you know you are hurried, then say that you value learning others' ideas and you would like to schedule another time to hear them. Making another appointment is important because it indicates that you respect other people's opinions and intend to follow through. You could say the following:

> I'm touched that you have gone to the effort of preparing some feedback for me on the in-service I gave. Could we schedule a convenient time to go over your views? I want to hear what you have to say when I'm not as pressed for time as I am today, so I can take it all in.

Make Sure You Understand the Feedback

Let feedback givers have the floor long enough to clearly state their views and then ask questions about anything that was unclear.

After your nursing instructor has given you feedback on your sterile technique, for example, you might respond as follows:

> I think I understand your comments. You noticed that I opened the tray before washing my hands and then I left the tray exposed to the air while I washed them. I also had the client's furniture placed in my way so I had to lean over the sterile field and I almost contaminated it. I think those were the main areas in which I need to improve, weren't they?

It is not only respectful to repeat the feedback to ensure that you understood it, but it is also a way of

once more outlining the points as a reminder for yourself.

Request Guidance on How to Change

If you would like to make changes in your behavior because of the feedback, then ask for directions for change—if you genuinely want to hear them. Consider this example:

Your student nurse colleague has given you feedback about your leadership style during your first week as team leader. Most of her comments were positive, but she also indicated that she occasionally felt slighted or put down when you unilaterally made decisions about the nursing care for her clients.

You are surprised to hear her reaction because you had assumed that it was up to you as team leader to take charge, but you feel bad that your leadership style may cause your team members to feel unimportant or left out. You want to change to a more respectful leadership style, so you could respond to your colleague as follows:

> Thank you for your comments. I'm pleased about the areas in which I seem to be doing well, but I really want to overcome being so autocratic. What could I do differently as team leader to make you feel more included in the decision making for your clients?

Show Appreciation for the Feedback

Thank others for their feedback. Even if you are not going to change, it has likely been of benefit to hear another person's point of view about your behavior, and you can express your gratitude for this information. Here is an example:

One of your nursing instructors tells you that she fears your habit of taking only half the allotted time for lunch will wear you out, and she worries about your health. You respond as follows:

> Thanks for your concern, Mrs. Brown. I find that the physical nursing care on this medical floor demands much more of me than the care on the ear, nose, and throat floor I just came from, where I had more than enough time. I'm slowly getting more accustomed to the pace in the 9 days I've been here, and I'm sure I'll soon be organized and relaxed enough to take the full break at lunchtime.

Think About the Feedback You Receive

You are the one who benefits from thinking over any feedback you have been given. Take the opportunity to consider the implications of feedback you receive. Here is an example:

One of your patients, uncomfortable because of her pain, often lashes out at others. As you start her bath one morning, she snarls at you:

> Oh! It's you! Miss Sugary Sweet Nancy Nurse! Your smile is sickening, and your cheeriness is just too much to take this morning! Go away and find someone else to gush over!

Your first reaction may be one of hurt. Or you may brush off her comments and rationalize that she spoke because of her pain and did not really mean them. As time passes, you might find yourself recalling her words and wondering if perhaps you are too cheery and bubbly with your clients; as a result, you might begin to keep your distance and not allow yourself to reach out to their sadness or fear. To be fair to yourself, you should really check out the answer to your concern about your possible insensitivity.

By reevaluating your ability to be warm and compassionate with your clients, you can learn about your strong points and areas in which you could be connecting more humanly with them. By making use of the feedback you receive, you can grow and develop, both personally and professionally.

> *One may find the faults of others in a few minutes, while it takes a lifetime to discover one's own.*
>
> **Author unknown**
>
> **WIT&***Wisdom*

How to Seek Feedback

As you become comfortable with receiving feedback, you may wish to seek out feedback from others before they offer it. To seek out feedback is to publicly announce that you are ready for self-growth; it implies that you have the confidence to look at your strengths and explore areas in which you could make improvements.

Be Sure You Are Ready to Receive Feedback

Before seeking feedback, check to see that you are really ready to receive it. When you are not fully open to receiving feedback, you convey that message either verbally or nonverbally. Verbally, you may become angry, get defensive, or make excuses to rationalize your behavior. Nonverbally, you may physically tune out feedback by losing eye contact, turning your body away, or folding your arms to create a barrier against the penetration of the feedback. Both these verbal and nonverbal responses are disrespectful to the person whom you are asking for feedback.

There are times when we are simply not ready to hear feedback. In those cases we should protect ourselves and not seek out others' reactions until we are confident enough to examine them. Receiving feedback with implications for change when we feel shaky or unconfident may serve only to make us feel worse about ourselves. It is a risk to ask for feedback; when we are ready to receive feedback, then it has great potential for enhancing self-growth.

 Moments of Connection . . .
Put It in Writing

One nurse manager, when asked for suggestions on how to build staff skills, talked about writing thank you or acknowledgment cards for staff when they were observed doing something extra for clients, family, or co-workers. During Nurse Week, this manager sends each staff member a card thanking the person for his or her contributions and mentioning at least one specific thing about that person. Staff report saving such cards and notes and reviewing them in tough times.

Be Specific in Your Request for Feedback

Clarify the aspects of your behavior about which you want feedback. Delineating those areas helps your clients and colleagues focus and ensures that you receive the information you want to hear. For example, after you complete a preoperative teaching session with your surgical client, you ask him the following:

> What did you think about the session?

This request for feedback is vague and does not help your client to address any particular area. The following request would help your client to focus his comments:

> I included this brochure, which I will leave with you. It reviews what you can expect to happen immediately after surgery. What other questions do you have at this time?

Use Feedback as Caring Communication

If you follow the guidelines for giving, receiving, and seeking feedback outlined previously, your feedback behavior will be assertive. Clearly, feedback is a responsible process because it allows participants to make use of all the information available. As you care for your clients you are part of an ongoing "cycle of exchange and interconnection" (Jasmine, 2009), giving and receiving feedback, and with each interaction striving to create a balance between a varied set of nursing functions and caring behaviors (Jasmine, 2009). Behavioral science tells us that whatever behavior we reward will be strengthened or repeated. Remember to take time to comment on what your colleagues do that makes your day easier. Commend clients for progress you see in their goals and encourage them to feel pride in their accomplishments and in their ability to cope and heal. In your development of interpersonal communication skills, feedback is a crucial factor.

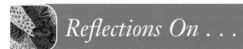

Reflections On . . .

Feedback

Consider what you read about the importance of feedback. Can you identify your own experience with seeking, receiving, and giving feedback? How can you be open to these communication skills? Answer the following questions.

What? . . .
Write one thing you learned from this chapter.

So what? . . .
How will this affect your nursing practice?

Now what? . . .
How will you implement this new knowledge or skill?

Think about it . . .

Practicing Giving and Receiving Feedback

Exercise 1
Read the following quote and discuss the relationship between feedback about your performance and professional and personal growth. "Insanity is doing the same thing over and over again and expecting different results."

Exercise 2 · QSEN
Sleep deprivation is a human factor that influences safe delivery of care. To practice the skills involved in accurately collecting information for feedback and discussing it with the team, maintain a sleep diary for 1 week. Record the number of hours you slept each night, your time to bed and time up, and contextual factors that influenced when you went to sleep each day and when you awakened. Use database searches to determine the evidence base for the appropriate amount of sleep for your age. Put the information into a graph. Develop a set of feedback questions. Present these to your clinical group and ask for feedback on the questions you developed to determine how effectively you have collected and presented the data as well as how you measure against the evidence-based sleep standard.

Reflect on the experience:

- How well did you document and communicate your data?
- How did you feel as you were receiving feedback?
- How can you apply the lessons from this experience to communicate information more effectively?

QSEN Competencies: Quality Improvement; Evidence-based Practice; Informatics

Exercise 3
Storytelling can help us learn from each other's experience. In a small group or with another student or colleague, share a story about a time when you received feedback, welcomed or unwelcomed, and what changes you made in response to the feedback. If you did not make changes, talk about why.

Exercise 4

Find a partner in the class. One of you takes the role of listener and the other the role of speaker. The speaker chooses any topic and talks about it for 5 minutes. The listener conveys interest in the speaker's topic and uses the communication behaviors learned in Part 1.

At the end of 5 minutes, the listener makes a specific request to the speaker for feedback on his or her listening skills. The speaker responds by giving feedback on the specific points requested by the listener. If appropriate, the speaker offers to give additional feedback on the abilities of the listener. The listener responds to the feedback given by the speaker.

After you have finished this exercise, take a few minutes to answer these questions.

As the speaker:

1. Was the listener's request for feedback specific?
2. Did the listener look as if he or she were open to receiving feedback from you?

As the listener:

1. How specific was your request for feedback on your listening skills to your speaker?
2. How openly did you respond to your colleague's feedback?
3. Was the speaker's feedback to you specific, clear, and tentative?

After you have answered these questions, switch roles and repeat the exercise. This exercise provides you with the chance to seek, receive, and give feedback. What have you learned about feedback from completing this exercise? Get together with the rest of the class and compare your notes about the important and delicate communication behavior of feedback.

Exercise 5

Over the next week, pay attention to how others give you feedback. What do they do to make you feel comfortable about receiving their feedback? What could they do differently to make their feedback more receivable?

At the end of the week, you may wish to meet with your colleagues and compare notes on your observations about effective and ineffective ways of giving feedback.

Exercise 6

Over the next few days, keep track of how often you seek out feedback from others. What factors make it comfortable for you to seek feedback? Observe how you receive feedback. What is your assessment of your ability to receive feedback from others?

After you have completed this exercise, join with the class as a whole and pool your ideas about what factors increase the possibility that people will seek out feedback and what factors increase the possibility that they will receive it openly.

References

Ambrose L, Moscinski P: The power of feedback, *Healthcare Exec* 17(5):56, 2002.

Anderson K: Don't worry, be happy, *Nursing* 32(1):69, 2002.

Carr-Ruffino N: *The promotable woman: advancing through leadership skills*, New York, 2001, Career Press.

Clynes MR, Raftery SEC: Feedback: An essential element of student learning in clinical practice, *Nurse Educ Pract* 8(6):405, 2008.

Eisenberg EM, Goodall HL Jr: *Organizational communication: balancing creativity and constraint*, New York, 2001, Bedford/St Martin's Press.

Gallagher RS: *How to tell anyone anything: breakthrough techniques for handling difficult conversations at work*, New York, 2009, AMACOM.

Jasmine T: Art, science, or both? Keeping the care in nursing, *Nurs Clin North Am* 44(4):415, 2009.

Merriam-Webster Online Dictionary: *Feedback* (dictionary entry). http://www.merriam-webster.com/dictionary/feedback. Accessed June 21, 2011.

Watkins R, Leigh D: *Handbook of improving performance in the workplace, vol 2, Selecting and implementing performance interventions*, San Francisco, 2009, Pfeiffer.

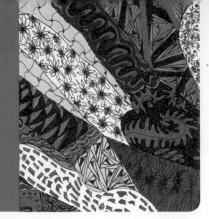

Chapter 20

Relaxation

> *One of the greatest necessities in America is to discover creative solitude.*
>
> Carl Sandburg

Objectives

1. Discuss the H.A.L.T. approach for resiliency and stress management
2. Discuss the importance of relaxation skills for the nurse
3. Identify stressors in nursing
4. Describe guidelines for beginning to practice meditation to elicit the relaxation response
5. Identify the steps of progressive relaxation for deep relaxation
6. Identify brief, practical strategies for immediate relaxation
7. Identify brief stretching exercises to promote relaxation
8. Practice relaxation techniques

H.A.L.T.!

Relaxation skills are tools for effective stress management that are a part of a proactive approach to taking responsibility for coming to your work strong and feeling emotionally and physically well. Resilience is the ability to adjust to change, to "bounce back." Relaxation strategies work best when you are not totally depleted. H.A.L.T. is an acronym for Hungry, Angry, Lonely, and Tired, introduced in Alcoholics Anonymous, to remind us of vulnerabilities that make us less resilient (Friedmann et al, 2003). To make the best use of relaxation skills, pay attention to your own self-care needs. Choose nutritious foods. Go off the unit to take lunch times and breaks, which are your allotted time to refresh yourself. Deal with fear, frustration, and hurt, which are emotions that lead to anger (Herring, 2011). Nurture relationships with others by scheduling time to be together, recognizing that although we may be connected electronically, we may become isolated. Interesting research about women is referred to as "tend and befriend," which addresses the differences in how women respond to stress. Men's response to stress is known as "fight or flight." Women tend to nurture their children and seek out companionship, especially with other women; this is related to the hormone oxytocin (Taylor et al, 2000). Women often eliminate time with other women friends, putting it at the bottom of their list of priorities. Commit to getting 8 hours of sleep when possible and allow yourself time to just rest!

Importance of Relaxing Your Body

As a student in nursing, balancing a full life with your academic responsibilities, you likely have experienced the unwanted effects of stress. As a graduate you balance a different set of stressors. There is no quick-fix to manage stress, because stress is a result of "an interaction between a negative environment, unhealthy lifestyles, and self-defeating attitudes and beliefs" (Micozzi, 2010). Exposure to noise and artificial light can be stressors for nurses and contribute to job dissatisfaction (Applebaum et al, 2010). Interruptions in the work environment of nurses can have a significant impact on client safety (McGillis Hall et al, 2010). Injuries can occur when we are "just not thinking." Consider a time when you were driving and suddenly realized that your mind was not on your driving and you don't remember how you got from one place to another. Geller (2010) uses mindfulness exercises in his work with job safety analysis (JSA) to promote prompt reaction to prevent industrial accidents. This chapter encourages you to take charge of your reactions to stressful situations in the workplace and develop a habit of daily relaxation, a letting-go technique, to eliminate the negative build-up of stress in your body. When you engage in relaxation practices you become more focused and alert, promoting safety for clients and for yourself. Other chapters help you prepare your mind for communicating effectively in your interpersonal encounters with clients and colleagues. This chapter focuses on preparing your body to relax during your workplace interactions. Worry can trigger tension in your muscles, resulting in soreness, headaches, or digestive upsets. In turn, bodily tension is an aggravating signal to your mind that you are not at peace and that something is "eating away at you." If you allow these physical symptoms of stress to build up, you are in danger of eventually damaging your body. In contrast, relaxation is "a state of consciousness characterized by feelings of peace and release from tension, anxiety and fear" (Ryman and Rankin-Box, 2001) that contributes to your general sense of well-being (Spencer and Jacobs, 2003).

Chronic tightened muscles, tension headaches, or digestive disturbances reflect your "disease" and register diminished well-being. Built-up stress reactions steal valuable energy and put you at risk of holding back or closing off in your interpersonal relationships. In a study of high school students who received relaxation training, state (transient) anxiety scores were reduced. This is important, too, for nursing students, because high anxiety adversely affects learning (Rasid and Parish, 1998). You can see that it is assertive to learn to minimize your tension and expand your relaxation response in the workplace. Your own self-caring strategies, meditation, and relaxation practices help you build self-awareness and resiliency in times of personal stress and illness (Anselmo, 2005; Tusaie and Edds, 2009; Irving et al, 2009). There are benefits for you, as well as for your clients and colleagues, when you are more relaxed.

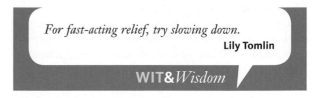

For fast-acting relief, try slowing down.
Lily Tomlin

WIT&*Wisdom*

Stress of Nursing as an Occupation

Occupational stress is a major health issue leading to anxiety, short-term and long-term physical problems, and counterproductive behavior at work (Spector, 2002). As a nurse, you navigate several organizational structures to ensure client well-being: the nursing hierarchy, the medical hierarchy, and the agency's bureaucracy. To survive this organizational maze, you need effective interpersonal communication techniques and efficient management skills. Increased acuteness of clients' conditions and a shortage of personnel contribute to increased stress.

Not only do nurses require a sound knowledge in their own areas of expertise, but to be effective in helping clients, they need to know the roles and functions of other healthcare professionals, how to communicate clearly with other members of the healthcare team, and how to coordinate the work efforts of all these disciplines. The changing exposure to different personnel demands that you quickly size up how to relate to colleagues effectively, which adds one more level of stress to an already complex working environment.

One of the most frequently cited sources of stress in nursing is the excessive workload, which gives nurses the feeling that they are always in a hurry, as if in a race with time. This factor is intensified by nurses' day-to-day encounters with distressing and anxiety-provoking situations, as well as insufficient resources in these times of healthcare restraint. As helping professionals, each of you has a vision of what your workplace, colleagues, and clients will be like, and these images may not prepare you for the reality you encounter. This chapter invites you to empower yourself by taking charge of your individual resourcefulness for increasing your relaxation response.

Part of your health teaching with any client is reviewing the basics of health promotion, such as eating nutritiously, exercising regularly, securing adequate sleep, engaging in supportive social encounters, and making time for solitude and/or spiritual contemplation. Your knowledge of the benefits of taking care of yourself physically, emotionally, socially, and spiritually is sound. With the investment you have in health, you likely try to incorporate these health behaviors in your own daily life. The return on your investment is an enhanced feeling of well-being and a readiness to handle the stress of working as a nurse. This chapter invites you to add three practices to help you relax and prepare for stress in your interpersonal relationships with clients and colleagues: daily meditation, progressive relaxation, and on-the-spot relaxation exercises. These techniques are designed to relax your body, putting it in a state in which the fight-or-flight response or the defense-alarm syndrome of arousal is greatly diminished or eliminated, so that your energy is available for communicating effectively (Luskin and Pelletier, 2005).

Meditation as a Way to Augment Your Relaxation Response

Meditation is a "mind body practice with many methods and variations . . . grounded in the silence and stillness of compassionate, nonjudgmental present-moment awareness. Although contemplative meditation practices are largely rooted in the world's spiritual traditions, the practice of meditation does not require belief in any particular religious or cultural system" (Fortney and Taylor, 2010, p. 81). Meditation has become a general term that includes a variety of practices to relax the body and still the mind. The word "meditation" comes from the root word *meditari*, which means to "consider" or to "pay attention to something" (Fontaine, 2010). Meditation is an experiential exercise you do by yourself and for yourself to benefit from the subjective sense of deep relaxation of the body's musculature; an added benefit is that you may possibly come to know yourself more fully. Meditation is psychologically and physically refreshing and energy restoring (Luskin and Pelletier, 2005).

Empirical study has confirmed that the meditative process relieves nervous system stress more efficiently than either dreaming or sleeping. It has been proven that marked physiological alterations accompany meditation: a reduction of the metabolic rate, a reduction

of the breathing rate to 4 to 6 breaths per minute, an increase in the number of alpha waves in the brain (waves of 8 to 12 cycles per second), the appearance of theta waves in the brain (waves of 5 to 8 cycles per second), and a 20% reduction in the blood pressure of hypertensive patients (Luskin and Pelletier, 2005).

The regenerating effects of meditation are experienced during the meditation itself and have a carryover effect into your daily activities (Luskin and Pelletier, 2005). Once you have learned the low arousal effect during the meditation practice, you can maintain this state of neurophysiological functioning in response to stressful situations. It is impossible to be relaxed and tense at the same time, and your enhanced ability to maintain relaxation during the day in the face of stressful interpersonal situations is what will help to minimize the effects of stress on you. With practice you will be able to call upon your low arousal state as needed during your working day. By itself this mechanism is helpful, and your heightened feelings of being able to cope with the pressures of everyday life will augment your good feelings (Luskin and Pelletier, 2005). When you learn to diminish your reaction to stressors, you free yourself to deal with aspects of the interpersonal situation more worthy of your energy. Being able to shift focus from being tight or nervous to feeling calm and in charge allows you to communicate more effectively with your clients and colleagues.

Mindfulness is an aspect of meditation that "reflects the basic and fundamental human capacity to attend to relevant aspects of experience in a nonjudgmental and nonreactive way, which in turn cultivates clear thinking, equanimity (composure under stress), compassion, and openheartedness" (Fortney and Taylor, 2010, p. 81). Mindfulness, which is developed through meditation, enables you to maintain a fluid awareness in a moment-by-moment experiential process that helps you disengage from a strong attachment of beliefs, thoughts, or emotions; this results in a greater sense of emotional balance and well-being. This evidenced-based practice holds the potential for many health benefits, including challenges such as increasing healthcare costs, chronic lifestyle-induced illness, healthcare provider burnout, client dissatisfaction, and stress in clients and caregivers (Fortney and Taylor, 2010; Ludwig and Kabat-Zinn, 2008; Deyo et al, 2009; Paul-Labrador et al, 2006; McCray et al, 2008; Eckleberry-Hunt et al, 2009; Chiesa and Serretti, 2009). Meditation teaches you to fix your attention firmly upon a given task for increasingly protracted periods of time, overcoming the habit of flitting from one subject to another. A chaplain working in a hospice setting made this remark about meditation: "When you are trying to still the mind, if a thought comes into your head, you need not invite it to tea."

Once you have truly tried to quiet your mind or to allow images to run through it without letting any particular one become distracting, you will understand why practice and perseverance are necessary if you are to be successful. Have you noticed how your thoughts seem to wander or race? It is not easy to still the mental chatter. When you attempt to become quiet, your mind may jump from one thought or concern to another. This is expected. Think "Oh well, a thought," and let it go. Begin with 10 minutes of meditation and increase it to 20 minutes at a time. Experiment to determine the best approach for you. You will find it gets easier to be still and be present for yourself. At this point, the subtle benefits of meditation become more pronounced (Luskin and Pelletier, 2005).

Guidelines for Beginning to Practice Meditation

The following guidelines are for a nonreligious form of meditation. It has a very simple form, requiring that you sit comfortably in a quiet place, that you focus your attention on the word "one," and that you adopt an accepting and unconcerned attitude. These conditions will help you experience what is called the relaxation response, a state that research shows is associated with reduced physiological activity. That means the heart rate will become slower and the blood pressure will fall. You'll notice that you feel calmer than usual and the whole sensation will be a pleasant one. At no time will you lose consciousness or be controlled by an outside force. The state you reach is one that you will have induced in yourself (Payne and Donaghy, 2010; Benson and Proctor, 2010). There are other forms of meditation, and you may wish to read about them or even take a course or individualized instruction in meditation.

> *Meditation is simplicity itself. It's about stopping and being present. That is all.*
>
> **Jon Kabat-Zinn**
>
> **WIT&***Wisdom*

Make Time to Meditate

To experience benefits from meditation, it is desirable to meditate for 15 to 20 minutes at least once a day. This commitment means consistently setting aside that time.

Many individuals say that they have an extremely busy schedule and simply do not have the opportunity to sit for such a long period of time each day. Very often a realistic examination of a person's schedule indicates that in fact there is sufficient time if the individual is conscientious and serious in his or her efforts. To some extent, the minor life reorientation necessitated by meditative practice may be responsible for its success. It involves a reordering of life priorities and behavioral patterns (Luskin and Pelletier, 2005).

Set the Climate to Meditate

Find a quiet place in which you will not be disturbed. Turn off your cell phone or silence the ringer on your telephone for the time you are meditating. Tell others that you do not wish to be disturbed for a specified length of time and assure them that you will be available after your meditation. Taking these precautions frees you to relax instead of tensing at sounds in your environment. Many people find it best to meditate the first thing in the morning when their home is quiet and the world has not yet started to intrude. For nurses doing shift work, other arrangements can be made. Some people choose a quiet place outside their home such as the hospital chapel.

Secure a Comfortable Position for Meditation

Find a position that is truly comfortable for you in which your body is supported by minimal muscular work. Support your back and feet if necessary. If possible adjust the room temperature so that you are comfortable. If you are warm enough, you are more likely to stay relaxed and not be distracted.

Develop a Passive Attitude

Distracting thoughts are likely to occur during your meditation, especially at first when you are learning to focus. Let these thoughts pass without becoming worried about their intrusion or your ability to meditate.

Select a Mental Device

To help you shift away from logical, externally oriented thoughts, select a mental device—a phrase, a word, or a sound—that you can repeat while you meditate. Repetition of this sound, called a mantra, assists in breaking the stream of distracting thoughts. Some suggestions for a mental device are single-syllable sounds or words such as *in*, *out*, *one*, or *zum* that can be repeated silently or in a low tone while meditating. Select a mantra that is not emotionally charged and is soothing to you. Make up a word if you prefer (Payne and Donaghy, 2010; Benson and Proctor, 2010) or use a word that is rooted in your belief system. A nonreligious person might use a word such as *one*, *peace*, or *love*, whereas a person from the Christian tradition might use the opening words of a comforting prayer such as "The Lord is my shepherd," from Psalm 23. A person of the Jewish tradition might use the word *shalom* (Micozzi, 2010).

Relax Your Body

When you are ready to begin your meditation, start by relaxing your body with a body scan. Begin with the muscle groups in the head and work down to the feet. Say to yourself: "Relax your face; now allow your neck muscles to thaw; let your head relax; take the tension out of your shoulders; let your chest muscles loosen; allow your abdomen to soften; let your back muscles unfreeze; take the tension out of your thigh muscles; let your calves melt; allow your feet to rest comfortably supported." As you tune into the difference between relaxation and tension in your muscles, you will be able to quickly release the tightness in your body in preparation for your meditation times. Wearing comfortable, loose-fitting clothing helps you assume a posture that is relaxing.

Focus on Your Breathing

Breathe through your nose and focus on, or become aware of, your breathing. This awareness helps you relax. Breathe easily and naturally, allowing the air to come to you on each inhalation (Payne and Donaghy, 2010; Benson and Proctor, 2010). Exhale slowly, allowing all the air out of the lungs. You will find that this focus on your breathing is very peaceful. When you are stressed, your breathing is quicker; by slowing your breathing and appreciating its rhythm, you begin to relieve tension. Remember not to control your breathing; you do not want to become light-headed. Just breathe easily and naturally.

While you are first focusing on your breathing, you can repeat your mental device silently on inhalation and exhalation. You can try saying to yourself as you inhale, "I am breathing in peace and calm." Upon exhalation, try thinking, "I am blowing out tension and negativity."

Meditate for 10 Minutes

Start by meditating for 10 minutes, then increase the time to 15 or 20 minutes as you gain experience in being still. Close your eyes during your meditation if this helps you focus on your breathing and on your mantra. Do not think of things or try to solve problems during this quiet time. Your meditation time is time out from running your life, managing time, controlling events, and performing as an adult in your hectic world. In this quiet time, for 10 to 20 minutes, you are free to just sit and breathe. Don't expend energy judging your thoughts or criticizing any distractions; simply let them pass by and remain focused on the present, on your breathing, and on your mental device.

Allow your images and thoughts to flow freely. Your mantra will come back to you. While you are meditating, you do not need to expend a great effort or concentrate. Enjoy this quiet, peaceful experience. If you need to open your eyes to check the time, arrange to have a clock in view so that moving is unnecessary.

Experience Your Unique Meditation

There are no rules or "shoulds" for what you will experience in your meditations. Enjoy the peaceful break in which you can unwind and experience the sensation of relaxation. You may discover sensations in your body that you were previously too busy to notice. It may happen that in addition to peacefulness, you achieve a level of stillness in which you might be overwhelmed with joy and a sense of unity with life. This powerful feeling is described as dissolving all fear, including the fear of death, and creating an inundation of warmth, joy, and harmony (Luskin and Pelletier, 2005).

Transcendental meditation, one form of meditation, has been found to be an effective tool for the following (Sheikh, 2002):

- Changing your time orientation to the "here and now"

- Increasing your behavioral motivation to be more inner-directed
- Developing sensitivity to personal needs and feelings
- Improving your ability to express feelings spontaneously
- Increasing your self-acceptance
- Raising your level of self-actualization

Such effects add to the nurse's ability to learn and maintain the perspective necessary to be able to stay connected to clients and family without becoming personally overwhelmed. A variety of relaxation and guided imagery techniques are useful with children (Allen and Klein, 2000; Klein and Holden, 2001).

End Your Meditation Peacefully

When it is time to end your meditation, pause before standing up and moving. It may be soothing to sit for a brief moment with your eyes closed before slowly opening them. Don't rush away; rather, gently leave your meditation and enter your world refreshed and relaxed.

> *Those who seek the truth by means of intellect and learning only get further and further away from it. Not til your thoughts cease all their branching here and there, not til your mind is motionless as wood or stone, will you be on the right road to the Gate.*
>
> **Huang Po**
>
> **WIT&***Wisdom*

Progressive Relaxation

Progressive relaxation is a method of decreasing muscular tension to promote the relaxation response. This process of progressively tensing and relaxing muscle sets in a systematic way can be useful for you and for your clients (Box 20-1). This technique helps clients with chronic tension become aware of the difference between a muscle that is tense and one that is relaxed (Fontaine, 2010). Progressive relaxation training has produced favorable results for conditions such as anxiety, hypertension, insomnia, asthma, dyspnea and anxiety in chronic pulmonary disease, and rheumatic pain (Payne and Donaghy, 2010).

Box 20-1	*Sample Relaxation Exercise Script*

- Find a quiet room with soft light where you are unlikely to be interrupted
- Sit in a comfortable chair, feet flat on the floor, arms supported at your sides
- Slowly begin to take several deep breaths, focusing on your breathing
- Tense your facial muscles, close your eyes tightly, and hold your mouth closed
- Relax your face, making the muscles feel as though they are sagging
- Clench your right fist and tighten the muscles in your right arm
- Open your right fist and relax the arm muscles, making your arm feel loose and heavy
- Clench your left fist and tighten the muscles in your left arm
- Open your left fist and relax the arm muscles, making your arm feel loose and heavy
- Tighten the muscles in your right leg and squeeze the toes on your right foot
- Relax your right leg muscles and toes
- Tighten the muscles in your left leg and squeeze the toes on your left foot
- Relax your left leg muscles and toes
- Tighten your buttocks
- Relax your buttocks
- Relax your entire body. Allow it to feel free and heavy. You are in a state of total relaxation
- Stay in this relaxed state for about 5 minutes. Pay attention to how your body feels in this state
- Gradually open your eyes and slowly stretch. Experience this relaxation

Adapted from Eliopoulos C: *Integrating conventional & alternative therapies: holistic care for chronic conditions*, St. Louis, 1999, Mosby.

On-the-Spot Relaxation Exercises to Relieve Tension Caused by an Interpersonal Stressor

Meditating on a daily basis will make you more relaxed and vital at work or school. Even with this new peacefulness, however, there will be times when a distraught client, an enraged family member, or an agitated colleague can raise your tension level. It would be ideal, but probably impractical, if you could leave the unit for some quiet time when clients and colleagues upset your peacefulness. What can help are some on-the-spot ways to regain your relaxation response. Techniques such as meditation or prayer can help you learn to maintain your perspective in the face of the complex demands of nursing. This chapter offers you creative techniques on which you can call to cool down when the heat is on. So when the unit is understaffed, the client population is on overload, and you are encountering interpersonal stress, here are some things you can do to relax your body.

Strategies for Relaxing Your Body When Your Stressor Is Immediate

Some stressful situations occur with no warning. In these instances, it helps to have on-the-spot methods for relaxing your body in your repertoire. Start by practicing a few abdominal breaths. Breathe in through your mouth, focusing on making your stomach bigger; breathe out though your nose, pushing your stomach in toward your spinal column. When working with pediatric patients, nurse researcher Sharlene Weiss (1998) calls these "belly breaths" and asks children to imagine blowing up a balloon in their tummies. She explains that this simple exercise halts the sympathetic nervous system's response during stress by stimulating the parasympathetic nervous system. Try a few abdominal breaths now and notice how you feel after in contrast to before the exercise. Stop reading now and try it. Many people report feeling light-headed. Did this happen to you? We are more accustomed to shallow breathing. More oxygen to your brain can provide quicker problem-solving responses!

Each of the following brief relaxation exercises can be done on a moment's notice with no need for privacy or special equipment. Each can be done as you walk down the corridor, ride on the elevator, or stand up to face the person who is stressing you.

Exercises to Help Cope with an Unexpected Stressful Interpersonal Encounter

Imagine that it is noon on the orthopedic unit, where you are in your third week of clinical work. The lunches have not arrived and the clients are hungry.

You are hungry. A physician strides out of the elevator, spies you, and heads in your direction. Her forceful walk, scowl, furrowed brow, and finger pointed in your direction give you clues that she is irate about something and, because you are the only nurse in the vicinity, you will likely bear the brunt of her aggression.

The following are some ideas about what you can do to relax your body before tension tightens your muscles in a fight-or-flight response. These techniques can be done in the moment while you are awaiting the approach of the irate physician (your stressor) and even while you are communicating assertively in the face of this threat.

Sprinkling Shower

The spray from an imaginary shower nozzle is above your head and you feel the water trickling through your hair, warming your shoulder muscles on its way down your back. Your hunched shoulders sag with relief from the warmth. You feel the warm soapy water caressing your muscles and heating your skin. The soapy lather massages your skin as it flows over you, warming your legs and feet before disappearing down the drain. As you lift your face to the nozzle, you are pelted with a clear stream of fresh water. Someone has adjusted the nozzle; you sense a firm staccato pressure on your face and over your neck and shoulders. You notice that this beating of water is simultaneously comforting and invigorating. You feel regenerated. The comforting relief you experience from the water surrounding your body makes you sigh deeply. The pressure of the water eases up to a refreshing sprinkle. As the shower turns off, you are suddenly dry, and you feel warm and refreshed. As you relax, say to yourself: "This is relaxation. This is how it feels to be loose. This is what I want."

Sunbeam

Picture a radiant ball of light just above your head creating a field of bright rays vibrating in a protective pyramid around your body. Feel its protective glow encircling your body to a diameter of 4 feet. Notice that the light feels warm and, as it envelops you, you are comforted by its penetrating rays. You find yourself raising your face to bask in the heat of the radiant sun. You can actually feel the light infiltrate your body, permeating your cells. This experience is comforting, and to your surprise, you can actually feel the warmth from the light circulating from your head to your toes. Now you notice that the light is twinkling, and as it touches your skin you feel unusually invigorated. The sparkling sunbeams dance over your skin, dissipating any tension you were feeling. Your energy opens up in response to the warmth and tingling. As you relax, your muscles are overwhelmed with a feeling of profound comfort and safety in the rays of your own special sunbeam. As you relax, say to yourself: "This is relaxation. This is how it feels to be loose. This is what I want."

Safety Shield

Picture a clear Plexiglas shield that rises up to surround you when you sense danger. Your protective shield is about 2 feet away from your body, and it allows you to move freely while it protects you on all sides. You can see quite clearly into the outside world, as if the shield were invisible. Inside your shield, the air is fresh and makes your skin tingle as it circulates around your body. This is your personal air supply, and when you breathe, you notice that the air penetrates your lungs, invigorating your cells as it circulates throughout your body. You feel energized and nourished by this special supply of air in your protected space. You also notice that you feel calm and well defended inside your shield, because you realize that the shield deflects tension away from you. You are relaxed and free from any tensions outside your shield, and you feel this assurance in your body. You notice your breathing is slowing down with the nourishing air, and you feel that your muscles are loose and fluidly mobile. You relax because you know you are safe. As you relax, say to yourself: "This is relaxation. This is how it feels to be loose. This is what I want."

Sweeper

A magic broom comes out of nowhere to sweep the tension from your body. It rakes through your hair, leaving your scalp tingling as the circulation is invigorated. Your head feels warm and free of tension after this stimulation. You notice that your neck moves easily and is relaxed instead of stiff. As the broom sweeps the stress from your shoulders, they relax and feel lighter. You stand less rigidly and notice that your back is free from any tension. This broom is powerful and thorough in its ability to brush the stress off and away from your body. You can feel its bristles brush away the tension from your abdomen and the fronts and backs of your legs. When your feet are swept, you feel lighter and more mobile; this sensation is energizing. You know you are tension free, and you feel safe when the stress is swept into a pan and thrown far away from your body. Without the encumbrance of stress and tension, you feel ready to handle anything. The sweeping has regenerated your batteries and renewed your energy. Your feet are moving with renewed energy, and you're tempted to get up and dance on the balls of your feet. You feel alive and free! As you relax, say to yourself: "This is relaxation. This is how it feels to be loose. This is what I want."

Massage

A pair of powerful hands comes out of nowhere and lays themselves across your shoulders. These large but gentle hands are unusually warm and radiate heat to your upper back. The motion is soothing, and the heat penetrates deep inside. You rotate your shoulders easily after these comforting hands have massaged away the tension. No effort is needed to stand or move. You are relaxed. The hands move up to knead the knots in your neck muscles. The touch is magical, as if by merely being there the hands can dissipate tightness from built-up tension. Before moving on, the hands shake the tension away from your body so that it is no longer a threat. Next the hands move to your lower back and massage the tightness out of your spine. The pressure is firm, and with each small circular stroke you notice that your breathing gets more relaxed; it slows down and you are totally soothed by the comfort and compassion emanating from the hands. You can feel the muscles in your neck, shoulders, and back filling with blood, becoming warm and supple under the gifted touch of the hands as they massage away fear and tightness. You feel release and a sense of freedom. You feel warm and protected. As you relax, say to yourself: "This is relaxation. This is how it feels to be loose. This is what I want."

Advantages of On-the-Spot Relaxation Exercises

Each of these brief but powerful relaxation strategies takes about a minute to experience. In that short time you can shift from tightness and fear to relaxation and a feeling of competence. Using these calming strategies will give you inner self-confidence. As you become aware of when your body is relaxed, you will become even more skilled at calming yourself in the face of tension. Relaxation is a skill, a coordination of mind and muscles, and it can be learned by anyone who wants to do so and is willing to spend the time and effort (Percival et al, 1977).

Stretches to Create Relaxation in Preparation for a Stressful Interpersonal Encounter

If you have more warning about an upcoming stressful interpersonal encounter, you can add soothing stretches to augment the benefits of meditation and on-the-spot exercises. Before encountering a stressor, or at any time during your hectic day, break away from the busy pace of the unit and find a quiet place in which to relax your muscles for a minute or so. Find some privacy in the bathroom or an empty office. Here are some stretches you can do that take little space and can be done from a standing position without any equipment.

These exercises involve tensing and relaxing the muscles until you feel the difference between the two sensations and learn to consciously relax any tense muscle. As your muscles learn the difference, they will develop a relaxation response (Percival et al, 1977).

High Stretch and Relax

Stand erect and stack your hands on top of your head. While taking a deep breath, reach high overhead, lifting your chest and moving your head back slightly. Stretch slowly until your hands are as high as they will go. Hold this for 3 seconds. Now exhale, letting the air out with a long, easy sigh, while dropping your arms slowly to your sides. Let your shoulders sag, your head fall forward, and your knees go loose and slightly bent. Remain in this relaxed position for 3 to 5 seconds. Allow all the tension to seep out of your neck, arms, shoulders, and chest muscles. Repeat this a few times before returning to work (Percival et al, 1977).

Shoulder Rotation

The shoulder rotation stretch improves shoulder flexibility and relaxes your shoulder girdle. Stand with your feet comfortably apart. Raise your elbows to shoulder height, allowing your forearms and hands to dangle loosely. Rotate elbows forward in large circles at a medium pace, keeping your hands and arms loose throughout. Move the shoulders in as large an arc as possible for about 20 rotations (Percival et al, 1977).

Shoulder Shrug and Relax

The shoulder shrug relaxation exercise can be done even while you are talking on the phone. Stand with your feet comfortably apart. As you take a deep breath, shrug your shoulders up to your ears and moderately tighten the muscles throughout your body. Hold for 3 to 5 seconds. Now exhale with a long, deep sigh, letting your shoulders drop down and your muscles go loose so that your knees bend slightly and your head drops forward to your chest. Repeat this several times (Percival et al, 1977).

Arms Out, Up, and Relax

Stand erect with your feet comfortably apart. Lift your arms out to your sides and up over your head, simultaneously pulling your stomach in and lifting your chest. When you've reached as high as you can, let your arms drop loosely down. Allow your head to sag so that your chin touches your chest and your knees go soft. Try to get as loose and limp as you can. Feel the tension drain out. Repeat this several times before returning to work (Percival et al, 1977).

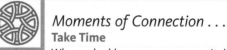

Moments of Connection . . .
Take Time
When asked how nurses can revitalize their practice, one nurse responded: "Take time to listen, to care, to share. Take time for yourself, especially. Life is too short to put it all into work. You have a lot to gain for yourself and can give more to others when you have energy and a meaningful life of your own."

With practice you will be able to call on your relaxation response at any moment. Being able to relax gives you the power to release tension in your muscles, reclaiming that energy for dealing with interpersonal stressors in your life. In the next few chapters, you will learn ways to change your mindset to handle difficult situations in your relationships with clients and colleagues.

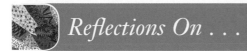

Reflections On . . .

Relaxation

Consider what you read about the importance of relaxation. What do you already do for relaxation? Which techniques in this chapter sound interesting to you? Answer the following questions.

What? . . .

Write one thing you learned from this chapter.

So what? . . .

How will this affect your nursing practice?

Now what? . . .

How will you implement this new knowledge or skill?

Think about it . . .

Practicing Relaxation

Exercise 1

During the next week, practice meditating for 10 minutes twice a day, perhaps once in the morning and once again in the afternoon. After each of your meditations, keep notes of what the experience was like for you. Here are some questions to think about (but do not be limited by them): *How does the experience of meditating make a difference to you? How does your mantra (sound) work for you? What thoughts or images occur? Are you able to let distracting thoughts float by and return to focusing on your breathing and on your mantra?*

Find an opportunity to talk about the practice of meditating with your classmates. Although meditation is a private event, you may feel comfortable exchanging ideas about how to make the process of meditation work more effectively so that it contributes to expanding your feelings of relaxation.

> *It's not easy taking my problems one at a time when they refuse to get in line.*
> **Ashleigh Brilliant**

WIT&*Wisdom*

Exercise 2

Dance and movement are being explored as part of the expressive arts in healing movement. Reflect upon your own experience with dance and movement and how these are related to your ability to relax. Try a walking meditation. Walk silently for 10 minutes, by yourself, without music, paying attention to all your senses. Reflect upon differences in your state of relaxation before and after the walking meditation. Experiment with moving to music you enjoy as another way to add to your repertoire of relaxation strategies, especially when you cannot quiet your mind enough to use more mental strategies.

Exercise 3

Reflect upon the following quotation from Elisabeth Kubler-Ross: "There is no need to go to India or anywhere else to find peace. You will find that deep place of silence right in your room, your garden, or even your bathtub." How long has it been since you spent time in a garden or a beautiful place in nature? Do you like to work with plants and/or have them in your environment? When did you last take a bath rather than a shower? Create a plan for relaxation based upon your response to the quotation and questions.

Exercise 4

Give the on-the-spot relaxation visualizations a try over the next few days. Focus on trying to stay with the relaxation that your visualization creates in your body. Notice when you get distracted and design a way of refocusing on your soothing internal technique. Note when you are able to distinguish the change from tension in your muscles to letting go in a relaxation response. As you practice, you will become more and more astute at recognizing the difference, and soon it will be within your power to quickly and simply allow the tension to escape from your body.

Exercise 5

The next time you are on one of your clinical units, take a moment away from the hectic pace to try out one of the relaxing stretch–release exercises. Time yourself to see how long it took to find a spot and complete a few relaxing stretch–releases. You will likely be surprised at
Continued

how little time it takes. Just breaking away from the unit with the anticipation and intention of doing something good for yourself is beneficial, and the stretching and releasing remind your body to relax. Note how refreshed you feel when you return to the unit.

Make time in your class to talk about creative ways to incorporate a stretch–release exercise into your workday.

> *The growth of the human mind . . . is the highest adventure on earth.*
> **Norman Cousins**
>
> WIT&*Wisdom*

References

Allen JS, Klein RJ: *Ready, set, relax: a research-based program of relaxation, learning and self-esteem for children*, Watertown, Wis, 2000, Inner Coaching.

Anselmo J: Relaxation: the first step to restore, renew, and self-heal. In Dossey BM, et al, editors: *Holistic nursing: a handbook for practice*, Sudbury, Mass, 2005, Jones and Bartlett Publishers.

Applebaum D, Fowler S, Fiedler N, et al: The impact of environmental factors on nursing stress, job satisfaction, and turnover intention, *J Nurs Admin* 40(7/8):323, July/August 2010.

Benson H; Proctor W: *Relaxation revolution: enhancing your health through the science and genetics of mind body healing*, New York, 2010, Scribner.

Chiesa A, Serretti A: Mindfulness based stress reduction for stress management in healthy people, a review and meta-analysis, *J Complement Med* 15(5):593, 2009.

Deyo R, Mirza SK, Turner JA, et al: Overtreating chronic back pain, time to back off? *J Am Board Fam Med* 22(1):62, 2009.

Eckleberry-Hunt J, Lick D, Boura J, et al: An exploratory study of resident burnout and wellness, *Acad Med* 84(2):269, 2009.

Fontaine KL: *Complementary & alternative therapies for nursing practice*, Boston, 2010, Pearson.

Fortney L, Taylor M: Meditation in medical practice: a review of the evidence and practice, *Prim Care* 37(1):81, March 2010.

Friedmann PD, Herman DS, Freedman S, et al: Treatment of sleep disturbance in alcohol recovery: a national survey of addiction medicine physicians, *J Addict Dis* 22(2):91, 2003.

Geller S: Industrial Safety and Hygiene News: *Are you mindful or mindless when working*, (website). http://www.ishn.com/Articles/Behavioral_Safety/1365afadc9fb7010VgnVCM100000f932a8c0. Accessed June 1, 2011.

Herring J: E-Zine Articles: *Stress management: never get too hungry, angry, lonely, or tired.* http://ezinearticles.com/?Stress-Management:-Never-Get—Too-Hungry,-Angry,-Lonely,-Tired,-or-Scared&id=68757. Accessed June 2011.

Irving AA, Dobkin PL, Park J: Cultivating mindfulness in health care professionals: a review of empirical studies of mindfulness-based stress reduction, *Complement Ther Clin Pract* 15(2):61, 2009.

Klein NC, Holden M: *Healing images for children: teaching relaxation and guided imagery to children facing cancer and other serious illness*, Watertown, Wis, 2001, Inner Coaching.

Ludwig DS, Kabat-Zinn J: Mindfulness in medicine, *JAMA* 300(11):1350, 2008.

Luskin F, Pelletier K: *Stress free for good: ten scientifically proven life skills for health and happiness*, New York, 2005, HarperOne.

McCray LW, Cronholm PF, Bogner HR, et al: Resident physician burnout, is there hope? *Fam Med* 40(9):626, 2008.

McGillis Hall L, Pedersen C, Fairley L: Losing the moment: understanding interruptions to nurses' work, *J Nurs Admin* 40(4):169, April 2010.

Micozzi MS: *Fundamentals of complementary and integrative medicine*, St. Louis, 2010, Saunders.

Paul-Labrador M, Polk D, Dwyer JH, et al: Effects of a randomized controlled trial of transcendental meditation on components of the metabolic syndrome in subjects with coronary artery heart disease, *Arch Intern Med* 166(11):1218, 2006.

Payne RA, Donaghy M: *Payne's handbook of relaxation techniques: a practical guide for the health care professional*, Edinburgh, 2010, Elsevier.

Percival J, Percival L, Taylor J: *The complete guide to total fitness*, Scarborough, Ontario, Canada, 1977, Prentice-Hall.

Rasid ZM, Parish TS: The effects of two types of relaxation training on students' level of anxiety, *Adolescence* 33(129):99, 1998.

Ryman L, Rankin-Box D: Relaxation and visualization. In Rankin-Box D, editor: *The nurse's handbook of complementary therapies*, Edinburgh, 2001, Baillière Tindall.

Sheikh AA, editor: *Healing images: the role of imagination in health*, Imagery and Human Development Series, New York, 2002, Baywood Publishing.

Spector PE: Employee control and occupational stress, *Curr Dir Psychol Sci* 11(4):133, 2002.

Spencer JW, Jacobs JJ: *Complementary and alternative medicine: an evidence-based approach*, St. Louis, 2003, Mosby.

Taylor SE, Klein LC, Lewis BP, et al: Behavioral responses to stress in females: Tend and befriend, not fight or flight, *Psychol Rev* 107(3):411, 2000.

Tusaie K, Edds K: Understanding and integrating mindfulness into psychiatric mental health nursing practice, *Arch Psychiatr Nurs* 23(5):359, October 2009.

Weiss S: Using relaxation imagery with children, paper presented at the 22nd annual seminar of the Florida Association of Pediatric Tumor Programs, Clearwater Beach, Fla, November 19, 1998.

Suggestions for Further Reading

Benson H: *The relaxation response*, New York, 2000, Harpers.

Google search: Search "relaxation techniques" on a search engine such as www.google.com

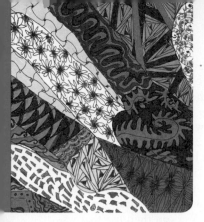

Chapter 21

Imagery

Objectives

1. Define imagery or visualization
2. Practice imagery, using the tart lemon exercise
3. Discuss the history of the use of imagery
4. Identify uses of imagery in clinical practice
5. Identify brief imagery exercises to cope with stressful situations
6. Discuss the use of imagery techniques to improve communication skills
7. Participate in selected exercises to build skills in using imagery to increase feelings of confidence and competence in communication

Definition of Imagery

When you use imagery you are deliberately using your imagination for success or wellness (Naparstek, 2008). An *image* is defined as a mental picture (Merriam-Webster Online Dictionary, 2011a). The term *visualization* is interchangeable with the term *imagery*. To visualize is to see or image mentally (Merriam-Webster Online Dictionary, 2011b). We use the term to mean creating an image of something invisible, absent, or abstract. As you read this chapter, begin to create an image of yourself as a confident, successful nurse, communicating assertively, gaining respect, and becoming a dedicated patient advocate.

Imagery or visualization is a process of mentally picturing an event we wish will occur in the present or future. It is a process of actually experiencing a picture that we hold in our mind's eye. In visualizing our picture, we may incorporate our senses to taste it, smell it, and feel it, and imagine the sounds and emotions associated with it. For example, when we visualize a freshly baked apple pie, we can actually smell it, taste the apples, and visualize eating the pie. We might evoke an image in vivid sensory detail of an absent loved one for extra emotional comfort. We might mentally rehearse a nursing procedure before performing it. As part of our fitness training, we might mentally rehearse running a 5K run or a marathon, envisioning being at the finish line successfully and proudly (Naparstek, 2008).

Try This Experiment: The Tart Lemon

Close your eyes and imagine that you are in your home. Picture yourself walking into your kitchen and looking at the refrigerator. In your mind's eye see the refrigerator. Open it and pull open the fruit and vegetable drawer. You see a large, bright, yellow lemon. Pick it up and notice the yellow, shiny, bumpy surface. Feel the weight of the lemon in your hand. Now take the lemon to a cutting board. Squeeze the lemon before you cut it. You can already smell the citrus scent. Cut the lemon and inhale its fragrance. Open your mouth. Now squeeze a few drops of the cold, tart lemon juice onto your tongue. Open your eyes. Did your mouth pucker? Could you see the lemon, smell it, taste it?

Everyone who is successful must have dreamed of something.

Maricopa Indian proverb

WIT&_Wisdom_

Note: Not everyone images the same way. Some people report being actively involved in the scene. Some see it as actors on a stage. Others get sensory impressions but not a clear image. Don't be concerned if you can't "see" things. Practice helps. This experiment helps you understand the behavioral applications of imagery.

When we visualize ourselves communicating, such as by listening actively, we can hear ourselves articulating empathic words; feel ourselves being warm, genuine, and natural; and enjoy observing a positive interaction between ourselves and our clients or colleagues.

Imagery is like a directed, deliberate daydream with purpose. It is much more than mere fantasy. The key to successful visualization is to be clear about what you want and then commit to that course of action in your imagery. This is a crucial step for producing successful results. In your mind's eye there need be neither limitations nor constraints.

How does imagery work? Research shows that the neurophysiology of the brain does not distinguish between an image and the experience of the imagined place or situation as demonstrated through dimensional brain studies (Sternberg, 2010). "The body does not know the difference between what one is thinking and what is actually happening. The image or thought is experienced with one or more of the senses with an associated emotion linking the mind with a feeling state and the body with a resulting physiologic change" (Reed, 2007, p. 262). For

example, beginning to worry about an examination, thinking about being unsuccessful, and thinking about the consequences cause the body to respond with a cascade of chemicals of the stress response, adrenaline and cortisol, interfering with immune function and our ability to cope (Reed, 2007).

This chapter focuses on how you can use imagery to positively influence your interpersonal communication. You will learn the steps required to formulate a clear image of how you want to communicate with your clients or colleagues. You can then use that visualization to help you actualize your vision in reality.

Imagery has been used in physical healing for a long time. You may be interested in the history of visualization in medicine.

History of Imagery

Imagery may be the oldest healing technique used by humans. Early records of this technique have been found on cuneiform tablets from Babylonia and Sumeria. Greek, Egyptian, Asian, and ancient Indian civilizations used visualization. Even today, Navaho Indians and Canadian Eskimos practice imagery for healing purposes (Johnston, 2002).

WIT&_Wisdom_

Just Imagine
Take me away
To a beautiful place.
Let's get away
From this awful rat race.
They say a vacation
I can take in my mind.
Close your eyes, relax,
Leave your tension behind.
Pay attention to each sense.
See, smell, hear, taste and feel.
Let your mind go, just travel.
Your own stress, you'll heal.
It's OK to daydream.
They always said, "NO!"
Now it's OK to daydream.
Just let your mind flow.

In all these cultures, disease was seen as a supernatural force that had incorporated itself into the ill person's being. The shaman, or physician-priest, would heal through rituals or ceremonies by confronting the disease-causing demon with a positive force and exorcising the demon from the patient. The shaman derived his power from visualization of a higher authority, god, or spirit. At that time, medicine was controlled by religion, mysticism, and magic (Johnston, 2002).

Paracelsus, a Renaissance physician, is known as the father of scientific medicine and modern drug therapy. A man opposed to the notion of separating the healing process from the spirit, he said: "The spirit is the master, imagination the tool, and the body the plastic material. The power of the imagination is a great factor in medicine. It may produce diseases in man and in animals, and it may cure them. . . . Ills of the body may be cured by the physical remedies or by the power of the spirit acting through the soul" (Hartmann, 2007). The views of Paracelsus differed from those of the early shamans because Paracelsus believed that people's own thoughts, as well as gods and spirits, could be healing (Samuels and Samuels, 1975).

The mind–body dichotomy was first conceived during the Renaissance. The French philosopher Descartes helped establish the split with his attempts to free scientific questions from arguments concerning God. Scientists could then be concerned about the body without theological debate, and the philosophers and theologians were left to study the spirit and mind (Flynn, 1980).

After the Renaissance, techniques of healing were divided into two systems: scientific and religious. Our Western society has adopted scientific healing—surgery and drug therapy. With increasing scientific investigation and medical specialization, the body–mind–spirit split continued into the twentieth century. By 1900, however, a number of medical scientists had begun investigating how the mind affects the body and healing (Samuels and Samuels, 1975).

Jacobson (1942), searching for effective methods of relaxation, demonstrated that the imagery we use in thought processes produces a muscular reactivity that resembles what occurs during the actual performance of the imagined act. That is, if we imagine ourselves in our mind's eye as running, the muscles we normally use when we run contract slightly.

Many scientists, as well as members of the medical profession, have continued to accept that the autonomic nervous system is unconscious, automatic, and not within conscious control. In the late 1960s,

physiologists DiCara and Miller demonstrated that parts of the autonomic nervous system can be conditioned and controlled. They determined that rats could learn how to alter their stomach acidity, brain wave patterns, blood pressure, and blood flow (Miller, 1969). Furthermore, in their work with humans, scientists have verified that yogis have the ability to control specific processes of the body such as metabolic rate and heart rate (Lauria, 1968).

Groundwork laid by these scientists has been revolutionary in the current shift away from the body–mind–spirit split to body–mind integration. The implications of these findings for nursing and medicine are extraordinary and exciting!

Application of Imagery in Healthcare

"Imagery creates a bridge between mind and body, linking perception, emotion, and psychological, physiological, and behavioural responses" (Apostolo and Kolcaba, 2009, p. 410). Helms describes guided imagery as a complementary intervention to help the mind "see" positive images of desired outcomes to influence health and well-being, part of the content in the development of the NCLEX-RN (2006). Imaging positive results can have the opposite effect of the stress response: promoting relaxation; helping control blood pressure; helping to control pain and anxiety; facilitating the action of medication and treatments; minimizing side effects; promoting coping with chronic illness; optimizing healing; and promoting comfort during and after procedures (Reed, 2007; Lewandowski et al, 2005; Mezies et al, 2006; Lewandowski, 2004; Lang, 2000; Kreitzer and Snyder, 2002; McCaffrey and Taylor, 2005; Wynd, 2005). Imagery techniques include end state, which involves the image of a healed state; process, which involves imaging step-by-step to a goal, such as successful, comfortable completion of a procedure; receptive, in which images for healing arise from the person's own mind; active, which involves a conscious choice of a healing image, such as a healing white light directed to the affected area; and anatomic, such as imaging of the opening of constricted vessels (Schaub and Dossey, 2009). Here is a specific example: a client with excessive gastric secretions was asked to gaze at the dryness and texture of blotting paper while imagining absorbent dryness. Tests indicated that after 10 days of performing these visualizations, the client's excessive secretions normalized (Luthe, 1969). The use of imagery empowers the client to promote wellness when disease produces a sense of loss of control.

One hypothesis is that the feelings of hope and anticipation are recorded by the limbic system in place of hopelessness and despair. Psychoneuroimmunology is the study of the "multidirectional interactions among behavioral, neuroendocrine, and immunologic process of adaptation. Thoughts, emotions, and information are reciprocal stimuli to sensory and motor neurons, glandular tissues, and immune cells via chemical transmitters" (Giedt, 1997). Clients who are enthusiastic about feeling better using imagery and who explicitly follow instructions show dramatic relief of their symptoms and marked improvement in their conditions.

There is evidence that visualization can influence a person's heart rate, blood flow, immune response, and total physiology. Visualization is a noninvasive, cost-effective intervention. Given this, what then are the implications of imagery?

Implications of Imagery

How does the knowledge that it is possible to voluntarily affect the autonomic nervous system using visualization influence us in our nursing care? First, we as nurses can adopt a holistic philosophy of body, mind, and spirit integration. A holistic perspective emphasizes the interrelationship of the parts that make up the whole person. It acknowledges that the mind affects the body and vice versa. Accepting this notion of interdependence means understanding the power that exists within our whole body–mind–spirit beings to heal ourselves. This internal power can be used to maintain and increase our level of wellness, either alone or in conjunction with an external source of healing (Samuels and Bennett, 1974). The American Holistic Nurses Association offers a forum for the discussion of the research and practice of holistic nursing, and nurses in other states conduct workshops on interventions such as therapeutic touch.

A simple application of imagery in nursing is the use of alternative language when performing procedures, language that, although still truthful, suggests a different sensation than anticipated. When giving an injection, say, "You may feel a stick." This language decreases anxiety and shifts the pattern from response to "pain" to response to "a stick" (Kron and Johnson, 1983). The use of imagery is also gaining increasing acceptance in the areas of corporate finance and sports. Researchers have discovered, for example, that a frequent characteristic of executives of major U.S. corporations is that "these

people knew what they wanted out of life. They could see it, taste it, smell it, and imagine the sounds and emotions associated with it. They prelived it before they had it. And that sharp, sensory vision became a powerful driving force in their lives" (Mayer, 1984).

In an experiment conducted at the University of Western Australia, one basketball team practiced 20 minutes longer a day, whereas a second team used this 20 minutes to imagine themselves playing the game and mentally correcting themselves each time they missed a basket. After a period of weeks, the group that physically practiced the game improved 24%, and the group visualizing themselves as practicing improved 23% (Mayer, 1984).

Professional golfer Jack Nicklaus uses visualization to improve the muscle memory and motor skills involved in golf. Nicklaus has said that good golf requires one-half mental rehearsal and one-half physical coordination. He never hits a shot without first seeing a sharp, clear picture of that shot in his mind's eye (Mayer, 1984).

Imagery has been used in medicine, athletics, and business. It is a process that can be applied by people in various walks of life to achieve success in whatever they value. We now look at how imagery can be used by nurses to improve their interpersonal communication skills.

> *"If you don't know where you are going any road will get you there."* [The Cheshire Cat's response to Alice when she asked how to get there. He asked her where she wanted to go and she replied she didn't know.]
>
> **Lewis Carroll's** *Alice's Adventures in Wonderland*
>
> **WIT&***Wisdom*

Relationship between Imagery and Interpersonal Communication

If we are clear about what is important to us, and if we are committed to creating what we value, imagery is an invaluable tool for self-direction (Mayer, 1984). This idea is the key to how imagery can be used by nurses to improve their interpersonal communication skills. If you are clear that it is important to be an effective communicator, and you are committed to creating that outcome, then imagery can help you achieve that goal. Silk and Norwood use the term "mental holography" to refer to the creation of mental images to enhance communication (2002–2003). A hologram is "a manipulation of light from different sources to create a very realistic, three-dimensional image of a person or object that is not physically present . . . the study of holograms is 'holography'" (2002–2003, p. 1). They suggest that when speakers learn to create sharp, vivid images in their mind, they can better communicate this image via language and body language.

As a professional nurse you want to implement the interpersonal communication skills you are learning in this book in a way that is beneficial to your clients, your colleagues, and yourself. Imagery grants you a visualization of yourself implementing these skills in a helpful and effective way. It provides you with a picture of yourself as a nurse who can handle a variety of interpersonal situations confidently and competently. These images act like a beacon, beckoning you to achieve the goal of being a competent communicator. Having a mental hologram of yourself that envisions how you want to act and be seen supports your success in projecting this image.

As you read about each of the interpersonal communication behaviors, you learn the correct way to implement each one with your clients and colleagues. You develop a vision of yourself executing the communication behavior you are studying. When using imagery, some people experience themselves participating, whereas others observe themselves as actors on a stage. Some people get impressions without clear images. Some clients report better success with the use of the word pretend rather than imagine. Your perception may be fuzzy and vague at first. It is essential that you work at making this image of yourself as clear as possible. You need to create an image that envisions you communicating in a positive, effective, and competent manner. The more detailed and specific you can make your visualization, the more effective it will be to guide your actual communication.

Imagining yourself being successful is much like a rehearsal. This mental dry run helps cement an image of yourself carrying out the skill correctly. When the dress rehearsal goes well, it gives you confidence that your live performance will also be positive. You may find that the actual visualization process takes you 1 minute or less. The more you use this process, the more proficient you will become.

Seeing yourself perform the way you want to is just one more step toward successfully carrying out your performance in public. Having an image of yourself communicating well makes the future reality of such an event a viable possibility. Imagery helps you become familiar with your desired outcome so that you start accepting the notion that achieving your ideal is possible and forthcoming. Imagery makes you believe that you can achieve your goals.

Imagery can be influential in helping us communicate in a way that is in keeping with our goals as a nurse. If golf scores and management strategies can be improved through visualization, so can nurses' interpersonal communication skills.

Consider, too, the use of imagery to explore how mental models, which are deeply ingrained, can negatively influence the nurse's performance. Krejci (1997) helps students examine their images in response to words such as *nurse*, *doctor*, *power*, and *caring*. Sometimes these mental models are outdated and can affect the ability of nurses to grow professionally. Krejci cites the example of students' imagery about the word power, which often depicts a female nurse as a bystander watching a male figure wielding power. By reflecting on the importance of the caring and advocacy roles of the nurse, nurses can reframe their views of power and claim the power of their role.

Brief Imagery Exercises to Cope with Stressful Situations

Consider one of the following brief images when you take a moment to put distance between yourself and the strong emotions of a situation that you want to face calmly. An intense emotional situation may impair your judgment and make you speak before you think. Being relaxed and focused will better enable you to respond rationally rather than react emotionally. Imagine one of the following that most appeals to you. Pay attention to all your senses as you mentally experience:

- A leaf floating downstream
- Clouds moving across the sky
- Helium-filled balloons rising
- Bubbles being blown away (Payne and Donaghy, 2010)

Use of Imagery to Improve Your Ability to Communicate

Here are some of the essential points of effective imagery. First, imagery requires discipline, that is, the willingness to briefly stop what you are doing and undertake the visualization process. Imagery is most effective when you are relaxed, so begin your imagery with three deep breaths to facilitate relaxation. (Refer to Chapter 20 for other relaxation exercises.) Relaxation helps you let go of the thoughts swimming around in your head. This enables you to focus on becoming clear about what you want to create with your imagery. Once you are clear about your goal or purpose, commit to creating it with no reservations and with complete faith that your goal or purpose will be attained. Using all your senses, allow yourself to feel the experience of your goal being attained as though it were happening at the very moment of your visualization.

Although this may sound complex at the outset, with practice, you will be able to go through these steps quickly and effectively.

You might think that the practice of visualization is quite abstract because it occurs unseen inside your head. On the contrary, there are concrete and specific things you can do to ensure that your visualization influences your future performance in the way you intend. The following are some systematic steps you can take to make sure that your visualization has the desired results.

Moments of Connection . . .
Just Imagine . . . Offering a Peaceful Pause for the People You Serve (You Can Try It, Too!)

A nursing student, already an RN going back to earn a bachelor of science in nursing (BSN) degree, wanted to begin to integrate guided imagery into her work in intensive care. She remembered the practical language her instructor had offered to help her clients use imagery in a simple way. Remind the client, "Your body stays here while you are in the hospital, but you can go anywhere you want in your mind. Think of a place you would rather be, a place of comfort, beauty, or a time, a memory which you would like to revisit." When the nurse offered this suggestion, her client said, "I'd rather be home cooking." The nurse reminded her to engage all her senses as she imagined being in her kitchen. "See what you are doing, smell the smells, taste the tastes, hear the sounds, experience the emotions you have here." The client became quiet and said she would try this. Later she laughed and reported what a wonderful relief this had been for her.

Be Clear about Your Desired Outcome

Before you envision how you will communicate, you must be clear about what it is you are trying to achieve. Is it your aim to be warm and comforting? Do you want to obtain specific information from your client or colleague? Is it your intention to get a point across? Whatever your purpose is in communicating, you must be clear about what you want to happen. The more your mental rehearsal is tailored to reality, the more positive an influence it will have on your subsequent performance.

It might be helpful for you to compare a poorly articulated goal with a clearer, more detailed one.

Barb and Jane are both nurses working on a burn unit. Both nurses are concerned about Mrs. Charter, who has become withdrawn and weepy in the last 48 hours. Each nurse decides on her own desired outcome for this unhappy client situation.

Barb makes it her goal to help Mrs. Charter overcome her blue mood. This goal is not as clear as it might be because it does not provide Barb with many clues about how to proceed. Not only is it not specific, but it is unlikely that it is a logical place to begin without more data.

Jane's aim is to determine if Mrs. Charter is aware of what might be causing her mood change and to discuss with her whether there is anything that can be done to lift her mood. Her aim is to put Mrs. Charter at ease so that she can talk more freely about her feelings. This clearer desired outcome provides Jane with some guidelines on how to proceed.

Mentally Outline the Whole Interaction from Beginning to End

You will feel more prepared for your interaction if you mentally outline it in your mental imagery. For instance, if you are going to be teaching a client to care for a colostomy, do not limit your visualization to the time when you will be talking. Bring into your vision your preparation time, postsession time, and the direct teaching time. When you visualize your preparation, you will anticipate all the equipment you will need and consequently will have it ready. You might become aware that you fear embarrassment in discussing the hygienic and sexual aspects of colostomy care with a male client. This awareness will prompt you to talk over your concerns with a more experienced colleague before the session so that you will feel less uncomfortable.

When imagining the actual teaching session, consider the beginning, middle, and end. Find out how much time you have and imagine yourself using the time effectively and productively for both you and your client. Envision the conclusion of the lesson: will you want time to debrief and discuss the session with a colleague afterward? Is it likely that you will have follow-up assignments after the session for which you must allow time—for example, making referrals, writing records, or securing information for the client? By mentally going through the whole encounter, you will be much better prepared.

Concentrate on Visualizing Details

Envision the most ideal environment for your encounter and take in all its details. In reality, try to approximate this environment in terms of privacy, lighting, warmth, accessibility to equipment, or whatever other criteria are important.

Visualize how you would like to be dressed for your interaction. If it is a play session with the children on the pediatric medical unit, you will likely envision yourself in a brightly colored pantsuit uniform. If you are mentally preparing yourself for your job performance interview with your manager, envision yourself wearing a uniform in which you feel your best. Pay attention to your posture and facial expressions. If you want to be businesslike with a serious middle-aged client, then picture how you will move to convey your intentions. If you wish to appear relaxed and confident as you present your case at your first nursing rounds, mentally see and feel yourself showing this composure.

As you direct yourself in your visions to create a positive impression, notice in your mind's eye that others are responding favorably. You may observe, for example, that you are being listened to and taken seriously and that your client or colleague seems interested in what you have to say.

In addition to visual imagery, use your other senses. For instance, listen to what you are saying and how you are saying it. If what you are saying does not come across in the way you intended, then roll back the reel and replay it. On the rerun visualize yourself communicating more in line with how you would ideally like to. The beauty of mentally rehearsing is that you can repeat it as many times as you like until you get it right! Tune into your words and the way you are saying them, striving to hear the content and quality you desire.

Envision how you want to feel during your communication and be sure to concentrate on the positive. Engender feelings of calmness, confidence, competence, or compassion—or however you want to be feeling in reality. It is important to pause and actually experience these good feelings in your rehearsal, so you will be more likely to recognize them and allow them to surface in the real situation. Also visualize your client or colleague having feelings that are appropriate for the situation.

Using your wide-angle lens, see the whole interaction going as you planned. For example, your bereaved colleague feels relieved to have shed a few tears with you after the death of her long-term client, your skeptical supervisor seems positively impressed with your suggestion for a new staffing schedule, and your once-worried client is able to drop off to sleep after your reassuring preoperative teaching session.

Envision the Best and Plan for the Unexpected

There are times when we are concerned about an interaction with a client or colleague for fear we will not be able to communicate in the way we want. Envisioning a positive rehearsal helps relieve some of that worry. To augment your confidence, it is wise to envision some of the unexpected turns of events you might possibly encounter in reality and practice how to cope with them. For example, if it is the first time you will be teaching prenatal classes and you are afraid that there might be questions about labor and delivery that you cannot answer, it would be wise to imagine a scene in which you are asked one of these questions and then rehearse the best way to respond. You may gain comfort with saying, "I don't know . . . but I'll find out for you," if you visualize it in advance. Or an angry colleague might unnerve you with her hostility. If you visualize her attack in advance, you can prepare yourself with effective ways to cope with the anger.

Practicing in this way expands your repertoire and prepares you for many contingencies. If you have prepared yourself for several versions of what to expect and rehearsed several options, you will feel more confident when you find yourself in the actual situation.

Rehearse Repeatedly When Necessary

Each of us has interpersonal situations in which we lack confidence. Some of us shudder at having to interact with angry, hostile people, whereas others remain calm and empathic with volatile clients and colleagues. Some of us dread taking charge of teaching sessions, whereas others love that opportunity. Some of us believe we relate better on a one-to-one basis, and others prefer groups. For those interpersonal situations in which you feel uncomfortable, it is wise to repeat your positive visualization several times. Repeatedly go over the picture of yourself performing successfully in your difficult area. A one-shot visualization may not allow you to register all the things you must do to make your communication successful. Seeing yourself handling things well in many visualizations will more thoroughly prepare you for the event. Repeating the scene in your mind's eye will prevent you from being caught off guard in the actual event—you will be able to act instead of react.

When we are concerned about a situation, we can lapse into forecasting the worst or we can choose to concentrate on seeing a positive picture. A positive visualization attracts like a magnet, getting you closer to your goal. If you repeat your positive visualization enough times, you will perform well in reality.

Review Your Live Performance and Update Your Visualization

After you have completed your interaction, take time to evaluate how the session went. If there were parts of your interaction with which you were less than pleased, think positively about how you could improve your next exchange and visualize that happening. For example, envision how you could rephrase your words, arrange the room differently, or include gestures such as touch. This rehearsal will prepare you for the next time.

Do not put yourself down for your errors. Instead, give yourself credit for your improvements. Remember that you are learning and consider that each practice will get you closer to the way you want to communicate to clients and colleagues. Think back to your rehearsal and notice where you met or even surpassed your ideals. Visualize patting yourself on the back and congratulating yourself on your successes. Taking time to commend yourself will increase your self-confidence.

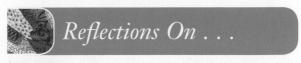

Reflections On . . .

Imagery

Consider what you read about the importance of imagery as a tool to build communication skills. Do you already use imagery techniques? Which techniques in this chapter sound interesting to you? Answer the following questions.

What? . . .
Write one thing you learned from this chapter.

So what? . . .
How will this affect your nursing practice?

Now what? . . .
How will you implement this new knowledge or skill?

Think about it . . .

Practicing Imagery

Exercise 1

Poetry creates powerful imagery and illustrates the power of the mind to create images with powerful emotion. Here is another of Howard Kirkman's poems. He has found meaning in life by "teaching nurses and nursing students for 30 years." Read this poem and then discuss the emotion the images evoke for you.

Hospital
Pans rattling
reflecting lights and pungent smells.
Quiet halls,
suddenly hurrying . . .
whispering,
then crying,
death just passed.

Copyright © Howard G. Kirkman. Used with permission.

Exercise 2

Take a few minutes to evoke a pleasant childhood memory. One example is a grandfather telling a story, sitting in a rocking chair on a front porch just as the lightning bugs come out at twilight. Silk and Norwood (2002–2003) describe such a scene and say the magic of the story and this memory depend on your senses and detailed images of the memory, which is linked to emotion. As you access a pleasant memory, write a few sentences in your journal. Describe the memory, sensory perceptions, and emotions evoked.

Exercise 3

In this chapter the following images are offered as distancing strategies, to help you relax and center: a leaf floating downstream, clouds moving across the sky, helium-filled balloons rising, bubbles being blown away. Take a few minutes now to experience each to identify what works best for you. Practice it often so it will be a readily available strategy when you need it.

Exercise 4

McKim (1972) has adapted a psychological test to help assess the vividness of your images. Rate the following items using the criteria given:

Rating: C = clear; V = vague; N = no image at all

- Face of a friend
- Rose
- Playful puppy
- Full moon
- Sound of rain on a window
- Taste of pepper
- Smell of peppermint
- Sound of fingernails scraping on a chalkboard
- Smell of coffee brewing
- Feeling of stretching to reach for an item on a tall shelf

Exercise 5

McKim (1972) suggests that it is even more important to be able to control imagery than to evoke clear pictures.

Rate your ability to control the following images using the criteria given:

Rating: C = controlled the image well; U = unsure; N = not able to control the image

- Rose unfolding into full bloom
- Flat rock skipping across the surface of a lake
- Pinwheel spinning clockwise, then reversing
- Car racing forward, then running backward
- Sofa moving unaided up to the ceiling and back to the floor
- Balloon drifting up into the sky and then returning to the ground
- Wave crashing onto the shore and then reversing itself
- Yourself sitting down in a chair and then standing
- Words appearing on a computer screen and then disappearing as if deleted
- Cake rising as viewed through a glass oven door and then going back to uncooked cake batter

McKim cautions you not to be disappointed if you do poorly but to repeat the exercises after you have practiced imaging. View this visualization as a pretest that is administered before you learn the course content.

Exercise 6

In your everyday life, take the opportunity to use imagery to help you communicate more effectively with others. For example, if you would like to invite a classmate to go shopping with you, visualize how you would like to extend the invitation and envision his or her enthusiastic response. Prepare yourself for a refusal by hearing the classmate extend regrets and watch yourself respond smoothly. Or you may have an upcoming test of your nursing care practice. Take time to see yourself successfully completing each part of the test and imagine your instructor giving you top grades.

Continued

After a few days of using imagery, take stock of the ways in which it has helped you. What personal adaptations to the process of imagery have you made that might be useful for your colleagues to apply? In the class as a whole, compare reflections on the benefits of imagery.

Visualize yourself as successful! As you practice imagery you will discover it is a skill that requires discipline and concentration. It is self-constructive to develop the power of concentration to visualize yourself communicating in an effective way. If we want to be self-destructive, we can let our thoughts take control of us by allowing thoughts of making mistakes, embarrassing ourselves, or failing to communicate effectively dominate our visions. If we permit negative and unproductive thoughts to worry and plague us, we might fall into the trap of acting out the failure. On the other hand, our chances for success are augmented by mentally rehearsing a positive outcome. If you have seen yourself succeeding in your mind's eye, it is but one more step to performing well in reality.

As you practice, you will discover that imagery does not require much time and can be done anywhere. In the shower, on the bus, as you walk to your meeting, at the nurses' station—you can visualize anywhere because your imagination is always active. What imagery emphasizes is taking control of your thinking so that you create positive, self-enhancing pictures of yourself that facilitate more hopeful and confident feelings. Because imagery can be done conveniently, you can repeatedly bring into your awareness the image of the successful you.

As you learn each of the communication behaviors in this book, practice a positive visualization of yourself using them correctly. Rehearsing with the valuable assistance of imagery will help you feel confident and facilitate the integration of the skill into your communications repertoire.

Exercise 7

In the opening paragraph of this chapter you were asked to begin to visualize yourself as a successful nurse. Take a few minutes to draw this image of yourself, write a journal entry describing yourself with the characteristics and behaviors of a successful nurse, or write a poem about yourself in this successful role.

> *The debt we owe to the play of imagination is incalculable.*
>
> **Carl Jung**

WIT&*Wisdom*

References

Apostolo JLA, Kolcaba K: The effects of guided imagery on comfort, depression, anxiety, and stress of psychiatric inpatients with depressive disorders, *Arch Psychiatr Nurs* 23(6):403, December 2009.

Flynn P: *Holistic health: the art and science of care*, Bowie, Md, 1980, Robert J. Brady.

Giedt JF: A psychoneuroimmunological intervention in holistic nursing practice, *J Holist Nurs Pract* 15(2):112, 1997.

Hartmann F: *Paracelsus: life and prophecies*, Whitefish, Mont, 2007, Kessinger Publishing.

Helms JE: Complementary and alternative therapies: a new frontier for nursing education? *J Nurs Educ* 45(3):1117, March 2006.

Jacobson E: *Progressive relaxation*, Chicago, 1942, University of Chicago Press.

Johnston SL: Native American and traditional and alternative medicine: *Ann Am Pol Soc Sci* (583):195(1), 2002.

Kreitzer MJ, Snyder M: Healing the heart: integrating complementary therapies and healing practices into the care of cardiovascular patients, *Prog Cardiovasc Nurs* 17(2):73, 2002.

Krejci JW: Stimulating critical thinking by exploring mental modes, *J Nurs Educ* 36(10):482, 1997.

Kron ER, Johnson K: *Visualization: the uses of imagery in the health professions*, Homewood, Ill, 1983, Dow Jones—Irwin.

Lang E, Benotsch E, Fick L, et al: Adjunctive non-pharmacological analgesia for invasive medical procedures: a randomized trial, *Lancet* 355(9214):1486, 2000.

Lauria A: *The mind of a mnemonist*, New York, 1968, Basic Books.

Lewandowski WA: Patterning of pain and power with guided imagery, *Nurs Sci Q* 17(3):233, 2004.

Lewandowski WA, Good M, Draucher CB: Changes in the meaning of pain with the use of guided imagery, *Pain Manag Nurs* 6(2):58, 2005.

Luthe W: *Autogenic therapy*, vol II, New York, 1969, Grune & Stratton.

Mayer AJ: Visualization, *En Route* 48(50):30, 1984.

McCaffrey R, Taylor N: Effective anxiety treatment prior to diagnostic cardiac catheterization, *Holist Nurs Pract* 19(2):70, Mar/Apr 2005.

McKim RH: *Experiences in visual thinking*, Monterey, Calif, 1972, Brooks/Cole.

Menzies V, Taylor A, Bourguenon C: Effects of guided imagery on outcomes of pain, functional states, and self-efficacy in persons diagnosed with fibromyalgia, *J Altern Complement Med* 12(1):23, 2006.

Merriam-Webster Online Dictionary. http://www.merriam-webster.com/dictionary/image. Accessed June 1, 2011.

Merriam-Webster Online Dictionary http://www.merriam-webster.com/dictionary/visualizing. Accessed June 1, 2011.

Miller N: Learning and visceral and glandular responses, *Science* 163:434, 1969.

Naparstek B: *Staying well with guided imagery* (Kindle edition), New York, 2008, Grand Central Publishing.

Payne RA, Donaghy M: *Payne's handbook of relaxation techniques: a practical guide for the health care professional*, ed 4, Edinburgh, 2010, Elsevier.

Reed T: Imagery in the clinical setting: a tool for healing, *Nurs Clin North Am* 42(2):261, 2007.

Samuels M, Bennett HZ: *Be well*, Toronto, 1974, Random House.

Samuels M, Samuels N: *Seeing with the mind's eye*, New York, 1975, Random House.

Schaub BG, Dossey BM: Imagery: awakening the inner healer. In Dossey BM, et al, editors: *Holistic nursing: a handbook for practice*, Sudbury, Mass, 2009, Jones Bartlett.

Silk G, Norwood MS: Mental holography: the power of imagery in communication, *J Imag Lang Learn Teach*, vol VII, 2002–2003. http://www.njcu.edu/CILL/vol7/silk-norwood.html. Accessed June 1, 2011.

Sternberg E: *The science of healing with Dr. Esther Sternberg*, PBS DVD, 2010.

Wynd CA: Guided imagery for smoking cessation and long-term abstinence, *J Nurs Scholarship* 37(3):245, 2005.

Suggestions for Further Reading

American Holistic Nurses Association (website). http://www.ahna.org. Membership includes a subscription to the *Journal of Holistic Nursing*.

Beyond Ordinary Nursing: *Nurses certificate program in imagery* (website.) http://www.integrativeimagery.com.

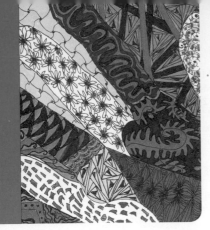

Chapter 22

Positive Self-Talk

It's not who you are that holds you back. It's who you think you're not.

Source Unknown

Objectives

1. Define self-talk and its influence on behavior
2. Discuss the relationship between self-talk and interpersonal communication
3. Discuss the use of affirmations as a strategy to create positive self-talk
4. Practice positive self-talk to develop confidence in communication skills and nursing practice

Definition of Self-Talk

Have you noticed that we have an ongoing internal dialogue? We speak to ourselves and we listen to ourselves. Self-talk is not unlike the conversation that occurs between two people. Self-talk is also known as inner thought, inner speech, self-instruction, or that "little voice" in your head that forms a self-communication system. In an in-depth review of the self-talk literature, Hardy delineates self-talk as instructional or motivational (2006). Self-talk can be rational, based on reasoning, logic, or facts, or irrational. It can be positive, offering encouragement or praise, or negative, offering discouragement and criticism (Mayo Clinic, 2009). What you tell yourself can affect your health. In a study by Levy and colleagues (2002) people who said they had positive views about aging lived an average of 7.6 years longer than those who had negative views.

A familiar childhood story tells us that this skill is time tested. Remember *The Little Engine That Could*, the tale of an old train that was being replaced by a shiny new model? The new train refused to climb a steep hill to deliver toys to the children (Piper, 1998). The old train met the challenge with positive self-talk. He repeated, "I think I can . . . I think I can . . . I think I can," and sure enough, he was successful. A search indicates that this well-loved children's story goes back to 1910. We have been encouraging our children to use positive self-talk for many years.

Casual remarks made unintentionally by those around us can become self-prophecies. In response to the book, *What Do You Say When You Talk to Yourself?*, which sold more than a million copies, thousands of letters were sent to the author by readers who related that they had believed something totally false about themselves throughout their lives based on something someone else had said (Helmsetter, 1990).

Turkington (1998) calls negative self-talk the "evil within" and points out that we would seldom talk to others the way we talk to ourselves.

Cognitive psychologists have learned that internal dialogue has a powerful influence on our behavior. Our thoughts are our interpretations of the world, our judgments about our own behavior, and our assumptions about others' reactions to us. Our feelings are directly influenced by our thoughts, and how we construe our world provides the blueprint for our actions. It is not what is happening to us that is so significant, but how we interpret what is happening to us and what we do under the influence of these thoughts.

For any situation or interpersonal encounter we have, our self-talk determines the following:

- Our attitude toward the situation
- What we see, hear, and attend to
- How we interpret what we take in
- What we think the outcome will be
- How we act (including what we feel, say, and do)
- How we appraise the consequences of our actions

It is important that our internal dialogue be in our own best interests, because it is a continuous and powerful influence on our well-being and performance. Cognitive psychologists believe our internal dialogue causes problems when it is irrational, unrealistic, or ineffective (Ellis and Powers, 1998).

Our internal dialogue can be constructive or destructive. Take as a simple example a person whose mother has always told her that she is clumsy. Because she believes it to be so, the woman's self-talk is not positive. She says, "I'm so clumsy. I'm always bruising myself." She finds that she truly seems to be clumsy. When she changes her self-talk to "I am graceful and move easily and carefully," however, her awkwardness decreases.

Following are several clinical examples of positive and negative self-talk. As you read the examples, think about their possible effects on the nurses in the situation.

Tanya and Deirdre are nursing students in their senior year. As they anticipate their forthcoming clinical placements in a public health department, these thoughts go through their minds:

Tanya: "I've heard that the new director of the agency is a tyrant. I hate people like that. They have miserable dispositions that grate on my nerves. I just know I'm not going to like working with her. Team conferences will be a pain. She's sure to pick on me, and knowing me I'll probably make some blunder that'll be a red flag for her to show me up. I'll be glad when this rotation is over."

Tanya has set herself up for an unhappy and unfruitful clinical placement. Her negative thoughts about the director have entrenched the notion that she will be miserable in the public health rotation. This negative self-talk is destructive. Thinking the way she does, Tanya will likely act defensively and be so on edge that she will make a mistake. Her attitude will probably isolate her from friendly sources of support from the staff.

Deirdre: "I've heard that the new director is a real stickler for good nursing care and demands a lot from her staff. It's great that I get to go to a health department in which the home care is so good. I'm sure I'll learn a lot. I'm looking forward to making home visits and seeing how nursing care is given there. I'm also nervous because this is new and I don't know what we'll face, but I know I'll have the best teachers and get a lot out of the experience. Too bad it's only a brief rotation."

Deirdre has mentally prepared herself for a happy and rewarding clinical experience. Her interpretation of the excellence of the nursing care makes her keen to observe the nurses and reap the benefits of their experience. Her positive self-talk sets her up to risk interacting with the staff, and she will most likely get a lot out of the experience.

Our self-talk goes on continuously in our heads and is so automatic that we have to listen carefully to hear whether it is exerting a negative or positive influence on our feelings and behavior. If we want to have control of this habitual process, we need to listen to our thoughts, decide how we want to change, and systematically convert our thinking so that it influences our behavior in the intended direction.

Here is an example of a typical situation many student nurses encounter in the clinical area. As you read the scenario, put yourself in the position of the student nurse and write down your reactions.

You are a nursing student just entering your senior year after your summer vacation. To date, your clinical experience has been on the specialty units of your hospital: ophthalmology, gynecology, and the day-stay surgical unit. You are assigned to the intensive care unit and will be working with more complicated equipment. You are sure the patients will think you are clumsy and are afraid you'll make a terrible mistake. You hear that the staff is discouraged because they have to cut back hours temporarily due to budget problems. You know the unit has a full census of clients, and you fear the staff will not have the time or energy to help you. Your clinical instructor told you the staff is looking forward to having the students, because last year's seniors were so eager to learn.

After you have written your reactions, put the list aside for the moment and review the following example of Suzanne's negative self-talk as she encounters the same situation.

Suzanne: "I'll never cope! Who can ever have enough experience to prepare for intensive care? I hear the patients are all so sick that most of them die. I can barely think of all the scary equipment. What about the families? They won't want a student when their family member is so sick. I'm nervous already thinking about it. I feel nauseated. Why did I ever come into nursing? I don't like the idea of being compared to last year's seniors. I know they had some real brains. I can see it now. I'll be feeling panicky the whole time. I'll go home depressed because of the deaths. I'll feel so inadequate."

Suzanne's self-talk is destructive. It is escalating her anxiety and focusing on all the things that could possibly go wrong. Suzanne is drowning in a flood of catastrophic thinking. With a mindset like hers, she will be tuned into anything negative and may force a self-fulfilling prophecy. Her self-talk dismisses any self-confidence and makes her anxious before, and likely during, the experience.

Take a moment to write down a constructive internal dialogue that Suzanne could use in the same situation.

Here is an example of positive self-talk for Suzanne. Compare your suggestions with this example.

Suzanne: "This is going to be difficult. There's a lot of new equipment to learn, but I know the prediction is that most inpatient beds will be in critical care, and I plan to work in a hospital. I need to learn this. This experience might help me get a good recommendation. Everyone has to learn something new sometime. I'm bright, and I'll just make it a point to let the staff know I'm eager to learn. This is the best time to learn to deal with dying patients. These nurses have so much experience. I'm sure they can give me some help if I ask them how they cope. I know I can do this. The staff nurses know that I'm a student and will not expect miracles from

me. They will be glad for the contribution I can make to the unit. I must find out more about the unit from Betty so that I can prepare myself as much as possible for the experience."

This self-talk is constructive. Suzanne's internal dialogue in this example is realistic and hopeful. By acknowledging her assets, Suzanne will go onto the unit feeling confident. She is likely to approach the staff in a friendly way, eager for new opportunities. Thinking about her situation as a challenge provides Suzanne with a positive goal for her career as a nurse. By deciding to seek out information beforehand, she is increasing her chances of success.

Now go back to your own internal dialogue that you generated earlier in this exercise. Determine whether it is positive or negative. Does your self-talk work in your best interests, or is it potentially destructive?

Positive Self-Talk: Assertive and Responsible

The previous examples demonstrate how self-talk can be harmful or helpful to us. Positive self-talk is helpful because it emphasizes our strengths and our ability to handle the situations confronting us. This mental preparation makes us feel hopeful and confident. We have the right to feel good about how we handle situations we encounter, and positive self-talk is one technique we can use to ensure that our rights are realized. It is assertive to keep our internal dialogue positive.

Positive self-talk is not unrealistic or wishful thinking. It involves an accurate assessment of our abilities and the situation we are facing. Not having the knowledge or skills to effectively handle an interpersonal situation is no reason to think less of ourselves or to put ourselves down. Admitting our lack of experience and acknowledging our willingness and ability to learn realistically prepare us to tackle the situation. This positive kind of mental assessment is responsible, because it takes into account the facts of the situation. Mentally putting ourselves down or discrediting our abilities is not responsible thinking.

Butler (2008) warns us that when our self-talk is negative, we are carrying around a toxic environment for ourselves everywhere we go. Negative self-talk is harsh and judgmental, demanding superheroic achievements, chastising us for failing, and generally making us feel tense and dissatisfied with ourselves. Butler encourages us to develop a positive, supportive way of talking to ourselves to cushion us from negative events. Chapman (1992) comments that "positive people are far more likely than others to face up to problems, make tough decisions, and refuse to look back." He says that those with a positive outlook are often mistaken for people who just let things happen as if by fate. "Not so! Positive people often have more problems, because they take more risks and live life more fully."

Moments of Connection . . .
Moving from "Not One More Patient" to "Make Time for Joy"

"Let's get this over with," the nurse thought to herself. After 15 hours of a 24-hour on-call day in the postanesthesia care unit (PACU) with only a brief break, the nurse was dreading the "one more" case, a dislocated hip. Expecting a long recovery time and an admission to the short-stay unit, the nurse was surprised to learn that the client was young, the procedure would be short, and he would be dismissed as an ambulatory client. The nurse was tired and crabby and wanted to "get this over with." After talking with the family, the nurse learned that they had all been headed to a special event: Mom and Dad's 50th anniversary party. They were to have had photos taken. Instead they missed the photo appointment and had to eat in the hospital cafeteria. The nurse was instantly humbled and got to work to create a celebration. The family was invited into the PACU, and the staff made punch and retrieved an instant camera from the operating room to take pictures. What a mental shift. This was an opportunity to remember that joy can come when you least expect it!

Becoming aware of our self-talk is the first step to discovering if it is in our best interests. Learning how to change our self-talk starts with such an assessment. Butler (2008) suggests we ask ourselves the following questions:

- What am I telling myself?
- What negative thoughts am I generating that are destructive to me?
- What positive thoughts am I generating that are constructive for me?
- Is my self-talk helping me?
- How can I change my self-talk so that it is more positive?

The answers to these questions can indicate times when our thinking works in our best interests and times when it does not. This assessment alerts us to whether we need to change our self-talk. Whenever you feel overwhelmed by negative self-talk and the accompanying anxiety, consider the thought-stopping technique of silently yelling to yourself, "Stop!" to interrupt the barrage and derail your negative thinking.

The next step is to specify how we need to change our internal dialogue so that it is more positive. At first this planning will require considerable effort, but then it will become part of our awareness, enabling us to tune in to our internal dialogue and adjust it quickly. Later in this chapter you will get experience in reformulating self-talk.

Relationship between Self-Talk and Interpersonal Communication

In Part 1 you learned about behaviors that are essential for caring communication. Parts of your self-talk will be about your ability to implement these behaviors with your clients and colleagues. How you construct your internal dialogue can enhance or diminish your skill level.

Here are examples involving the communication behaviors of empathy and confrontation.

Example 1: Self-Talk about Empathy

Here is what one nurse said to herself about empathy:

> I can't be empathic and sound natural. I'll trip over my words. If I try using empathy, I'll sound artificial. My colleagues will laugh at me if I change my style and try to be empathic. I don't think I can think up an empathic response fast enough in a real conversation to make it sound sincere. I'll look and feel awkward trying to be empathic.

Examine this nurse's self-talk.

1. *What is she telling herself?* She is telling herself that she will feel uncomfortable, silly, and unnatural if she attempts to be empathic. She is convincing herself that her friends will not admire her attempts and that she will lose their respect.
2. *What negative thoughts is she generating that are destructive?* She is convincing herself that she will not be effective in her use of empathy. She expects that she should be perfect the first time she is empathic. She is not permitting any failure, nor is she hopeful that her colleagues will support her.

3. *What positive thoughts is she generating?* This nurse is not generating one positive thought that might give her the hope and encouragement to try being more empathic.

4. *Is her self-talk helping her?* This self-talk will likely stop her from including empathy in her communication strategies. These thoughts will make her feel bad on two counts: she will miss providing the benefits of empathy to others, and she will feel disappointed in her lack of willingness to try. She is left feeling convinced that neither she nor her colleagues have confidence in her ability. Her thoughts are nonassertive and irresponsible and not in any way helpful to her.

5. *How can she change her self-talk so that it is more positive?* Here is an example of how her self-talk could be more positive:

I'm going to try to use empathy even if I am a little stilted and awkward at first. I am convinced of the importance of empathy and know that my colleagues and clients will appreciate my efforts to show them that I understand, even if I am not perfect in my attempts. Some of my colleagues may teasingly comment on the change when I try to be more empathic; I will not let them deter me from including empathy in my communication. It may take me awhile to find the right words, but that's OK. It will likely seem longer to me than to the other person. I really want to improve my communication, and I know that something new takes time to learn. I can be patient with myself until empathy comes more naturally in my interactions with others.

This positive self-talk is assertive and responsible. It emphasizes the importance this nurse places on being empathic and gives her encouragement to try being more understanding. It is not a glib dialogue, but rather a realistic assessment of her ability to weather the struggle of trying something new until it becomes a natural part of her communication. This positive self-talk is helpful because it boosts confidence and facilitates the incorporation of a new skill into her repertoire.

Example 2: Self-Talk about Confrontation
Here is one nurse's self-talk about confrontation:

I think it's better to keep peace by not saying anything to the boss about his abrasive manner to me these past few days. If I confront him, he'll think

I'm being too sensitive and he'll be wary of me after this. He'll pull rank on me and get angry if I confront him. The more I think about it, the crazier it seems for me to be upset about his manner; he's probably got something on his mind and doesn't realize he's taking it out on me. What if I get all upset and mix up my words? I'd really look like a fool then.

Examine this nurse's self-talk.

1. *What is she telling herself?* She is convincing herself that she would be better off not to confront her boss about an issue important to her. She is arguing that her feelings are not as important as those of her boss.

2. *What negative thoughts is she generating that are destructive?* This nurse is denying her own feelings by deceiving herself that it might be better to let this episode pass. This self-deception undermines her judgment. She is creating bad feelings about herself by suggesting that being sensitive or expecting to be treated politely is undesirable. She attempts to frighten herself with the assumption that her boss will get angry and, furthermore, that she would not be able to handle his anger. She imagines the worst scenario and tries to convince herself that she is likely to fail.

3. *What positive thoughts is she generating?* This nurse's self-talk is entirely negative and contains nothing positive for her.

4. *Is her self-talk helping her?* This negative self-talk would only deter her from standing up for something that is important to her: her desire to be treated with respect. This approach makes her doubt her ability to confront and to handle one possible consequence of a confrontation: her boss's anger. Her negative self-talk is nonassertive and irresponsible in that she is allowing herself to be mistreated and refuses to accept her responsibility for letting the behavior continue.

5. *How can she change her self-talk to make it more positive?* Here is an example of how her self-talk could be more positive:

I don't like to confront my boss, but I don't like to be treated disrespectfully, so I will confront him. I know I can make my points clear to him without seeming like a whiner. My boss may become angry or hostile when I confront him, but I can handle this reaction without backing off or becoming defensive. I have practiced confrontation and feel confident that I can carry it off. If my confrontation isn't perfect, it doesn't matter; that I make my point as clearly as possible is what counts. Just because he's my boss is no reason for him to treat me so badly. I have the right to be treated with respect. He is more likely to respect me in the future if I set limits now.

This positive self-talk is assertive and responsible. It encourages the nurse to stand up for herself, and it takes into account her ability to handle several possible outcomes. It is encouraging and supportive and would give this nurse the comfort and confidence to carry out her confrontation.

In Part 4 of this book you will learn how to communicate assertively and responsibly in the following situations in which nurses are known to have difficulty:

- When clients or colleagues are distressed
- When clients or colleagues are aggressive
- When there is team conflict
- When evaluation anxiety is experienced
- When unpopular clients are encountered

In all these situations, positive self-talk is important. Here are examples of self-talk in two of these situations.

Example 3: Self-Talk When Colleagues Are Distressed

Here is one nurse's self-talk when encountering a colleague who is distressed and crying:

I hate it when colleagues cry; I mean, with clients it's OK, I expect them to be upset. I don't know what to do when staff at work cry. Whenever anyone at work cries, I get tearful, too, and I'm useless to them. If anyone cries, I don't know what I'll do. I just can't cope when grown people cry. I don't know what to do to make her feel better. What if she won't stop crying? If I can't help her to calm down, then I'm not much good.

Examine this nurse's self-talk.

1. *What is she telling herself?* This nurse is telling herself that staff members do not have the same feelings and reactions as clients. She is telling herself that a lot is expected of her and that if she does not perform adequately by calming her upset colleague, she is not an effective person. She is convinced that if she cries too, it will be detrimental to her colleague.

2. *What negative thoughts is she generating that are destructive?* She is putting considerable pressure on herself to perform in the only way that she thinks is acceptable. She is assuming that she will not be helpful to her colleague and gives no credit to herself. Her denial of a normal range of feelings in her colleagues prevents her compassion from surfacing in a way that would be helpful. Her impending sense of failure if she does not perform perfectly is likely making her tense.

3. *What positive thoughts is she generating?* This nurse is not saying anything comforting or encouraging to herself.

4. *Is her self-talk helpful?* Her self-talk is nonassertive because it downplays her potential to be helpful. It is not responsible because it distorts reality. Her self-talk would hinder her ability to reach out to her colleague and communicate in a helpful way. The restrictions imposed by this negative thinking would leave her feeling inadequate.

5. *How can she change her self-talk so that it is more positive?* Here is an example of how her self-talk could be more positive:

Everybody gets upset, and staff are no exception. I may not be able to stop her from crying, but I think I can comfort her. I always cry when any other staff member cries; but that's OK. It just shows how compassionate I am. My crying doesn't interfere with my ability to be helpful. She may not respond to my efforts to calm her down, but that doesn't mean I'm a bad nurse. Each of us has someone special to whom we can relate when we are upset. I don't have to do a lot to be helpful. Just listening and being there is often enough.

These inner thoughts are reassuring and confidence building. They are responsible because they do not distort the reality of the situation. They are assertive because they acknowledge the nurse's desire and ability to help. This positive self-talk is helpful.

Example 4: Self-Talk When There Is Team Conflict

Here is an example of one nurse's thinking about a conflict situation on her nursing unit.

All I want is a peaceful place to work. Wherever I go there are power struggles and I hate it. I just know this conflict is going to drag on; I wish I worked in Dr. Session's office. They never have any conflicts there. Maybe I should apply for a position in another office; I can't do anything about the conflicts between the support and clinical staff. I thought we had dealt with this conflict once and for all; I just hate these drawn-out disagreements. Whenever we discuss upsetting issues, my stomach gets in a knot and I feel like exploding; I don't know how much more I can take. I'm useless when there's conflict. I just let it tear me apart, and that's no good. I'm afraid I'm going to give the office manager a piece of my mind. She should get this conflict under control.

Examine this nurse's self-talk.

1. *What is she telling herself?* This nurse has the erroneous notion that conflict is brief, easily resolved, and nonrecurring. The false expectation that there are some places in which conflict does not occur is self-defeating. She is trying to convince herself that there is little she can do about the conflict. She believes that the office manager or the doctor should magically control the conflict.

2. *What negative thoughts is she generating that are destructive?* Her unrealistic ideas about the nature of conflict are causing her grief. Her image of herself as someone with little control in conflict situations makes her feel hopeless and ineffective. Her anticipation of unpleasant physical signs and symptoms in conflict situations initiates her anxiety at the slightest indication of conflict.

3. *What positive thoughts is she generating?* There is nothing reassuring and hopeful about her thinking.

4. *Is her self-talk helpful?* Her self-talk is nonassertive because it does not grant her any power to contribute to the resolution of the conflict. Her distorted perception about her lack of influence to effect change is irresponsible. These thoughts are not helpful because they immobilize her and increase her tension about the conflict.

5. *How can she change her self-talk so that it is more positive?* Here is an example of how her self-talk could be more positive:

Every office staff has conflict; it is an unavoidable part of working with others. Sometimes creative and effective ways of handling situations can come out of conflict. Maybe there are some positive benefits to this conflict. I can keep my cool to express my feelings about the conflict on our unit. My ideas will have more impact if I remain calm. Each thing I do to diminish the conflict goes a long way toward resolving our problems. No one person can eliminate the conflict alone, but each contribution is significant. I get anxious when there's conflict on the unit, but it is not overwhelming. I can keep it under control.

This positive self-talk is assertive and responsible. Admitting that conflict is a normal part of working with others removes the sting of disagreement and makes her more apt to tackle the problem. Believing that whatever steps she takes to manage the conflict are significant promotes positive action on her part. Putting her anxiety in perspective allows her to function without being ashamed or overwhelmed. She is responsible in her assessment of the situation and her ability. This positive internal dialogue is assertive in its acknowledgment of her desire to handle situations effectively.

In his book *Pulling Your Own Strings*, Dyer (1994) challenges us by suggesting that several concepts that we take for granted do not exist in reality. Some examples are "disaster," "a good boy," "a stupid person," and "a perfect person." Each of these concepts represents a judgment about reality. Negative self-talk about our ability to communicate or handle interpersonal situations is our destructive and self-defeating judgment. Dyer advises us not to be victimized and encourages us to subscribe to thoughts that are reality based and self-enhancing. If we can apply this advice to our intrapersonal communication, it will stand us in good stead for our interpersonal encounters with clients and colleagues. Talking to ourselves in encouraging, realistic ways increases our ability to communicate with others in assertive and responsible ways.

Bach and Torbet (1986) assert that we have two voices in our inner life: our "inner enemy" and our "inner ally." Our inner enemy keeps a running inventory of our weaknesses, maintains a certain misery level, and keeps all joyless, negative information on file and can display it at a moment's notice. Our inner ally is interested in action, growth, and change and prevents us from getting bogged down in doubts and fears. Our ally reassures us of the benefits and rewards of success and the pleasures of trying, encouraging us to take risks that will help get us where we want to go. When we make mistakes, it is our inner ally that comforts us and helps us view our mistakes in perspective.

As you practice enhancing and augmenting your interpersonal communication skills, focus on what your inner ally tells you. Allow comforting and realistic thoughts to support and encourage you while learning.

Consider using the skill of positive self-talk as you grow your career when preparing for an interview, when you are going back to school, and when you are preparing for public speaking (McConnell, 2009; Schaeffer, 2006). Effective self-talk focuses on encouraging yourself and can build self-esteem and help you perform better (Sutton, 2010).

Use of Positive Self-Talk to Enhance Your Interpersonal Communication

Positive self-talk can help you at three phases of interpersonal communication: before, during, and after.

Before your interaction with a client or colleague, you can take control of your thoughts and focus on realistic and encouraging inner dialogue that will make you feel more confident about your forthcoming encounter. This preparation makes you focus on your strengths rather than worrying about potential catastrophes. When you feel prepared, you will likely act more competently.

For some encounters you have hours or days to prepare your positive self-talk. At other times you get little preparation time. Even for surprise encounters, however, you can quickly tune into your internal dialogue (it is continuously active) and talk to yourself in encouraging ways.

For example, when you take a call from an angry family member, you can be saying these words to yourself:

Positive self-talk: The unit secretary tells you there is a call from an angry family member. Tell yourself: "He's impatient and angry, and it could get me upset. But I will stay calm and collected." Slow down, relax your breathing, and loosen up your shoulders. You will find out what is troubling him and be able to handle it. Haste makes waste, so just remain steady and pay attention to each thing he says.

This preparation primes you to handle this aggressive client situation calmly and effectively.

During your conversation you can tune into your inner voice and concentrate on supportive dialogue. For example, if the caller's voice is getting louder, and his language is getting more hostile, you can say to yourself:

Positive self-talk: "He's getting angry. That's OK. I can handle his outburst. I will remain calm and

find out what is so upsetting for him. My breathing is regular, my posture is relaxed, and I will keep my voice steady. There's no point in getting upset. I can take this professionally, not personally!"

This positive self-talk reminds you to stay in control and handle the situation effectively. The comfort provided by your own supportive thoughts helps you to act the way you want.

After an encounter you can use positive self-talk to constructively review your performance. Noting your successes and the areas in which improvement is needed are both important. This example of a constructive review may be helpful:

Positive self-talk: "I thought I controlled my fear of his hostility really well. I actually remained calm and kept my voice tone on an even pitch. I think what I said to him helped to calm him down, but next time I'd like to achieve a relaxed body posture. My fists were clenched, and my shoulders were pretty tight, and I could feel that my knees were locked. When I can relax my body, that will be one more positive message going out that I am in control and confident."

Affirmations as a Strategy to Create Positive Self-Talk

Affirmations are self-talk statements of what you want, written in the positive tense, as if they have already happened. Affirmations can help you to take an optimistic point of view about your life and work. People who are optimistic hold generalized favorable expectations of the future. Optimism versus pessimism, negative expectation about the future, has been related to a better sense of well-being in the face of life challenge, higher levels of coping, health promotion behaviors, and more success in interpersonal relationships (Carver et al, 2010) (Box 22-1 and Box 22-2).

When nursing students in a holistic self-care course write a plan for one behavior change to be worked on throughout the semester, they include one or two affirmations. For example, a student who contracts to run for 30 minutes three times a week, writes: "I look forward to running three times each week and accomplish it easily" (Riley, 2010).

Box 22-1   *How to Create and Use Affirmations*

1. Use the present tense. You want your mind to know it has already happened.
2. Be POSITIVE. Avoid negative words. For example: "I choose healthy foods" rather than I do not eat high-calorie foods. "There is always enough time" rather than I will not be late.
3. Write them. Keep them short and very specific.
4. Believe. Always believe that what you are saying is happening.
5. Repetition. Being repetitive and persistent helps to set them in your head and in your unconscious mind.
6. Time. Have a specific time set aside daily for your affirmations or link the affirmation to an activity you do each day. This will help set a pattern.

Box 22-2   *Examples of Affirmations*

I am at peace with my life.
I love and accept myself.
I feel energetic and enthusiastic today.
I love and care for my body.
I am healthy.
I respect my abilities and work to my full potential.
I spend money wisely.
I am a forgiving and loving person.
I am worthy of love.
Centered and poised in the presence of God, I move through the activities of the day, easily and gracefully.
I am in the right place, at the right time, doing the right thing, in the right way.

A Final Thought

Consider how you name your experiences. Could you reframe a "life crisis" into a "life challenge?" Many people find that difficult times offer the most possibility for growth in life. Reflect on your own life and the times of the "dark night of the soul." How would your life change and how could you change the way you partner with clients on their healing journeys if you could make this shift? Consider this affirmation: "Within every problem there is a lesson. Release the problem and embrace the lesson." Positive self-talk, the attitude you choose, is a tool you carry with you and is available at a moment's notice. When you have yourself on your side, you are never alone and you always have an encouraging supporter on whom to call.

 Reflections On . . .

Positive Self-Talk

Consider what you read about the role of self-talk in communication. Do you already pay attention to your self-talk? What messages do you find that you give yourself? Answer the following questions.

What? . . .
Write one thing you learned from this chapter.

So what? . . .
How will this affect your nursing practice?

Now what? . . .
How will you implement this new knowledge or skill?

Think about it . . .

Practicing Positive Self-Talk

Exercise 1   QSEN

Emotional intelligence is a developmental process that helps build confidence through improving self-awareness and how our actions impact others. By reflecting on our experiences we can learn from them. Teamwork behaviors are dependent on our awareness of how our actions impact others. The stories we tell ourselves become our reality. How can we use stories of our success to improve self-awareness and confidence?

- Write an example of a time you felt your actions were successful.
- Describe the event. What steps did you take?

- What about the event made you feel successful?
- How can you apply these same strategies to have confidence when you face future challenges?
- How does "confidence" in your "competence" influence quality and safety?

QSEN Competencies: Teamwork and Collaboration; Safety

Exercise 2

Monitor your own self-talk for one work or student day. Positive self-talk offers praise. Negative self-talk offers criticism. Assess areas for change. Any time you encounter a difficult interpersonal situation, whether in practice or in real life, try talking positively to yourself to augment your ability to communicate assertively and responsibly. Now, select a recent upsetting experience, describe it briefly, and ask yourself if it could be given a positive name. For example, "This is a learning experience." Try a humorous approach. For example, "Another example of God's great sense of humor." Mother Teresa used this strategy. She said, "I know God will not give me anything I cannot handle. I just wish he didn't trust me so much."

> *Man is disturbed not by things but by the views he takes of them.*
>
> **Epictetus**
>
> WIT&*Wisdom*

Exercise 3

As a class, compare your experiences with employing positive self-talk after you have practiced using it as suggested in Exercise 1. What difficulties did you encounter in employing positive self-talk? What successes did you achieve by keeping your internal dialogue positive?

> *In tough situations, where self-talk moves between the encouraging and discouraging, follow the Nike shoe manufacturer's slogan: "Just do it."*
>
> WIT&*Wisdom*

References

Bach G, Torbet L: *The everyday slow torture of self-hate*, New York, 1986, Berkley Publishing Group.

Butler PE: *Talking to yourself*, New York, 2008, BookSurge Publishing.

Carver CS, Scheier MF, Segerstrom SC: Optimism, *Clin Psychol Rev* 7(30):879, 2010.

Chapman EN: *Life is an attitude: staying positive during tough times, how to control your outlook on life*, Menlo Park, Calif, 1992, Crisp Publications.

Dyer WW: *Pulling your own strings*, New York, 1994, Harper Mass Market Paperbacks.

Ellis A, Powers M: *A guide to rational living*, Hollywood, Calif, 1998, Wilshire Book Co.

Hardy J: Speaking clearly: a critical review of the self-talk literature, *Psychol Sport Exerc* 7(1):81, January 2006.

Helmsetter S: *What do you say when you talk to yourself?* New York, 1990, Pocket.

Levy BA, Slade MD, Kunkel SR, et al: Longevity increased by positive self-perceptions of aging, *J Pers Soc Psychol* 83(2):261, 2002.

Mayo Clinic: *Positive thinking: reduce stress and enjoy life more* (website). http://www.mayoclinic.com/health/positive-thinking/SR00009. Accessed September 1, 2011.

McConnell CR: Effective oral presentations: Speaking before groups as a part of your job, *The Healthcare Manager* 28(3):261, 2009.

Piper W: *The little engine that could*, New York, 1998, Grosset & Dunlap.

Riley JB: Nursing 430: *Holistic self-care: complementary and alternative therapies for professional self-care and practice*, University of Tampa, Tampa, Fla, 2010.

Schaeffer K: Facing down the fear factor in interviews, *Wall St J*, December 12, 2006.

Sutton B: Tricks for taking charge, *The McKinsey Quarterly* 3:240, 2010.

Turkington CA: *Stress management for busy people*, New York, 1998, McGraw-Hill.

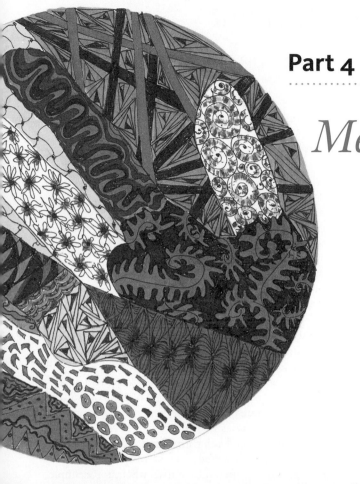

Part 4

Meeting Challenges

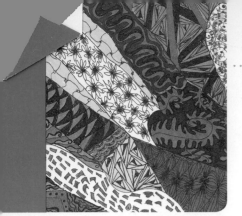

Chapter 23

Confrontation

> *Unless you stop the crack you will rebuild the wall.*
>
> **African proverb**

Objectives

1. Identify the benefits of confrontation skills
2. Discuss the steps of the CARE (Clarify, Articulate, Request, Encourage) model of confrontation
3. Identify the relationship between confrontation skills and empowerment
4. Practice confrontation in selected exercises to build confidence in the skills

Different Kinds of Confrontation

Confrontation skill is "being able to identify and to respond—communicate—provide feedback—regarding those discrepancies in another person's behavior in such a manner that the other person can grow" (Tindall, 2008). Setting feelings aside and focusing on problem solving, using a calm approach, invite cooperation (Northam, 2009; Gallagher, 2009). Patterson and colleagues (2005) say that to confront is to hold someone accountable, to offer an opportunity to solve problems and build relationships. Their research demonstrated that leaders throughout an organization were successful because they held colleagues, co-workers, and bosses accountable. An example of one type of confrontation is a nurse's deliberate invitation to clients and colleagues to examine incongruities or distortions between feelings, beliefs, attitudes, and behavior (Egan, 2009). This type of confrontation, designed to make others aware of incongruity, can be offered by nurses when, for example, clients or colleagues are saying one thing and doing another, or obviously feeling one way and exhibiting the opposite emotions. Pointing these discrepancies out can be an invitation to expand their self-awareness. This dimension of confrontation is a gift of feedback, which is covered in Chapter 19.

Here is an example of a confrontation to expand self-awareness:

John tells you that he smokes only a few cigarettes a day. He has yellow stains on the fingers of his left hand, smells of smoke, and wheezes on inspiration. His wife says he smokes two packs a day.

Nurse: "John, I'm concerned about conflicting information concerning your smoking. The stains on your fingers, the smell of smoke on your clothes, and the sound of your breathing indicate that you smoke more than a few cigarettes a day."

Confrontation that involves an explicit request for a change in behavior along with feedback is the focus of this chapter.

Situations in Which Confrontation Is Appropriate

Confrontation has two parts: the first is making others aware of the destructiveness or lack of productiveness of their behavior, and the second is making a suggestion about how they could behave in a more constructive or productive way. Two situations warrant confronting clients or colleagues: when their behavior is unproductive or destructive to them and when their behavior invades our rights or the rights of others. In confronting others, we are attempting to get them to change in a way that protects their self-interests or is more considerate of others. One note of warning: be aware that the problem belongs to the other person and it is not our role to "fix" other people to meet our standards of behavior (Cox, 1998).

Some nurses shudder at the thought of confronting another person and do not want to discuss their differences. We think about people we know who have a tendency to be argumentative when confronted. We are concerned about the impression others will have if we confront them about an issue (Shih, 2002). Confrontation conjures up images of a heated argument. For most nurses, verbal attacks conflict with their images of themselves as level-headed professionals. Yet confrontation can be a time-saving strategy (Davidhizar and Cathon, 2002).

To avoid being labeled aggressive, we often refrain from saying anything about others' unproductive or destructive behavior. Later, we watch our clients or colleagues get into trouble because of their misdirected actions and then we feel guilty and regret that we did not take the opportunity to speak up. In other situations we fume because we do not quite know how to confront those who have violated our rights or the rights of others and we stew in frustrated helplessness. The next time you hesitate to confront others when you believe it needs to be done, remember this: short-term gain, long-term pain. Being nonassertive may get you off the hook for now, but in the long run the problem will only escalate.

Patterson and colleagues (2005) write about crucial confrontations to avoid silence or violence. Neither of the two extremes—nonassertion or aggression—is acceptable to nurses who want to feel confident and act competently. There is a way to confront others, however, that makes you feel as if you are effectively doing something about troublesome behavior. People can be confronted in such a way that they are unlikely to be offended. Moreover, they may appreciate your perspective and opinions.

 Moments of Connection . . .
A Caring Confrontation
"During a series of electrical treatments for myofascial pain, the client and I had an opportunity to talk. She was concerned about her diabetic husband, who refused to eat properly, exercise, or take care of his health in any way. She tried hard to prepare the right foods and motivate him, but his health was deteriorating rapidly. Based on my own experience, I suggested to her that she might need to focus on herself, developing friendships and working on improving the quality of her own life. We talked about her getting her finances and other business in the best of order in preparation for the time when her husband might not be there. She was silent and thoughtful. On her next appointment, she thanked me for my insight and said she knew she had done all she could for him and that it was now time to help herself."

The CARE (Clarify, Articulate, Request, Encourage) Confrontation

Elements of the CARE Confrontation

When you confront your clients or colleagues, it is important to do so in a caring way that shows concern for both your feelings and theirs. The following CARE approach is a caring way to confront others. (The format for this comprehensive confrontation is adapted from Bower and Bower, 2004.)

- **Clarify** the behavior that is problematic. Be specific about the aspect of your client's or colleague's behavior that is self-destructive or destructive to others. The behavior to be changed should be the focus so that it is clear that you are attaching no hurtful labels to others.
- **Articulate** why their behavior is a problem. Your articulation may include how their behavior is likely

to hinder them or irritate others or how it makes you feel.

- **R**equest a change in your client's or colleague's behavior. Your suggestions should be offered tentatively and respectfully.
- **E**ncourage your clients or colleagues to change by emphasizing the positive consequences of changing or the negative implications of failing to change.

Remember, too, not to expect a negative response, to use neutral words without blame, and to stay open to the person's response rather than jumping to conclusions (Ryan et al, 1996). Respect that the clients' values may be different from yours and be careful not to take a lecturing tone when you confront them (London, 1998).

Examples of CARE Confrontations

The three situations outlined in the following sections demonstrate how you can confront someone in an assertive way without being aggressive.

Situation 1

Your roommate is untidy. He leaves his clothes strewn around the bedroom you share, and the bathroom looks like a pharmacy. Frequently his notes and textbooks are laid out all over the apartment. Although he does a major cleanup about every 2 weeks, he slides back into his messy ways and you have to put up with his disarray for the rest of the time. Not only is this mess aesthetically displeasing to you, it makes you hesitant to invite friends over. You confront your roommate with the following:

Clarify

John, you have your clothes spread out over the bedroom, and all your notes and articles for your paper are strewn around the living room and on the kitchen table.

Articulate

I'm feeling annoyed that you are messing up the shared space in our apartment.

Request

I'd like you to keep your personal belongings in your area of our den.

Encourage

That way it'll be more spacious for both of us in the apartment, and I'll feel free to invite friends over without worrying about whether the place is a mess.

Presented with this respectful and assertive confrontation, John will most likely comply and change his behavior. If such a confrontation does not result in the desired behavior change, you have the option of indicating a negative consequence, such as, "If you don't become neater, I will . . . " (and give a possible consequence, such as hire a cleaning service and charge him, find another roommate, or move out).

Situation 2

Your colleague Janet is upset. She has been trying to lose weight for the past 6 months. You notice that she has a pattern of starting off successfully on Mondays and going back to binging on high-calorie foods by the end of the week. Afterward she fasts for several days and then overeats again. You think that these feasts and famines are not helpful for Janet and that it would be better if she distributed her calories more evenly. Janet knows you struggle with the same issue and you have often shared your challenges.

After you have asked her permission to express your views, you confront Janet about her unproductive behavior in this way:

Clarify

Janet, I notice you do well on your diet at the beginning of the week and then you have ups and downs of eating more than you want to or eating so little that you are starving.

Articulate

I think one reason you are unsuccessful in losing weight is because you don't have an adequate intake of calories on a consistent basis.

Request

I'd be interested in attending Weight Watchers again and I just learned there will be a class at lunchtime here at work. Perhaps we could go back together and support each other. If we stick to their meal plan you might not be as hungry and will be less likely to binge.

Encourage

If you can cut out the overeating, you won't feel guilty and have to starve yourself. What do you think?

The respectful and clear way this confrontation is delivered is likely to invite Janet to consider your idea and possibly implement it. An accusatory confrontation would only be ignored.

Situation 3

You are a nurse manager. It has been reported to you that one of your staff has misused the hospital e-mail, sending jokes to an in-house distribution list. You understand that e-mail is often seen as a casual rather than formal way of communication and assume incorrectly that e-mail is protected from company access (Falcone, 2009).

Clarify

Susan, it has come to my attention that your have been using hospital e-mail to forward jokes to other staff.

Articulate

I can understand wanting to use humor to help others relieve stress, but e-mail is not an appropriate way to share jokes even though it is easy and quick. It may seem like a casual form of communication, yet the purpose of e-mail in the hospital is for business-related correspondence. Remember, too, our e-mail here is not private. It can be accessed and reviewed.

Request

I suggest you share humorous e-mails through personal accounts but not on company time or through company e-mail addresses.

Encourage

I enjoy your sense of humor. You have often helped us regain our perspective in meetings and I welcome your sharing your comic vision.

This approach acknowledges the benefit of Susan's sense of humor and offers an alternative, more appropriate venue for sharing it.

Confrontations with Clients or Colleagues

We can often see how other people's behavior is not safe or in keeping with their goals. Each of us has blind spots about how some of what we say or do is predisposing us to emotional or physical harm, or is incongruent with our professed values or attitudes. As nurses we can offer an objective perspective on how others can change and act in a way that will serve their best interests. The following examples use CARE confrontations to offer clients and colleagues ways to enhance their goals and avoid emotional or physical dangers.

Situations in Which Your Client's Behavior Is Self-Destructive or Unproductive

Mr. Jones, a finance officer for a large corporation, is a 35-year-old client who has suffered a massive myocardial infarction. Yesterday he was moved from the intensive care unit to the cardiac step down unit. You overhear him asking his wife to bring his laptop computer to the unit so he can keep up with his e-mail.

Your nursing knowledge alerts you to the fact that Mr. Jones is escalating his work schedule too quickly and that his workaholic habits may delay his heart's healing or even put him at risk for another heart attack. You want him to slow down his reentry into the business world and gradually build up his stamina. You strongly believe that a gradual increase in his workload will increase his chances for a successful recovery. You confront Mr. Jones this way:

Mr. Jones, I overheard you making arrangements for your wife to bring your laptop to the hospital. I can imagine that you must be eager to keep up with things at work. However, jumping in too quickly and taking on too much responsibility at this point in your recovery will likely make you tense, and the stress on your heart may increase. Your chances for a successful and complete recovery will be better if you ease back into work more slowly. I suggest that you put off asking for your computer and limit your work with your secretary to 15 minutes a day by phone for this week and then gradually increase the time. If you build up your stamina slowly, you'll reduce the risk of another heart attack. What do you think?

John, an 18-year-old client, has just had a torn Achilles tendon repaired. After his lesson on using crutches, you notice that John is bearing too much weight on his affected leg. In doing so, he is increasing the chance of his sutures weakening and putting strain on his tendon, thus preventing healing. You confront John as follows:

> When you put any weight on your injured leg, you are risking further injury to your tendon. If you weaken your tendon, you may not recover full use of your leg. I'd like you to practice using your crutches so that you place weight only on your good leg. That way you'll ensure maximum healing of your injury. Will you try that please, John?

Situations in Which Your Colleague's Behavior Is Self-Destructive or Unproductive

On the medical unit in your hospital, you and Judy have been working together on the evening shift for the past three evenings. Judy has been complaining of a strained back, which she has attributed to turning, positioning, and transferring the heavy clients on the unit. You have noticed that Judy takes few or no precautions to protect her back. After you have received her permission to express your views, you decide to confront her about her negligence in the following way:

> Judy, it sounds as if your back is bothering you quite a bit. I've noticed that when you are turning our heavy patients, you tend to take the clients' full weight on your own without help from one of us or the Hoyer lift. I think you could save your back from a lot of discomfort and injury if you took the precautions of getting help and using protective devices. What do you think?

Note the different order of elements in this CARE confrontation. The reordering makes it sound more natural in this case, yet it still contains the essential components.

Your classmate, Toni, has not been achieving the grades to which she has been accustomed on her nursing examinations. Toni is complaining about the severity of the examinations and the tough grading of her instructors. You are aware that Toni has not been studying as much since she began dating two men at the same time and that she has been going out almost every night. She asks you what she should do. You decide to confront her about her recent unproductive behavior:

> Toni, I know you always do well even if the teachers are tough. It's just since you've been dating on weeknights that your grades have been lower. I'd have the same problem if I couldn't have extra time to review my class notes. It's a tough call. You know that when we go over the notes several times, we see a difference in the test grades. Maybe if you took a few minutes after classes to review, you'd see a difference, but that's not easy to do when it's tempting to go out. What do you think?

In each of these four situations the client or colleague has been confronted about something he or she is doing or not doing that is causing physical or emotional problems. The confrontation points out the specific behavior that is problematic and proposes a clear alternative, which is checked out with the client or colleague.

Let us examine some situations in which the skill of confrontation is used to deal with behavior that violates your rights or the rights of others.

Situations in Which Your Client's or Colleague's Behavior Is Bothersome to You or Others

Mr. Wars is a 53-year-old cardiac client who has been aggressive in the 3 days he has been on the unit. He has complained about the food, the room, and the other clients, and today he has been angry and abusive with you in the corridor. He complains that you are the slowest nurse he has ever encountered and that you don't know what you are doing. He has picked on your appearance, questioned your credentials, and repeatedly insulted your nursing care. His aggressiveness is embarrassing, time consuming, and unpleasant for you. You recognize that he is feeling out of control and assess that a referral to the psychiatric clinical nurse specialist might be of help to you and to him. You confront him when you are in the privacy of his room:

> Mr. Wars, we need to talk about how things are going for you. I know you are not happy with your care, and I want to talk about what we can do. I would like to help you be as comfortable as possible during these tough times for you. It upsets me to be unable to make things better for you. We have a nurse that we can call whose job it is to

evaluate such situations. She could spend some time with you to help you sort things out. I hope you are willing to let me call her so we can work together to turn things around for the better. How does that sound to you?

Miss Debris is a colleague with whom you share an office. She often moves your paperwork and leaves the desk in disorder. Yesterday, you could not find any pens or the stapler. Today, Miss Debris has left a dirty coffee cup and the wrapper from her sandwich on the desk. She is about to leave without cleaning it up when you confront her:

> When you leave the desk we share cluttered, I have to search for the things I need to do my work. I know you get busy, but this time I see trash, too. If we both are aware of keeping the work space clear, it will be ready when each of us needs it. How about taking a few seconds to dump the trash and make sure the papers and supplies are handy? It would make it easier for me to face my work, and I would appreciate it. Does that sound fair?

Situations in Which Your Colleague's Behavior Is Unpleasant for You or Others

You have been working the night shift for the past five nights. In the three previous mornings your nurse relief has been about 15 to 25 minutes late. You are not free to leave the unit until she arrives because there is only one nurse on duty. Her lateness leads to your being late getting home to see your family before they head off to school and work. You decide to confront her:

> Rena, I want to speak to you about your coming in 15 to 25 minutes late in the mornings. Since I can't leave until you get here, I've been getting home too late in the mornings to see my family. I would like you to arrange to be here, ready to receive report, at 7:00 AM when the shift begins from now on so that I can report without being too rushed and still get home on time. Can you do that?

Margaret is a new graduate working on a psychiatric unit with you. You notice that each time Margaret has an interview with a client she goes into the session with coffee only for herself and then puts her feet up on the desk. You know this casual behavior makes clients feel insulted and not respected and gives them the

impression that Margaret is less than interested in their cases. Because the clients have not had the nerve to challenge Margaret, you decide to say something to her about her behavior.

> Margaret, I couldn't help notice that when you interview some of the clients, you have a very casual style, with a coffee cup in your hand and your feet up on the desk. I think your manner may give the impression to some clients that you aren't taking them seriously. We don't wear uniforms, so it is important that our behavior send a clear message that we are caring professionals. Because I know you are interested in your work and like to do a good job, I thought you'd want to know if your behavior might be misinterpreted. (Await approval from Margaret before continuing.) Perhaps if you offered your clients a cup of coffee, too, and didn't put your feet up you would show your clients your real interest in them. What do you think?

The CARE confrontation provides a way of approaching others when either their best interests or yours are threatened. CARE confrontations allow you to take action in a calm, controlled, assertive way. They prevent you from being immobilized in a situation in which you want to be confrontative but not aggressive.

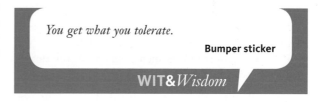

> *You get what you tolerate.*
>
> **Bumper sticker**

WIT&*Wisdom*

The Magic of a Little Word

Try using the word *and* instead of *but* when offering criticism or a differing opinion. The word *but* may put the person on the defensive. Berent and Evans (1992) give some examples of the use of this style when offering advice or criticism:

- "I appreciate the intensity of your feelings about this, and I think if you were to hear my side of it you might feel differently."

- "I can understand your reasons, and I think my reasons for doing it differently are also understandable."
- "That's an interesting idea, and here's another way to think about it."

Confrontation as One Part of Empowerment

Confrontation is an important skill to learn and is one aspect of many that you will use as you move forward as an empowered professional nurse. (Did you notice the use of *and* rather than *but*? Using *but* would have diminished the importance of the skill of confrontation.) As you feel more confident with your own nursing skills, the necessity for the skills of confrontation will be more obvious. Murphy (1994) admonishes nurses not to be doormats and discusses the personal responsibility of nurses who want to be more effective in conflict resolution. Dealing with conflict constructively helps us create the work environment we want (Cox, 2005). Nurses need to do the following:

- Make self-improvement a priority
- Pay attention to feelings of anger and fear as signals to deal with a situation
- Speak up respectfully and before an angry blow-up occurs
- Commit to treating others respectfully
- Be honest and confront colleagues when friction first occurs rather than letting it escalate
- Practice self-care skills such as exercise, relaxation, and recreation

Later chapters discuss self-care skills that help you to be responsive, rather than reactive, to colleagues and clients. This means being able to take time to sort out which situations require confrontation and which can be tolerated or are simply an overreaction due to fatigue or personal stress. Noddings (1994) concludes that "everywhere—in personal, social, political, and even professional life—people misunderstand one another." Confrontation takes thought, energy, and a caring attitude. In nursing, "in the caring orientation, we are more concerned with connecting, feeling—with responding positively to expressed needs, and understanding ourselves well enough to be able to summon the attitude of caring."

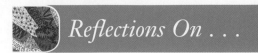

Reflections On . . .

Confrontation

Consider your own experiences with confrontation and how they affect your willingness to try on these new behaviors. Answer the following questions.

What? . . .
Write one thing you learned from this chapter.

So what? . . .
How will this affect your nursing practice?

Now what? . . .
How will you implement this new knowledge or skill?

Think about it . . .

Practicing Confrontation

Exercise 1

Make a list of examples when confrontation with a client or colleague is inappropriate. Discuss your list with another student or nurse.

Exercise 2

In your journal, keep a list of incidents in which you would like to have confronted someone and the potential or real consequences for not having done so.

Exercise 3   QSEN

Safety is a shared responsibility among all team members. How should you respond when you observe a team member engaging in unsafe behavior? CUS is an easy-to-remember method to raise the team's safety awareness with three statements. When all members of the team are taught to use CUS, it can be used to help "get everyone on the same page" and also "stop the line" to clarify actions. Uncertain actions when the team is not clear on the goals can lead to error. Assume someone is about to change a dressing without first washing their hands. Practice using the CUS communication:

C: I am concerned . . .
U: I am uncertain . . .
S: I feel safety is at risk . . .

QSEN Competencies: Teamwork and Collaboration; Safety

Exercise 4

For each situation below, attempt a CARE confrontation. After you have prepared a response, get together with your classmates as a group and discuss your different approaches. Compare your suggestions with those at the end of this exercise.

1. Mr. Steiger, your 38-year-old client, suffers from chronic bronchitis. You have noticed him smoking outside the building before he comes for his clinic visits, and as you enter the examining room his clothes smell of smoke. Your nursing knowledge tells you that his smoking is self-destructive. How would you confront him?
2. Your client, 60-year-old Mrs. Cantor, has severe pitting edema of the ankles. She has been taught to raise her legs on a chair when sitting and to wear elastic stockings from toe to mid thigh. You have observed that Mrs. Cantor is not wearing her stockings, and each time you have seen her in the chair, her feet have been on the floor. How would you confront her about her self-destructive behavior?
3. You and Jane started working in an emergency center 6 months ago, after your graduation from nursing school. Jane confides to you that she feels she does not have the respect of her team members and that she believes that others do not listen to or act on her opinions. You have noticed that Jane takes a passive stance: she is overly cautious about her suggestions and speaks quietly. When she presents an idea, she often puts it down first. You are reasonably certain that some of her nonassertive behavior accounts for the fact that her ideas are not being considered by the team. How would you confront her about her unproductive behavior?

Suggested CARE Confrontations

1. "Mr. Steiger, I have observed you smoking on several occasions in the past few days. Smoking causes you to produce more phlegm, and that makes you cough more and become short of breath. I would like to give you some information about help available to you should you choose to stop smoking. If you were able to do this, your lungs would have a chance to clear and your breathing would become easier. If you don't stop smoking, then you are at risk for a serious lung infection. I know it is tough, but I think you'd be surprised to hear about the successful outcomes of people using a nicotine patch. May I tell you more about it?"

2. "Mrs. Cantor, I notice that you aren't wearing your elastic stockings and your feet are on the floor instead of being raised on the stool. Wearing your elastic stockings helps prevent blood clots from forming. I strongly recommend that you wear your stockings and raise your legs on a stool so that you can prevent any more serious complications of your heart disease."

3. "Jane, I think you have some sound ideas about how we can be more efficient. I notice that when you present your ideas, you seem to hesitate and speak softly and uncertainly about your views. When you start off by saying, 'This idea may not work,' it's almost as if you've set the team up to discount your suggestions before the members have heard them. I think your suggestions might be considered if you would present your ideas in a more positive way. Then you and the team would both benefit."

For more examples, see Exercise 2 in Chapter 3 for situations in which clients have broken a mutually arrived-at agreement.

Exercise 5

Attempt to practice confrontation in real life, whether at school, on the units, or in social situations. How effective are you at making CARE confrontations? Have you discovered that by using this format you avoid both aggression and nonassertion? Do these guidelines for confronting people provide you with more confidence?

Exercise 6

Reflect on a time when you did not confront someone and you were not pleased with that decision. Close your eyes and imagine the situation and the resulting emotion. Think about that feeling as if it had color, line, shape, and form. Open your eyes and using colored markers or crayons, draw the image in your journal. Now close your eyes again and imagine successfully confronting this person and the resulting emotion. Again think of an image that reflects the emotion and draw it. Look at your art and write a reflection about it in your journal including differences you might see in yourself if you risked a caring confrontation. (For more expressive arts invitations for self-discovery see Riley, 2010.)

References

Berent IM, Evans RL: *The right words: the 350 best things to say to get along with people*, New York, 1992, Warner Books.

Bower SA, Bower GH: *Asserting yourself: a practical guide for positive change*, New York, 2004, De Capo Press.

Cox S: Nixing fix-it syndrome, *Nursing* 28(6):61, 1998.

Cox S: Taking the "con" out of conflict, *Nursing* 35(12):57, 2005.

Davidhizar R, Cathon D: Strategies for effective confrontation, *Radiol Technol* 73(5):476, 2002.

Egan G: *Skilled helper: a problem-management and opportunity-development approach to helping*, Pacific Cove, Calif, 2009, Brooks Cole.

Falcone P: *101 difficult conversations to have with employees*, New York, 2009, AMACOM.

Gallagher RS: *How to tell anyone anything: breakthrough techniques for handling difficult conversations at work*, New York, 2009, AMACOM.

London F: Improving compliance: what you can do, *RN* 61(1):43, 1998.

Murphy SZ: Don't be a doormat: personal empowerment in nursing, *Revolution* 2(2):66, 1994.

Noddings N: Learning to engage in moral dialogue, *Holist Educ Rev* 7(2):5, 1994.

Northam S: Conflict in the workplace, part 2: strategies to resolve conflict and restore collegial working relationships, *Am J Nurs* 109(7):65, July 2009.

Patterson K, Grenny J, McMillan R, et al: *Crucial confrontations: tools for resolving broken promises, violated expectations, and bad behavior*, New York, 2005, McGraw-Hill.

Riley JB: *Art in small spaces . . . (art at the bedside*, Ellenton, Fla, 2010, CS Publications. www.constantsource.com.

Ryan KD, Oestreich DK, Orr GA III: *The courageous messenger: how to successfully speak up at work*, San Francisco, 1996, Jossey-Bass.

Shih C: Confrontation: when does counterargumentation occur and when do people's thoughts predict their actions? *Dissert Abstr Int A Human Soc Sci* June 2002.

Tindall J: *Peer power: book one, becoming an effective peer helper and conflict mediator, Workbook*, New York, 2008, Routledge.

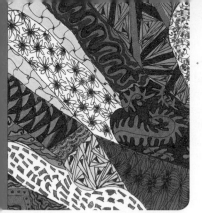

Chapter 24

Refusing Unreasonable Requests

Objectives

1. Discuss the importance of the right to refuse unreasonable requests from clients and colleagues

2. Distinguish between assertive, nonassertive, and aggressive refusals

3. Participate in exercises to build skills to refuse unreasonable requests

Defining Unreasonable Requests

As nurses, we receive requests from others for information, emotional support, and assistance. Daily, we are asked to carry out activities that help our clients and colleagues. Each request seems reasonable to the person making the request. In most instances, requests from our clients and colleagues seem legitimate when we think about the request in an objective way. When a request is made of you, however, you must consider how it affects you personally, as the person being asked to fulfill the request. You need to determine whether a request is reasonable. R. Creel, a professional organizer, created a list of "20 Ways to Say No," teaching that overcommitment can contribute to our inability to satisfactorily organize our personal and professional lives for success (Creel, 2011). With assertive communication skills, you learn how to refuse requests, but you choose whether to refuse the request depending on the situation.

A request may be unreasonable if it affects your right to provide nursing care in a way that is consistent with your ethics, values, or beliefs. Unreasonable requests are ones that escalate your negative feelings and encroach on your right to feel good about the work you are doing. You may be asked to perform tasks that are disrespectful of your safety or physical capabilities. It is unreasonable to respond to requests that put you in the position of hurting yourself, such as physically and emotionally stretching yourself to a point at which you feel stressed, overloaded, or irritable. However, it is important to note that sometimes you choose to fulfill a request even though you would prefer to decline. You may be asked to work an extra hour because of an emergency situation. A friend may ask a favor that is inconvenient. In these cases, you make your own decision as to whether to comply. In other cases, a request may seem unreasonable to you, and yet complying with it seems prudent. You may ask yourself not whether the request is reasonable, but whether it may be reasonable to fulfill the request.

WIT&*Wisdom*

Refusing Unreasonable Requests

You may ask of me.
I may ask of you.
We share our needs
And give our due.
I have my own needs.
My time I must measure.
I'll meet you halfway
Each other we'll treasure.
But some things you ask
I must refuse.
Please don't your own power
With mine confuse.
Please listen to me
When I say no.
It's not an issue
Of friend or foe.

As nurses, we have the right to work in a way that allows us to give our best nursing care to our clients, promotes positive relationships with our colleagues, and gives us feelings of satisfaction, safety, and comfort in doing our jobs. In Chapter 1, basic assertive rights were introduced. Chenevert (1997) puts our rights as nurses in perspective: "Nurses are responsible people. We have dwelled so long and so hard on our responsibilities we are often surprised at the prospect of having rights ourselves." Review your basic assertive rights listed in Box 1-2.

When you consider these rights, you need to use common sense. Of course, if you are a new graduate and your manager instructs you to give a pain medication at once, it would be inappropriate to say you prefer to bathe another client first. If you refuse a request, you may need to provide a rationale for the refusal.

Requests for our information or ideas, attention or affection, or physical power or skills all take time, energy, and commitment to fulfill. We need to check our resources before agreeing to any request. When we

take on a request that overtaxes us, we lose out because we become overloaded, and others lose out because we are ineffective when we are feeling burdened. Before saying yes to a request, we need to check to see if it is reasonable for us to accept it. If we decide it is unreasonable, then we must refuse. It is far better to refuse than to capitulate and risk a serious error. Failure to refuse can end up making you a sorry excuse for a nurse (Chenevert, 1997).

Mackay (1996) reveals that successful business people tap into their own states of mind before saying yes to important requests for their time, money, or expertise. "In the final analysis, what your inner voice tells you is the best advice you can get."

Saying No Assertively

The skill in saying no is to refuse the request in an assertive manner, rather than in an aggressive or a nonassertive way. Paskin (2005) advises you to begin by staying calm, realizing that your first reaction to an unreasonable request may be outrage. By being assertive, we protect ourselves by declining a task we cannot comfortably handle and we respect the other person's rights by refusing in a polite, matter-of-fact manner. Our desire to help our clients and colleagues and our wish to be seen as helpful nurses often interfere with our ability to say no clearly and simply.

Ellis and Powers (1998) discuss irrational beliefs that keep us from acting in our own best interests. Review the irrational beliefs listed in Box 1-3. Consider two such beliefs: "I must be approved of at all times" and "If I don't do everything people ask of me, they will reject me." Such beliefs escalate to "awfulizing." "It would be awful and I couldn't stand it if someone thought I considered my own needs." "They would think I am selfish" (Ellis and Powers, 1998). Get the idea? It sounds like an exaggeration, but sometimes we base our decisions on such faulty thinking. Assertive communication is based on a consideration of both parties' needs and recognizes that we have the right to set our own priorities for our actions and time allocation. This is difficult for some people. Jokingly, workshop participants are told that they can be taught how to say no but that they will have to get counseling like everybody else to deal with the guilt (Balzer Riley, 2002). You may at some time consider counseling if you have difficulty acting in your own best interests and find that this difficulty interferes with your ability to feel good about your work and yourself.

We sometimes fumble with weak excuses in attempts to avoid accepting a request. This nonassertive behavior makes us feel guilty and helpless, and we offend the asker with our irrelevant attempts to justify our refusal. A simple no would suffice and save both people embarrassment.

Sometimes our unnecessary or irrational guilt feelings about saying no make us refuse a request in a hostile, defensive manner. This aggression makes us feel ashamed that we have behaved unprofessionally, and the other person feels put down or hurt by our explosive response. Clearly, refusing a request in a nonassertive or aggressive way does not protect our interests or those of our clients or colleagues. The assertive refusal to an unreasonable request is the only way to show respect for ourselves and others.

Saying no to unreasonable requests is a way of saying yes to yourself. Just as clients are unique individuals and you struggle to consider their individuality when providing nursing care, when you protect your rights by refusing unreasonable requests, you are respecting your own uniqueness. You are saying yes to your values, yes to your style of doing things, yes to your ways of perceiving situations, and yes to your ways of judging and deciding. It is freeing to refocus your energy, shifting it from unreasonable requests to an investment in your visions and goals.

Examples of Refusing Requests Assertively

Here are several examples of effective, assertive ways of saying no, contrasted with ineffective aggressive and nonassertive ways.

Example 1

It is Tuesday. Your colleague Elsa asks you to be on call for her this weekend. Your in-laws are coming to visit, and you have made plans to take them on a tour of the excellent countryside restaurants. Your family has been looking forward to this visit, and it is unreasonable for you to work on this particular weekend. In the past, Elsa has been on call for you.

An assertive refusal:

Elsa: "Could you please be on call for me this weekend? Rob phoned long distance, and he's invited me to go to New York to spend the long weekend with him. I'm so excited! Can you do it?"

Assertive you: "No, Elsa. I'm not able to switch this weekend. My in-laws are visiting from out of town and we've made reservations to do things. I hope you can find someone to switch with. I can see you're really looking forward to going to New York to visit Rob."

This refusal is direct and clear. You are definite, yet you soften the refusal with the inclusion of the explanation for your refusal and your empathic hope that she can secure a replacement.

Elsa is determined, however, and persists in her attempt to persuade you to switch.

Elsa: "I know you've got company coming, but they're just in-laws and you get to see them often. I haven't seen Rob for 3 months. I know it's last minute, but Rob just found out he could be free and he called me as soon as he could. Oh, please, won't you be on call for me?"

Assertive you: "No, Elsa. I'm not available to switch with you this weekend."

You continue to be clear and definite. Elsa is pleading and trying to make you feel guilty so that you will give in to her. Your response successfully protects your rights to have a weekend with your family and attends to her rights to be treated respectfully.

Elsa does not stop. She wants you to switch so she plies you with more guilt.

Elsa: "Remember, I switched weekends with you in the spring when you wanted to go to your cousin's wedding? You agreed then that you owed me one. Well, now I'm collecting! I need you to pay me back this weekend."

Assertive you: "Elsa, I'm unable to help you this weekend."

This response continues to be clear and unwavering so that Elsa is given a definite, matter-of-fact answer that is congruent with your desire to avoid becoming hostile or weakened. Although you hope Elsa will find a replacement, it is unreasonable for you to be that person this weekend.

Elsa is starting to get your assertive message.

Elsa: "OK, OK. I see you've got plans you can't break. It's just that I'm desperate. I'll ask one of the other nurses if she can switch with me."

By being assertive, you have prevented yourself from doing two things you did not want to do: be on call this weekend and come across as defensive or indecisive to your colleague Elsa.

A nonassertive refusal:

Elsa: "Could you please be on call for me this weekend? Rob phoned long distance, and he's invited me to go to New York to spend the long weekend with him. I'm so excited! Can you do it?"

Nonassertive you: "Gee, Elsa. I don't think so . . . I'm sorry."

This response does not sound convincing. Elsa gets the message that you are not really sure you can't switch with her. It sounds like you are still debating with yourself, and Elsa will likely try to convince you to switch.

Elsa: "I haven't seen Rob for 3 months. I know it's last minute, but Rob just found out he could be free and he called me as soon as he could. Oh, please, won't you be on call for me?"

Nonassertive you: "Gee, Elsa, I don't think I can. I'm sorry. I've got my in-laws coming and we've made plans. I don't think so, Elsa."

You still have not given a definite no, and Elsa will likely keep asking you as long as she believes that there is hope.

Elsa: "Remember, I switched weekends with you in the spring when you wanted to go to your cousin's wedding? You agreed then that you owed me one. Well, now I'm collecting! I need you to pay me back this weekend."

Nonassertive you: "Yes, that's true. I guess I owe you one. OK, I'll switch with you for this weekend."

By being nonassertive and indefinite, you have agreed to a request that is unreasonable for you to take on. Giving in will most likely leave you feeling angry, and your in-laws will be disappointed you have let them down. When we are nonassertive, we forfeit our rights.

An aggressive refusal:

Elsa: "Could you please be on call for me this weekend? Rob phoned long distance, and he's invited me to go to New York to spend the long weekend with him. I'm so excited! Can you do it?"

Aggressive you: "Don't you know I've got my in-laws coming to visit this weekend? There's no way I can switch with you."

This abrasive, offensive reply shows no understanding of Elsa's predicament. Whereas a simple refusal would have sufficed, this response makes you appear unfriendly and inconsiderate.

Elsa is not put off and continues to try to convince you to change.

Elsa: "I haven't seen Rob for 3 months. I know it's last minute, but Rob just found out he could be free and he called me as soon as he could. Oh, please, won't you be on call for me?"

Aggressive you: "I can't help it if you haven't seen Rob for 3 months. That's your problem. I've got my own problems with my in-laws coming."

Elsa: "I know you've got company coming, but they're just your in-laws and you get to see them often."

Aggressive you: "They are just as important to me as your absentee boyfriend is to you. Maybe if you got together more often, you wouldn't be so desperate now."

Your insensitivity to Elsa's predicament and your judgmental, accusatory remarks will considerably damage your relationship with your co-worker. Aggressive responses are often disproportionate and fired by our irrational anger and guilt.

Elsa persists!

Elsa: "Remember, I switched weekends with you in the spring when you wanted to go to your cousin's wedding? You agreed then that you owed me one. Well, now I'm collecting! I need you to pay me back this weekend."

Aggressive you: "I gave you plenty of notice—not 3 days like you're offering me. If you think I can drop my plans, you're crazy!"

Elsa: "Well, I'll never do you a favor again. Some friend you are."

You may have won the battle by refusing an unreasonable request, but you have lost the war of conducting yourself in a considerate and professional manner. If the bad feelings created by being aggressive can ever be resolved, it will take an inordinate amount of energy and time.

Example 2

You are making a home visit to a client who has right-sided weakness. You are late in visiting two clients to whom you must give extensive diabetic teaching. Your child needs a ride home from school, and you think you can just make it on time. Mr. Gowers, your 70-year-old client, is right-handed and has not been very successful using his left hand to write. As you are about to leave, he asks you to write a letter for him to his nephew.

An assertive refusal:

Mr. Gowers: "Could you help me write a letter to my nephew tonight? I just remembered it's his twentieth wedding anniversary, and I want to let him know I'm thinking of him. He is like a son to me. I'd do it myself, but I can't get the hang of using my left hand."

Assertive you: "Mr. Gowers, I won't be able to help you to write your letter today because I'm running behind schedule. I can see it is important for you to get your best wishes off to this special nephew of yours in time for his anniversary. I saw your neighbor outside. How about if I ask him to come over and write the letter?"

This definite response makes it clear to Mr. Gowers that you are unable to do what he wants. Your expression of understanding about his urgency and your suggestion of an alternative solution would make him aware of your concern. You have protected your rights not to take on a task when you are already overloaded, and you have shown your client you are interested in his situation.

A nonassertive refusal:

Mr. Gowers: "Could you help me write a letter to my nephew tonight? I just remembered it's his twentieth wedding anniversary, and I want to let him know I'm thinking of him. He is like a son to me. I'd do it myself, but I can't get the hang of using my left hand."

Nonassertive you: "Uh . . . well, um, I'm not sure I can, Mr. Gowers. I'm pretty busy today, but I'll try. Maybe I can come back here on my lunch hour."

You know that you are so busy that you will be lucky to get the teaching done and pick up your son. You know you should not take on this extra task, and you are already feeling more tense because it is one more thing on your long list of things to do. You have not protected your rights for a reasonable workload, and you have conveyed a lot of ambivalence to Mr. Gowers, perhaps leaving him feeling that he is imposing on you.

An aggressive refusal:

Mr. Gowers: "Could you help me write a letter to my nephew tonight? I just remembered it's his twentieth

wedding anniversary, and I want to let him know I'm thinking of him. He is like a son to me. I'd do it myself, but I can't get the hang of using my left hand."

Aggressive you: "If you think I've got time to sit down and take dictation, Mr. Gowers, you're mistaken. I'll be lucky to get my real work done today."

This hostile rejoinder protects you from doing an unreasonable assignment, but it leaves Mr. Gowers feeling devastated. He is likely feeling guilty for asking you and embarrassed at your angry refusal. Neither of you wins with an aggressive refusal.

Example 3

A physician arrives late to the afternoon prenatal clinic. Today is especially busy because more expectant mothers have kept their appointments than usual. One of your nurses is ill, which leaves you short-staffed. In addition, you are responsible for all the prenatal teaching. The physician tells you he has missed his lunch and asks you to get him something to eat.

An assertive refusal:

Dr. Watts: "Will you go across to the deli and pick me up a salami on rye? I missed lunch because I was so busy this morning."

Assertive you: "No, Dr. Watts, I can't go across to get you lunch. Like you, today I am swamped with the workload."

This assertive response clearly conveys your refusal. It is polite and matter-of-fact. You have upheld your rights to do your job and treated your colleague respectfully.

A nonassertive refusal:

Dr. Watts: "Will you go across to the deli and pick me up a salami on rye? I missed lunch because I was so busy this morning."

Nonassertive you: "Um . . . uh, well, Dr. Watts, we're kind of busy here today, but, well, I suppose if I do it fast, it won't take too much time. Do you want it toasted or plain? Pickles? Mustard?"

Being nonassertive is probably leaving you feeling pretty angry and disappointed in yourself. It is clear to everyone that you do not wish to get your colleague's lunch. Being nonassertive this way means you lose time and lose face.

An aggressive refusal:

Dr. Watts: "Will you go across to the deli and pick me up a salami on rye? I missed lunch because I was so busy this morning."

Aggressive you: "Nurses aren't handmaidens anymore, Dr. Watts. You'd better get with the times. We're all busy, yet we managed to get our own lunches. I'm not being paid to go and fetch food for you."

Wow! You protected your rights with this response, but in the process you were rude to a colleague by overreacting and attacking him. Such accusatory aggressiveness only serves to escalate bad feelings. A simple refusal would have been in order.

Saying No Effectively

Quite likely these examples have made you aware of some do's and don'ts when refusing unreasonable requests. Here are some suggestions to add to your observations.

Do:

- State your refusal very near the beginning of your reply so that your requester hears a clear, direct answer right away.
- Indicate concisely the reason for saying no if it strengthens your refusal.
- Communicate your understanding so that the requester realizes that you are aware of the predicament even if you cannot solve it.
- Suggest an alternative source of help if it seems appropriate.
- Think about your response, then speak in a forthright, calm, polite manner.
- Maintain a matter-of-fact, consistent way of refusing in the face of an aggressive requester.

Don't:

- Begin your refusal with a list of lengthy excuses against which an aggressive requester will argue so logically that you will be forced to concede.
- Stammer, pause, hem and haw, hesitate, or burst out your refusal; this will reveal that you are unsure of your response.
- Lose eye contact for lengthy periods, shift uncomfortably, or convey other nonverbal discomfort that reveals your hesitancy.
- Raise your voice or give other bodily clues of being enraged. It is your right to refuse, and you

do not need to become hostile to protect this privilege.

Daring to Hold Fast to Your Principles

Sometimes it is difficult to find just the right words to express your refusal even when you are convinced of your opinion. Berent and Evans (1992) offer some phrases that might be helpful:

> *"No!"*
> *"No, thank you, I don't care to. I've never done that and don't want to start."*
> *"I can't do that."*
> *"I make it a habit never to . . . "*
> *"I make it a habit always to . . . "*
> *"As a matter of principle, I . . . "*

Sometimes healthcare consumers believe the recommended treatment regimen is unreasonable. How can they "just say no" (Box 24-1)?

Peter Drucker, a well-known leadership expert, at age 95 reflecting on lessons learned, advises that leaders are purpose driven, can establish a mission, and can say no to requests that do not support their mission (Karlgaard, 2004).

Box 24-1 | *When the Client Wants to Refuse*

Buying time to learn more: Gastric bypass surgery has been recommended for weight loss. "Surgery sounds so drastic to me. Can you refer me to some other people who have had this procedure, or is there a support group I could attend to learn more?"

Getting a second opinion: "I'm just not sure about all this. For my own peace of mind, I would like to get a second opinion."

Saying no to medication: A woman with some discomfort from osteoarthritis reads about the side effects of the medication and decides that sometimes the cure is worse than the symptom. "I think I'll hold off on medication for now and try the aquatic arthritis class at my club first."

From Breitman P, Hatch C: *How to say no without feeling guilty*, New York, 2000, Broadway Books.

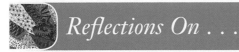

Reflections On . . .

Refusing Unreasonable Requests

Consider what you read about the right to refuse unreasonable requests and the skills to do so. Think of an unreasonable request you would like to refuse as you respond to the following questions.

What? . . .

Write one thing you learned from this chapter.

So what? . . .

How will this affect your nursing practice?

Now what? . . .

How will you implement this new knowledge or skill?

Think about it . . .

Practicing Refusing Unreasonable Requests

Exercise 1

If refusing requests is a recurrent issue with you consider the notion that "you can't improve what you don't measure" (Hedberg, 2010). If this is true, then consider making a brief entry each day in your journal to track your progress on refusing unreasonable requests.

Exercise 2

Reflect upon a situation in which you complied with an unreasonable request. Using colored markers, colored pencils, or crayons, choose the first color that comes to mind and draw an image or color shape that reflects how you feel. Examine your drawing and embellish it with other colors if you choose. Reflect upon a situation in which you were able to refuse an unreasonable request or imagine yourself doing so. Repeat the exercise. Compare the two and write a journal entry about the differences.

Exercise 3

For each of the following situations, write an assertive refusal. Compare your responses with those of your colleagues and pool your suggestions to come up with the most assertive refusal.

1. A client asks you for your home number so that he can call you "if he needs any follow-up advice." In the interests of your privacy, it is your policy not to give out your telephone number to clients.
2. A colleague with whom you are working the night shift asks you to keep an eye on the clients and an ear out for the telephone and night supervisor while she has a nap. You think this request is unreasonable because you are both being paid to do the job and if any trouble occurs, two staff members will be needed.
3. A client is being observed for withdrawal from street drugs. She asks you if she can go down to the cafeteria with her visitor to have a cup of coffee. Your preference is for her to remain on the unit, where you can have frequent contact with her.
4. A client who comes once a week to receive an injection from you asks you if he could come 15 minutes later in the future. Moving back his appointment would inconvenience you, because it would mean you would be late leaving work and would not make your bus connections.
5. A colleague who lives in the same area of the city asks you if he can get a ride to and from work with you. That quiet time in the car by yourself is your only peaceful time in the day. You would find it stressful to have to make conversation with another person during the commuting time.

You can also use the last scenario to verbally practice making refusals. One person can role-play the manager in the vignette and another the nurse, and a third can give feedback to the manager on her ability to refuse assertively.

Exercise 4

For this exercise, work in groups of three. One person makes a request, another refuses the request, and the third gives feedback. The requester can ask for
Continued

anything and should persist in his or her attempts to get what is wanted. Aggressiveness in the requester is encouraged for the purposes of this exercise. The refuser attempts to give an assertive refusal and tries to maintain that stance in the face of the requester's aggressiveness. The observer gives feedback to the refuser about his or her ability to refuse in an assertive way. The observer points out where the refuser could have been more assertive or less aggressive. In debriefing, these questions can be used as a guide.

As the refuser:
1. Were you able to achieve and/or maintain an assertive refusal?
2. Where did you have difficulty being assertive?
3. What could you do to overcome these blocks and be more assertive in your refusals?

As the requester:
1. In what ways did the refuser convince you of a firm no?
2. Where and how could the assertion be improved?

Make sure each person takes a turn in each role, and debrief after each role change.

Exercise 5
To reflect on words that may be useful as you work to refuse unreasonable requests visit http://www.onlineorganizing.com/ExpertAdviceToolboxTips.asp?tipsheet=16 for Creel's "20 Ways to Say No." One example is: "I'm not comfortable with that." Record in your journal the ones you want to remember.

Moments of Connection . . .
Refusing to Hurry in a Managed Care World

"In this day of health maintenance and preferred provider organizations, insurance dictates what we as healthcare providers are allowed to do for our clients. I try to be a patient advocate and go beyond my nursing duties to make sure the procedures are authorized. Even though it takes more time to teach the client and family about the financial end of healthcare, they are appreciative and often tell me how special they feel that I cared enough to help them answer reimbursement questions or put them in touch with someone who can. They see it as another demonstration of caring."

References
Balzer Riley J: Saying what you mean and meaning what you say. Workshop presented at the Faculty Development Institute, Scottsdale, Ariz, 2002.

Berent IM, Evans RL: *The right words: the 350 best things to say to get along with people*, New York, 1992, Warner Books.

Chenevert M: *Pro-nurse handbook: designed for the nurse who wants to thrive professionally*, St. Louis, 1997, Mosby.

Creel R: *20 ways to say no*. http://www.onlineorganizing.com/ExpertAdviceToolboxTips.asp?tipsheet=16. Accessed June 1, 2011.

Ellis A, Powers M: *A guide to rational living*, Hollywood, Calif, 1998, Wilshire Book Co.

Hedberg AG: Strategies and tools for personal growth and health awareness. In Hedberg AG: *Forms for the therapist*, St. Louis, 2010, Elsevier Inc.

Karlgaard R: Conversation with a giant, *Forbes* 174(12):45, 2004.

Mackay H: *Beware the naked man who offers you his shirt*, New York, 1996, Ballantine Books.

Paskin J: How to handle a crushing deadline, *Money* 34(11):44A, 2005.

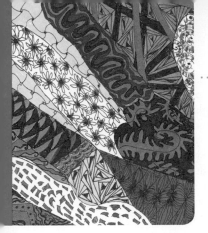

Chapter 25

Communicating Assertively and Responsibly with Distressed Clients and Colleagues

> *My bath was too hot, I got soap in my eyes, my marble went down the drain . . . the Mickey Mouse night light burned out and I bit my tongue. The cat went to sleep with Anthony, not with me. It has been a terrible, horrible, no good, very bad day. My mom says some days are like that.*
>
> **Judith Viorst,** in *Alexander and the Terrible, Horrible, No Good, Very Bad Day*

Objectives

1. Discuss the effect of distressed behavior of clients or colleagues on the nurse
2. Assess the situation and choose the assertive response for a variety of situations
3. Participate in exercises to build strategies for assertive communication with distressed clients and colleagues

Mad, Sad, Glad, and Scared . . . Nurses Bear Witness to All the Human Emotions

Watson (2008), who introduces the science of human caring, calls us to be present to and support the expression of positive and negative feelings (Gallagher-Lepak and Kubsch, 2009). When clients and colleagues are distressed we work to respond in helpful ways, yet we can be stressed by their distress. We are beginning to study the experience of suffering and how people find meaning in the illness experience (Pollock and Sands, 1997). Nurses witness suffering and distress. They must deal with the moment-to-moment lived experience of illness. Clients convey their anguish verbally and nonverbally. Changes in health status, illness, and hospitalization are just some sources of distress in clients. Their loss of composure is a signal that they are disturbed by what is happening to them.

The changing healthcare climate causes stress for us as nurses and for our colleagues. In addition, nurses may pick up the sadness of clients, called shadow grief (Smith-Stoner and Frost, 1998), which can lead to burnout. We may find that we have less energy, experience no zest for living, and talk about our clients continuously, even on our off hours. How we respond and how our clients respond to distress depend on personal history, culture, and experience. We experience the constraints of time, the emergent nature of a situation, and unanticipated change (Sheldon et al, 2006). We need to develop ways to relate to distressed colleagues

273

and clients that soothe their distress without upsetting ourselves. Maintaining our sensitivity to others so that we can respond in a caring way without being overcome and losing our objectivity is one of a nurse's most inviting challenges—the gift of your presence without giving yourself away.

Interpersonal problems experienced by health professionals clearly reveal that our reactions to emotionally laden situations interfere with our ability to act effectively. Nurses may ignore their responses to being overwhelmed with emotional demands, called compassion fatigue (Vaughn, 2001). Untoward reactions can come from within ourselves (feeling unsure or inadequate about how to act), the situation (feeling overcome or impotent), or the distressed person (feeling distress ourselves).

Moments of Connection . . .
Rx: Knowledge

"We had an 11-year-old boy having a nonmalignant tumor removed from his spine. He was labeled a 'brat' due to his demanding behavior. One day, I had a few extra minutes and went and sat with him. We took out his science book and talked about what was happening with his surgery and about his fears. From that time on, he was much less anxious and became one of our favorites."

The suggestion has been made that nurses develop a protective barrier against others' pain, or become insensitive to the discomfort of others, because they encounter so much suffering in the course of their daily work. If we become too involved with others' distress, we overload ourselves emotionally and become ineffective. If we avoid the distress of others by ignoring or belittling it, we are left with the feeling of not giving the attention and support that are expected. Some nurses feel helpless about how to be therapeutic with distressed persons. Others feel annoyed or irritated that clients or colleagues cannot solve their own problems. Thoughts about our own inadequacies, or judgments about the appropriateness of others' behavior, prevent us from acting in the best interests of the distressed person.

Kaufman and Wetmore (1994) suggest four common events that can cause stress: loss of control, change, sense of threat, and unrealized expectations. When nurses face distressed clients, these are the issues. Remember that it is not the situation itself that causes problems, but our reaction to it. The teaching of communication skills implies that if we say the right thing, clients or colleagues will have an "Aha!" experience, that is, they will immediately see our point of view and become both compliant and grateful. Consider a new view; that is, the extraordinary set of circumstances, the distress, is not a failure or a lack of compliance, but an opportunity. This is the opportunity for nurses to learn from others' experiences and to build new skills that increase communication effectiveness.

Ideally, we need to remain calm enough to be able to understand the reason for another person's distress, to remain nonjudgmental so that we can convey appropriate compassion for the situation at hand, and to remain clearheaded enough to act responsibly on behalf of the other person. Ascher (1994), in her memoir of grief at the death of her brother from acquired immunodeficiency syndrome, paints a picture that demonstrates the complexity distress can present. She defines grief as a "landscape without gravity." Of her family she says:

> My husband does not know I'm here, afloat. . . . They continue to communicate through normal channels as though we were all here together on the steady plane of everyday life. Grief is outside the scope of language. I can only speak in signs. The furrow of my brow, the tightness of my lips. But when they who love me entreat, "Do you want to talk about it?" I say, "no," and turn away. I could say "ouch," I could say "it hurts." But language seems slight. Grief is physical and it hurts.

Ascher called it a "journey into paralysis." We must remain humble at the pain and anguish of suffering clients and their families, and yes, of suffering colleagues, too, to whose stories we may have no access.

How to Improve Your Communication Skill with Distressed Clients and Colleagues

In the rest of this chapter you are given situations involving distressed clients and colleagues. Assess each situation, determine the request being made, and choose the most assertive and responsible communication strategy.

WIT&*Wisdom*

Poetry is a way some people share their distress. Ken Saulter, coping with early memory loss, and his wife spoke at Innovations in Dementia Care (2010), where he shared a poem his wife identified as important in their relationship. As you read "Between Us," think about offering writing as an expressive outlet for distress.

Between Us

Losing my memory,
Losing my memory to a terminal disease,
Is getting to be a problem.
Like when I'm in a group
And people talk to me and then,
Suddenly I fall silent,
While my brain skips a beat.
We know it's not a simple senior moment.
Eyes divert to shoe laces or thereabouts,
Anywhere else but the ceiling.
The moment becomes one of deep discomfort.
And here I am, a fraction of a person,
A clown without make-up or costume,
Waiting giant seconds to recover.
I'm told I will not remember
These bricks of separation
In the wall that is, regrettably,
Being built between us.
I worry a lot about forgetting habits, like
My locker combination, after 20 years of use.
And then, someday maybe, remembering where
   I live;
Or, luckily, maybe not.
But, against our will,
The wall keeps getting higher and higher.
Yet I keep on living, accepting the losses and
Focusing on what I've got, and you.
And trying to lower the wall between us
Or slow it down,
Or build a gate,
Or do something.

© Ken Saulter. Used with permission.

A critique of all the response choices for each situation is listed at the end of the chapter, beginning on p. 284. It is worthwhile to read the advantages and drawbacks of each option.

Communicating with Upset Clients

Step 1: Assessment of the Data

1. Review the following situation and formulate your own assessment of the client's thoughts, feelings, and requests.

Mr. James is a 58-year-old avid outdoorsman who has been hunting in the woods near your rural hospital. While climbing steep terrain, he slipped and fell 50 feet down a ragged incline. In addition to suffering multiple bruises and scratches, he broke his glasses. Today he was admitted to your hospital for overnight observation. As you make your first round on the evening shift you go into his room to introduce yourself:

> *You:* "Good afternoon, Mr. James. Welcome to our hospital. I'm sorry you have to be here under such unfortunate circumstances. How are you?"
>
> *Mr. James:* "How long am I going to be here? Can you get me the phone? I need to reach my wife. Somebody's got to bring me my extra glasses. I can't drive. . . . I can't do anything without them. You can have your damn hospital. Just get me a phone so I can make arrangements to get out of here."

Mr. James raises his voice as he is talking and turns away from you. He squeezes the bed sheet in his hands and looks exasperated.

2. On a separate sheet of paper write down your assessment of Mr. James's thoughts and feelings. Indicate what request Mr. James is making of you, his evening nurse.
3. Compare your assessment to the assessment that follows:

Thoughts: Mr. James thinks that he cannot manage without his glasses. He is aware that he must reach his wife so that arrangements can be made to get his spare glasses.

Feelings: He is upset that he cannot read, write, or see to drive. He feels trapped in this remote rural hospital. He desperately wants to talk to his wife about arranging to get home.

Request: Mr. James wants you to understand how frustrating it is for him to be stuck in this unfamiliar hospital. He is trying to get you to comprehend how dependent and immobile he is without his glasses. He wants you to help him contact his wife. Indirectly, he may be asking to be comforted; that is, to be helped to feel more at home in this strange place.

4. Did your assessment reflect an accurate analysis of the facts as they were presented? If not, return to the original data presented in the vignette and reassess the cognitive and affective messages. If so, proceed to Step 2.

Step 2: Communication Strategies and Desired Outcomes

5. You have determined that Mr. James needs understanding, action, and comfort. On a piece of paper write which communication behaviors you would use to show Mr. James how you intend to respond to his request. Indicate the desired outcome(s) of your suggested strategy.
6. Compare your suggested strategy with this one:

It is appropriate to meet Mr. James's request for understanding and action. A warm, genuine, respectful manner would convey that you care about him. An empathic response would ensure that he knows you understand his predicament and would reduce any embarrassment he might feel for displaying his upset feelings in such a volatile way. If his upset behavior agitates you, then you can calm yourself and focus on his distress, using positive self-talk and imagery to prepare yourself to communicate assertively and responsibly.

This strategy would help Mr. James relax and feel accepted. He would likely look calmer and feel more patient with his circumstances. Your compliance with his requests contributes to the development of a trusting rapport.

Step 3: Implementation and Evaluation of Your Communication Strategy

7. Now you must reply to Mr. James. Develop your own response and write it on a separate sheet of paper. Keep it handy so that you can refer to it later.
8. At this point you get the chance to compare your suggested response to the following options. Look over each of the response choices and turn to p. 284 at the end of the chapter to read a critique of each.

As you review the following choices, look for those that are congruent with your assessment of Mr. James's requests and your desire to communicate in an assertive

and responsible way. (Notice that the choices are not listed alphabetically. This is to prevent the temptation to quickly scan all the answers without giving yourself the benefit of evaluating each response.)

Choice A: "You should be grateful to be alive. If that farmer hadn't heard you yelling and pulled you out of the ravine, you'd be out there freezing at this very minute. You don't need to snap at me. I can hear. I'll get you the phone."

Choice Z: "It's hard to be in a strange place where nothing is familiar. I know that feeling. I'll bring you the phone."

Choice J: You get red in the face, clench your fists, then turn on your heels and head down the hall to get the portable phone for Mr. James.

Choice S: "I'm sure you're eager to talk to your wife and make arrangements to get your glasses and go home. I'll get our portable phone for you right away. I can imagine that it must be frustrating to be without your glasses, so please let us know how we can help you manage until you get the spare ones."

9. After you have found the most satisfactory strategy and discovered why the other options are unsuitable, go back to the response you suggested earlier in this exercise. Evaluate your response in terms of how assertive and responsible it was.

Communicating with Upset Colleagues

Step 1: Assessment of the Data

1. Review the following situation and formulate what you think are your colleague's thoughts and feelings. Indicate what you think your colleague is requesting from you.

Joe is the intern on the medical unit where you have been a student for the past 6 weeks. Because you are both students working on the unit at the same times, you have become good friends. This day Joe looks preoccupied and you have noticed that he is not his usual good-natured self. He snaps at you for not having your client ready for his physical examination, even though he had not warned you about his plans. Later he approaches you with the following:

Joe: "Shirley, I'm sorry for snapping at you earlier. I'm just not myself. Dayle just found out she's pregnant, and it's all I can think about. I just can't imagine being a father. I can barely cope with being a husband and an intern. It's been the only thing on my mind since I found out 2 days ago. I can't think straight. I can't sleep. . . . I still can't believe it. I don't know what I'm going to do. We want kids, but why now?"

2. On a separate sheet of paper write down your assessment of Joe's thoughts and feelings. Indicate what you think Joe is requesting from you, his colleague.

3. Compare your assessment to the assessment that follows:

Thoughts: Joe knows his wife is pregnant and is aware that his preoccupation with this unexpected, and not yet welcome, news is causing him to be short-tempered with you. He wants to be a father but does not think the timing is good.

Feelings: He regrets that he snapped at you. Joe is shocked by the news of his wife's unexpected pregnancy and is worried about how he can cope with the added strain of being a father when he is having difficulty juggling the two roles of intern and husband. He likely is tired because he has not been sleeping, and he is upset that he cannot think straight.

Request: Joe is asking you to accept his apology for snapping at you, and he wants you to understand how the news about the pregnancy is turning his life upside down. Indirectly, he may be asking for some comfort for his predicament.

4. Did your assessment reflect an accurate analysis of the facts as they were presented? If not, return to the original data presented in the vignette and reassess the cognitive and affective messages. If so, proceed to Step 2.

Step 2: Communication Strategies and Desired Outcomes

5. You have determined that Joe wants you both to demonstrate your understanding of the shock he is experiencing and to accept his apology. Identify which communication behaviors you would use to meet these two reasonable requests. Indicate the desired outcome of your suggested strategy.

6. Compare your suggested strategy to this one:

Warmth would show that you feel kindly toward Joe and you do not hold a grudge. An empathic response would convey your understanding to Joe. A self-disclosure about adjusting to the news about your own pregnancy (or another major event) would

provide him with hope that getting used to the idea comes in time.

It is appropriate to meet Joe's requests. This strategy would make Joe feel relieved that you understand the reason for his outburst and that you forgive him. The hope you might give him—that he will work things out in time—would be comforting.

Step 3: Implementation and Evaluation of Your Communication Strategy

7. Now you must reply to Joe. Develop your own response to Joe and write it on a separate sheet of paper. Keep it handy so that you can refer to it later.

8. At this point you get the chance to compare your response to the following options. Look over each of the choices and turn to p. 284 at the end of the chapter to read a critique of each option.

As you review the following response choices, be looking for those that are congruent with your assessment of Joe's requests and your desire to communicate in an assertive and responsible way.

Choice T: "It's OK, Joe. We all get upset at times."

Choice F: "Joe, I forgive you (smiling). I can see that you are preoccupied and upset with the unexpected news of Dayle's pregnancy. It seems overwhelming right now to imagine trying to squeeze in being a father when you are busy enough being a husband and getting your career launched. I, too, felt shocked when I first found out I was pregnant, but after several weeks I began to accept the idea. By the end of term I was even looking forward to Sarah's birth."

Choice V: "It's OK this time, Joe, but don't let it happen again. You really threw my whole schedule off this morning. That's great news about Dayle. So you're going to be a father, eh? I love being a parent, and I know you will too, once you get used to the idea. It just takes a few weeks to get over the initial shock and then you'll be fine."

Choice O: "Apology accepted, Joe. It's easy to see that you're upset with your news. Things will turn out, Joe. You'll get used to the idea."

9. After you have found the most assertive and responsible choice and checked out why the other options are not suitable, go back to the response you wrote earlier in this exercise. Evaluate your suggestion in terms of how assertive and responsible it was.

Communicating with Clients Who Are Sad or Depressed

Step 1: Assessment of the Data

1. Review the following situation and formulate what you think are your client's thoughts and feelings. Indicate what you think your client is requesting from you.

Jim is an 18-year-old client on your unit. He has just had a surgical repair after breaking his leg in a football game. Jim is an all-star athlete who knows he won't be playing any more sports this year, his senior year. He is worried about getting behind in his schoolwork because of the advanced placement classes he is taking. Every day counts if he is to keep up with the fast pace of the class. This is Jim's final year in high school, and he is worrying that his grade point average may slip, because a football scholarship is now out of the question. He is tearful and seems embarrassed.

You: "Good morning, Jim. How's it going?"

Jim: "It's not . . ." (looking away from you and sighing).

You: "What's wrong?"

Jim: "Oh . . . what's the point? I've got nothing to look forward to. All my plans have gone down the tube." (Jim's voice is flat, and he makes no eye contact with you.)

2. Take a piece of paper and write down your assessment of Jim's thoughts and feelings. Indicate what request Jim is making of you, his nurse for the day.

3. Compare your assessment to the one that follows:

Thoughts: Jim thinks that his academic and athletic hopes are not going to be realized. At this point in his life this injury seems like a total disaster.

Feelings: Jim probably has mixed feelings. Right now he feels discouraged and hopeless about his future. It is likely that he is frustrated that his plans have been thwarted, angry that his life has been so affected, and apathetic about doing anything.

Request: Jim wants you to understand how he is feeling. He may also want some help to lift himself out of his depression.

4. Did your assessment reflect an accurate analysis of the facts as they were presented? If not, return to the original data presented in the vignette and reassess the cognitive and affective messages. If so, proceed to Step 2.

Step 2: Communication Strategies and Desired Outcomes

5. You have determined that Jim needs understanding and information. On a separate sheet of paper, identify which communication behaviors you would use to respond to Jim's requests. Indicate what desired outcomes you expect by using the communication behaviors you have suggested.

6. Compare your suggested strategy to this one:

Jim's concerns are reasonable, and it is appropriate to respond to them. Warmth and genuineness would convey that you care for Jim. An empathic response would demonstrate that you really understand the unhappy situation he is in. When you talk to Jim, you should stop whatever physical activity you are doing, face him, and give him your full attention. If his despair generates negative feelings in you (such as hopelessness or anger), relax before you respond. Visualize yourself responding to Jim in a caring and constructive way. If necessary, use your positive self-talk to remind yourself that you can be therapeutic when one of your clients is sad.

This strategy would make Jim feel cared for and give him a chance to talk. This planned intervention might lift his mood.

Step 3: Implementation and Evaluation of Your Communication Strategy

7. Now you must reply to Jim. On a separate sheet of paper write down the response that you have developed. Keep it handy so that you can refer to it later.

8. At this point you get the chance to compare your suggested response with the following options. Look over each of the response choices and turn to p. 284 at the end of the chapter to read a critique of each option.

As you review the following response choices, look for those that are congruent with your assessment of Jim's requests and your desire to communicate in an assertive and responsible way.

Choice K: "You're young, Jim. It won't be that long before you'll be up and getting back in shape again. Come on, Jim, chin up. There's no point in getting depressed. You might as well make the best of it. We all have disappointments in life. I've had plenty, and you just have to make the best of things and ride through the bad times."

Choice B: "I'm worried about you, Jim. You're not thinking of doing anything like harming yourself, are you?"

Choice Q: "You're really feeling down, aren't you? Breaking your leg is a big disappointment and enough to get anyone down. Maybe you're afraid you'll have trouble catching up with things in your life. You may not think so, but you'll be back to school soon. It takes time to get adjusted to the idea of something so unexpected happening to you. With all the visitors you've had, I bet it wouldn't be hard for you to find a friend to fill you in on what's happening at school. Would it help to call someone to chat?"

Choice X: "I'm sorry you feel that way, Jim."

9. After you have found the most satisfactory strategy and discovered why the other options are not suitable, go back to the response you wrote earlier in the exercise. Evaluate your response in terms of how assertive and responsible it was.

Communicating with Colleagues Who Are Sad or Depressed

Step 1: Assessment of the Data

1. Read over the following situation and formulate your own assessment of your colleague's thoughts, feelings, and requests.

Petra is a fellow student whom you have come to know and like. The two of you have been in the same classes in nursing and, coincidentally, have had the same clinical rotations for the past year and a half. Now you are working on an oncology service where many of the clients are dying of cancer. Petra has been quieter and has kept more to herself in the past week. She looks pale and lethargic, in sharp contrast to her usual witty and spunky self. At your coffee break one morning, you ask Petra how she is feeling and she responds as follows:

Petra: "I didn't think it was that noticeable. It's working with cancer patients. . . . I don't think I can take much more of it. My visions of being a nurse are to cure people—to get them well again. It seems all the people we are working with now are dying, and there's no way around it. It's so depressing. How can you stand it? I go home every night, and all I can think is, 'Is this all there is to life?' All we do seems so pointless if this is how things end."

2. On a separate sheet of paper write down your assessment of Petra's thoughts and feelings. Indicate what request Petra is making of you, her classmate.

3. Compare your assessment to the assessment that follows:

Thoughts: Petra thinks it's pointless to prolong people's lives for a short time if they are going to feel sick from chemotherapy or radiation and die anyway. She wonders how you cope with the seeming futility of it all, and possibly she wonders if she can continue in nursing with such a hopeless attitude.

Feelings: Petra is feeling discouraged and sad about the death and dying she sees every day on the wards. She is shocked about the apparent hopelessness of nursing, since people end up suffering and dying anyway. She cannot seem to focus on those clients who do get better or those who choose to prolong their lives even for a short time. She is worried about coming to terms with her feelings so that she can continue nursing. She is frightened about the whole notion of dying. She is dispirited and wants to know how you handle similar feelings.

Request: Petra wants you to understand and accept how she is feeling. She is also asking you for information about how to handle her feelings so that they do not interfere with her ability to nurse effectively. Indirectly, she is asking to be comforted by having some of her sad feelings dissipated.

4. Does your assessment reflect an accurate analysis of the facts as they were presented by Petra? If not, return to the original vignette and reassess the cognitive and affective messages. If so, proceed to Step 2.

Step 2: Communication Strategies and Desired Outcomes

5. You have determined that Petra needs understanding and information. Identify which communication behaviors you would use to show Petra how you intend to respond to her requests. Indicate the desired outcome of your strategy. Write down your suggestions.

6. Compare your suggested strategy to this one:

It is quite a risk for Petra to reveal her feelings and questions about nursing and her fears of dying; therefore, it is important to respect and accept the issues she is trying to work through. It is appropriate to respond to Petra's requests, and warmth and respect need to be conveyed to show Petra that you do not harbor negative feelings about her questions about the purpose of nursing. Accurate, genuine empathy shows her that you understand her fears about dying. To show her you are willing to share how you handle similar feelings, you might use an appropriate self-disclosure. If you wish to invite her to explore the topic of the meaning of life, you might make a gentle suggestion about how to begin.

This strategy would make Petra feel understood and possibly get her started on finding answers to some crucial questions for her personal and professional life. Her sadness is not likely to lift immediately because she is facing some major philosophical questions, but this strategy may give her some direction about how to find some answers.

Step 3: Implementation and Evaluation of Your Communication Strategy

7. Now you must reply to Petra. Develop your own response to Petra and write it on a separate sheet of paper. Keep it handy so that you can refer to it later.
8. At this point you get the chance to compare your suggested response with the following options. Look over each of the response choices and turn to p. 284 at the end of the chapter to read a critique of each option.

As you review the following choices, look for those that are congruent with your assessment of Petra's requests and your desire to communicate in an assertive and responsible way.

Choice W: "You're wondering what's the point of nursing if clients end up dying on a unit like this one where everyone is terminally ill. When I feel discouraged, like you are now, I try to adjust my perspective. I have to remind myself that the people we see in here are a small sample of the people in our city. There are lots of older healthy people out there living active lives. Something else I try to do, even though I need to work at it more, is to strengthen my belief that dying is part of living. I think we have control over how we adjust to our dying, and I like to think I can help some of our clients live each day until they die. I think of their time with us as a very special part of their lives. They look to us to be able to listen to them without having to worry about what they say. Their family and friends can't always be helpful. These thoughts help me feel more hopeful, anyway. What do you think?"

Choice C: "Well, your sadness does show, Petra. Those clients are sad enough without having us add

to their misery. Everyone has to die, Petra. You must accept that."

Choice L: "Boy, you are down about this rotation, Petra. Let's talk about something more pleasant that'll cheer you up. Are you and Gary going to the hockey game on Friday?"

Choice P: "Petra, I should have picked up that something was really getting to you on this rotation. I knew there was something, and I thought it might have to do with Gary. Gee, I don't know what to say, Petra. These are issues you have to sort out. I know it's hard to accept, but some of our clients are going to die. Yet some do get better, too. Keep that in mind. You'll feel better when we're on the next rotation in pediatrics."

9. After you have found the most satisfactory strategy and discovered why the other options are unsuitable, go back to the suggested response you wrote earlier in the exercise. Evaluate your response in terms of how assertive and responsible it was.

Communicating with Clients Who Are Crying

Step 1: Assessment of the Data

1. Review the following situation and formulate your own assessment of the client's thoughts, feelings, and requests.

Mrs. Urst is a 35-year-old woman who has just given birth to her second child. Both she and her baby are healthy, and her husband and their 8-year-old son are thrilled with the new addition to their family. You have just entered her room and found her weeping. She has gone through several tissues, and her eyes are red and swollen.

You: "Oh, Mrs. Urst. You are really upset. What's troubling you?"

Mrs. Urst: "Ohhhh . . . (sobs and blows nose; laughs and then starts crying again). I can't stop. It's just dawned on me that I'm now a mother of two. It's ridiculous . . . (sobs) . . . I've known for 9 months, but now I wonder how I'll cope. I've forgotten all the stuff mothers need to know, and if I stay at home I'll forget all the stuff secretaries are supposed to know. Why did we get ourselves into this predicament? Oh, I'm sorry to burden you. I guess I've just got the 'baby blues' (blows nose and bites lip to keep from crying anymore)."

2. On a separate sheet of paper write down your assessment of Mrs. Urst's thoughts and feelings. Indicate

what request Mrs. Urst is making of you, her nurse for the day.

3. Compare your assessment to the following one:

Thoughts: Mrs. Urst thinks she is going to have difficulty being a mother of two. She wonders if she has made a mistake by having another child. She thinks she might be overburdening you with her disclosure.

Feelings: Mrs. Urst is upset and confused. She is overwhelmed by the new responsibilities she will have as the mother of a newborn, and she is worried that she will get out of practice while she is away from her job as a secretary. She is somewhat embarrassed by her outburst and tries to pass it off as "baby blues" to save face.

Request: Mrs. Urst wants you to understand her fears of being overwhelmed, but she does not want to delve into her personal life in any great detail, as indicated by her referral to "baby blues" and her apology that she might be burdening you. She may be indirectly asking you for reassurance that she will manage.

4. Did your assessment reflect an accurate analysis of the facts as they were presented? If not, return to the original data presented in the vignette and reassess the cognitive and affective messages. If so, proceed to Step 2.

Step 2: Communication Strategies and Desired Outcomes

5. You have determined that Mrs. Urst needs understanding and comfort. Identify which communication behaviors you would use to show Mrs. Urst that you are prepared to act on her reasonable requests. Indicate the desired outcome of your suggested strategy. Write down these plans on a separate piece of paper.

6. Compare your suggested strategy to this one:

Warmth would be appropriate to show Mrs. Urst that you care that she is upset. Respect for her privacy could be demonstrated by a nonjudgmental, empathic reference to her struggle to be both a mother and a working person. It would be appropriate to express your agreement that some of her feelings are related to her postnatal hormonal imbalance. Your opinion that she will likely work out a satisfactory schedule would reassure her, once you have convinced her that you understand her feelings. This strategy would make Mrs. Urst feel understood and diminish her embarrassment. In addition, your reassurance would make her feel hopeful that she can and will manage.

Step 3: Implementation and Evaluation of Your Communication Strategy

7. Now you must reply to Mrs. Urst. Develop your own response to her and write it on a separate sheet of paper. Keep it handy so that you can refer to it later.

8. At this point you get the chance to compare your suggested response to the following options. Look over each of the response choices and turn to p. 284 at the end of the chapter to read a critique of each.

As you review the following response choices, look for those that are congruent with your assessment of Mrs. Urst's requests and your desire to communicate in an assertive and responsible way.

Choice D: "There, there, Mrs. Urst. It's natural for most women to have a crying spell after giving birth. Things will work out; they always do. Most mothers get the 'baby blues.' I see it all the time. Don't feel embarrassed."

Choice I: "It's too late to be crying over spilt milk, Mrs. Urst. You must have thought about all this when you discovered you were pregnant. You'll feel better when you are home."

Choice R: "I'm sorry you're so upset, Mrs. Urst. I'll come back later."

Choice Y: "It's likely that your tears are in part due to 'baby blues,' Mrs. Urst. But your whole world has been upset with the arrival of your new daughter; that's bound to take some adjustment. Working out a schedule between two important roles like motherhood and career is complicated. Given time to adjust to your new schedule, I'm certain you can work out something that suits you. I have some time now if you'd like to talk."

9. After you have found the most satisfactory strategy and discovered why the other options are unsuitable, go back to the response you generated earlier in the exercise. Evaluate your response in terms of how assertive and responsible it was.

Communicating with Colleagues Who Are Crying

Step 1: Assessment of the Data

1. Review the following situation and formulate your own assessment of your colleague's thoughts, feelings, and requests.

Don is a nurse on the rehabilitation unit in the long-term care facility where you are working. When you go into the office to collect your purse, you find him sitting in a chair with his head in his hands. When he sees you coming in, he quickly rubs his eyes and turns in his chair so that you cannot see his face. He gets out a tissue and blows his nose and says the following:

Don: "Come on in, Kathy. Guess you caught me crying. It's the news about Mr. Kent that's got to me. (Looking at you.) I really thought he would make it. I can't believe he's dead. He was making so much progress. I never thought I'd say it, but I'll even miss the way he used to act like the king of the unit."

Don is referring to Mr. Kent, an elderly resident of your rehabilitation unit, who was transferred yesterday to an acute care hospital after a cardiac arrest. Mr. Kent had been on the unit for 8 months, during which time he made himself known by his lively and sometimes overbearing involvement with all the staff. He was a well-liked, integral part of the life of your team. Your colleague Don had often been assigned as Mr. Kent's nurse because of Mr. Kent's request for a male nurse. Don and Mr. Kent had enjoyed friendly arguments about politics.

2. On a separate sheet of paper write down your assessment of Don's thoughts and feelings. Indicate what request Don is making of you, his co-worker.
3. Compare your assessment with the assessment that follows:

Thoughts: Don is having difficulty believing that Mr. Kent is dead, in view of his progress just before his transfer. It doesn't seem possible that after all that, he would die from a heart problem.
Feelings: Don is shocked and saddened by his client's death. He feels confused and amazed because Mr. Kent seemed to be improving. He misses Mr. Kent, and even longs for his more unpleasant habits.
Request: His invitation for you to enter the room, and his self-disclosure, are evidence that Don is asking you to listen to him. He is asking for understanding and some comfort.

4. Did your assessment reflect an accurate analysis of the facts as they were presented? If not, return to the original data presented in the vignette and reassess

the cognitive and affective messages. If so, proceed to Step 2.

Step 2: Communication Strategies and Desired Outcomes

5. You have determined that Don needs understanding and comfort. Identify which communication behaviors you would use to show Don how you intend to respond to his reasonable requests. Indicate the desired outcome of your suggested strategy. Write your ideas on a separate sheet of paper for future reference.
6. Compare your suggested strategy to this one:

An empathic response would show your understanding of Don's bereavement. Expressing your opinion about the comfort Don provided Mr. Kent would be respectful and give Don some comfort. Coming into the room and being with Don would be a warm gesture showing your respect for his feelings. If it felt genuinely comfortable for you, then a gentle touch would also convey your warmth and comfort to Don.

This strategy would make Don feel understood and comforted.

Step 3: Implementation and Evaluation of Your Communication Strategy

7. Now you must reply to Don. Develop your own response to Don and write it on a separate sheet of paper. Keep it handy so that you can refer to it later.
8. At this point you get the chance to compare your suggested response to the following options. Look over each of the response choices and turn to p. 284 at the end of the chapter to read a critique of each.

As you review the following response choices, look for those that are congruent with your assessment of Don's requests and your desire to communicate in an assertive and responsible way.

Choice G: (You sit down beside Don.) "I can't believe Mr. Kent is dead either, Don. You two had such a close relationship that I can see why you are so sad. You gave him a lot of pleasure with those heavy political discussions. It's so hard to just keep on working when you lose someone as special as Mr. Kent. Can I help you out with your assignment in any way today, Don?"

Choice N: (Continuing to get your purse in the locked drawer.) "I'll be out of your way just as soon as I get my purse, Don. It's awful news, isn't it?"

Choice U: "I can see that you're upset, Don, but we've got to get used to these old people dying. It's true the unit won't be the same without him, but another resident will come along and we'll all get attached to him. Do you want to come to lunch with us? We're going to try that new deli, you know, the one Johnson's took over. It would do you good."

9. After you have found the most satisfactory strategy and discovered why the other options are not suitable, go back to the response you generated earlier in this exercise. Evaluate your response in terms of how assertive and responsible it was.

How the Nurse Can Address Compassion Fatigue Proactively

We are called to create a sacred space for distressed clients and colleagues. Here they can be at ease, be themselves without fear, let down their guard, take off the masks, and just be (Fuimano, 2005). This is a place without judgment, what Fuimano describes when she calls acceptance a management tool. She says acceptance, being nonjudgmental, begins with you as a nurse, as a person being compassionate with yourself. When we accept our own uniqueness and the lessons we can learn from others, we can approach distressed people with an interest in learning about their perspectives and their journeys. But how can you hold this space for others and maintain your own ability to be compassionate? Think of how you begin your day.

How do you prepare yourself emotionally and spiritually to begin your day? Some nurses say a silent prayer. Some take deep cleansing breaths. Some mentally determine to bring their best selves to the people whose lives they touch. It is less important what strategy you choose than that you take the responsibility to find a way to center yourself before you enter into what can be the chaotic world of healthcare. Review chapters in Part 3 for strategies for self-care and see Chapter 30 for ideas about maintaining your commitment to healthcare.

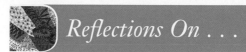

Reflections On . . .

Communicating Assertively and Responsibly with Distressed Clients and Colleagues

Consider what you read about assertive communication with distressed clients and colleagues. What experience have you had? Answer the following questions.

What? . . .
Write one thing you learned from this chapter.

So what? . . .
How will this affect your nursing practice?

Now what? . . .
How will you implement this new knowledge or skill?

Think about it . . .

Practicing Communicating Assertively and Responsibly with Distressed Clients and Colleagues

Exercise 1

Identify a difficult conversation you had in which the client or colleague was sad and one in which he or she was angry. Write a brief, reflective journal entry describing what happened and how you responded. Include your assessment of what you said and did and anything you would have done differently. Identify who you can talk with to support you and offer suggestions after these conversations (Sheldon et al, 2006, 2009).

Exercise 2

Identify a time when you were distressed and someone responded to you in a way that offered you comfort. Write a brief reflective journal entry identifying what brought you comfort. Think of what the other person did or did not do and said or did not say. Consider the person's body language, tone of voice, and the amount of time offered you. Reread what you have written and identify at least three things you learned from this that could help you be more fully present for a client or colleague who is distressed.

Critique: Choices of Responses to Distressed Clients and Colleagues

Choice A: You are defensive and hostile in this response. You have taken Mr. James's remarks as a personal insult, when they were only a release of his intense frustration and worry. By responding so aggressively, you have escalated bad feelings between you and your client and not respected your right to communicate in a caring way. You have not shown Mr. James that you understand his feelings and that you care about his predicament. Although you did not meet his request for understanding, you did meet his request for the action of getting the telephone. This response is not assertive; it is aggressive. Mr. James would likely feel angry and embarrassed by your outburst, not understood or comforted. The only responsible part of this retort is your offer to get the telephone.

Choice B: Your opening words show that you are concerned about Jim's behavior; however, by beginning this way, you have put the emphasis on yourself instead of on Jim. It is an aggressive approach because it puts your feelings first, at the expense of your client's feelings. Your implication that Jim is not like his old self is aggressive in its undertone of disappointment and scolding. By asking Jim if he is contemplating harming himself you are reading more into his symptoms than he presented. Jim might suspect that you are more worried about yourself (should he seriously be considering harming himself) than you are about his misery. As well as being aggressive, this answer is not responsible because it does not pick up on the data Jim presented; it exaggerates and goes beyond the facts. Jim would likely not feel understood or helped by this response. He would likely be cautious about revealing any further information to you because your words suggest that you do not want to get involved if there is any sign of trouble.

Choice C: Petra is likely to feel judged and reprimanded by this approach. Your confrontation would likely sting. It is judgmental and puts down your colleague. You proceed to lay on a lot of guilt about how she should hide her feelings to protect her clients, without giving her the right to have the feelings that she does. This approach is aggressive and uncaring. By not picking up on both her requests, you have used an irresponsible strategy.

Choice D: This strategy is not responsible because it tunes in to neither the information Mrs. Urst gave about her conflict between career and motherhood, nor to her stark realization that she is now the mother of two. Your patronizing choice of words is aggressive and demeaning. Mrs. Urst would not likely feel understood or comforted by this response. She might feel that you are insensitive to her concerns. She might feel like a child that has just been dismissed.

Choice F: This response is assertive and responsible. Your warmth and slight teasing shows Joe that you forgive him for his lack of consideration. By quickly focusing on his reason for being upset, you show him that you understand his situation. Your empathic remarks about his feelings are accurate and specific, leaving Joe no doubt that you understand him. Your self-disclosure is appropriate because Joe wants to be a parent, and your own experience will likely give him hope that he will adjust. Joe would probably feel accepted and reassured by these words.

Choice G: By sitting down, you show respect for the importance of Don's feelings. Your self-disclosure lets Don know that you understood his feelings of shock at the news of this resident's death. Your acknowledgment of the joy that Don brought to Mr. Kent would be pleasing to Don. Your offer to help him with his work for today is respectful because of the gentle phrasing. Your response is assertive because it offers Don helpful communication while respecting your right to be helpful, and it is responsible because it tunes in to all the data Don presented.

Choice I: This choice is aggressive because it judges and punishes Mrs. Urst for having normal doubts and fears. It is not a responsible strategy because it misses out on the data about her conflict concerning her roles and her shock about being the mother of two. Mrs. Urst would likely feel insulted that you question her decision making and angry that you did not give her a chance to respond. Your insensitive suggestion that she will see things differently when she gets home is arrogant and would likely frustrate Mrs. Urst. You have not respected your right to communicate in a caring way.

Choice J: By not saying anything, you have lost the opportunity to show Mr. James that you understand how he feels about his situation. Your nonassertive actions of blushing and looking flustered make you feel disappointed that you concentrated on your feelings without conveying any compassion to your client. Although you failed to meet his request for understanding, you did offer him the telephone. Mr. James would likely be more discomfited, and possibly embarrassed, that he upset you. This response is not assertive and is only minimally responsible.

Choice K: This choice is irresponsible because it does not acknowledge Jim's feelings of lethargy and disappointment in a therapeutic way. This response is judgmental and demanding. Jim is not accepted for feeling the way he does. This aggressive approach bulldozes over Jim's sadness. It protects neither his right to feel the way he does nor your right to relate to your client in a sensitive and caring way. Jim would not feel understood by this strategy, and it is unlikely he would look to you for advice on how to get himself out of his unhappy state. He has received the facile message from you that it is easy to stay happy: just keep your chin up in the face of any troubles.

Choice L: Petra would likely feel ignored by this strategy. By diverting the conversation from your classmate's important self-disclosure, you have minimized the importance of what she is saying, and you have overruled her right to be understood and respected. By avoiding the sensitive area of her feelings, you have been nonassertive; neither her rights nor yours have been attended to with this reply. This retort is irresponsible because it does not pick up on the information embodied in Petra's plea.

Choice N: This is a nonassertive and irresponsible response. By not pausing to show consideration for Don's reaction, you evaded giving him the support he could have appreciated. Your opening remarks are inappropriately focused on you, and they could indicate that the whole situation is embarrassing. This self-centeredness is not helpful. Your vague references to Mr. Kent's death are disrespectful in their lack of specificity. This strategy would leave Don feeling uncomfortable and hurt by your lack of respect for both him and his client.

Choice O: You have met Joe's request for forgiveness, and you have made an attempt to reassure him that you think he will adjust to the situation. Your attempt is nonassertive because it does not acknowledge the specific feelings that Joe raised when he related his troubles to you. This choice is glib and is not responsible because it is not a specific reflection of the data presented. Joe would probably feel you really didn't understand the depth and turbulence of his reactions.

Choice P: Petra would likely feel understood but somewhat admonished by this strategy. At the beginning your focus is more on your guilty feelings about

not picking up on Petra's changes. This self-disclosure is irrelevant. It is aggressive because it suggests that Petra's sadness is so blatant that it would be obvious to anyone. Your suggestion that she needs to work out her concerns is obvious and unhelpful. It is glib to suggest that she will feel better in the next rotation. She is likely hoping for a more personal disclosure about how you, a colleague, would handle these important issues in a similar situation. Your reply is only partially responsible.

Choice Q: This strategy is responsible because it picks up on all the data presented in Jim's opener. His feelings are acknowledged. It is assertive to ask if he wants to call a friend. This response is assertive because it meets his request for help and employs your skills in a helpful way. It is responsible because it attends to the verbal and nonverbal data about Jim's thoughts and feelings. Jim would likely feel that you understand his situation.

Choice R: This self-disclosure could have been a beautiful introduction to an empathic response; however, by itself it is inadequate. Mrs. Urst would be left to wonder why you are sorry. Is it because you do not know how to handle her crying, or because you think she should be able to snap back to her happy self, or because you care about her and are sad that she is distressed? It is nonassertive to leave Mrs. Urst without asking if you could be of some help. This response is not responsible because it does not reflect the data Mrs. Urst supplied.

Choice S: This response is the most assertive and responsible. It shows respect for Mr. James's thoughts about having to reach home and secure his glasses, and you have conveyed your understanding of his frustration at being in a strange place. Furthermore, you have offered to help him cope until his glasses arrive. Your offer is respectful because it allows him to dictate when he will need help so that he can maintain maximum independence. You offered to bring the telephone early in the response, thereby showing him you understand the importance of having contact with his wife. You can feel good about your response. You have met your client's requests and responded in keeping with your professional and caring image of yourself. It is likely that Mr. James would feel comforted by your words.

Choice T: Joe is likely to feel dismissed by this reply. You have forgiven Joe and thereby met his request for action. You have not demonstrated your understanding of his situation with your vague reference to the fact that we all get upset at times. This response would not lead Joe to feel you understand his serious and important situation. This communication strategy is nonassertive because it does not meet your colleague's right to be understood, and it does not demonstrate your ability to communicate in a caring way. Accepting his apology is responsible, but failure to act on all the data is irresponsible.

Choice U: This reply is aggressive and irresponsible. It indicates that you see Don is upset, but you neglect to show any compassion for his feelings. Your aggressive style of rushing him to consider new residents at this point is premature and disrespectful. Your invitation for lunch is intended to convey kindness, but your judgmental authoritarian approach takes the caring out of it. Your style is aggressive and would likely make Don feel angry and misunderstood. Your reply is partially responsible because you understand that he is sad, but you have not shown understanding for the depth of Don's feelings in his bereavement.

Choice V: Although you forgive Joe for his thoughtlessness, you are somewhat stern given his special circumstances and considering that it was not his usual way of doing things. Your warning about the future is aggressive and detracts from your forgiveness. Your exuberance about the news of the pregnancy is insensitive, given Joe's reaction. Your enthusiasm is aggressive because it puts pressure on Joe to feel happy when he really feels quite desperate. This communication strategy is aggressive and irresponsible. Joe would likely feel misunderstood and judged.

Choice W: Petra would likely feel understood and accepted by your reply, and have some alternative and more hopeful ways of viewing the situation. Right at the beginning you acknowledge Petra's feelings of despair so that she knows that you understand her. This approach is assertive because it attends to her right to receive helpful communication, and it meets your expectations that you will reach out to your colleagues in a caring way. By responding to her request for respectful understanding and offering her some insights about how you sort out your feelings, you are responding to the information she gave you. In doing so, you are communicating in a responsible way. You do not force your coping methods on her; rather, you reveal how they are helpful for you and ask for her opinions. This approach is respectful of her individual style of handling events. Your self-disclosure—revealing that you have not sorted out all your thoughts on these important issues—would likely make Petra feel that she is

not alone in trying to come to terms with the purpose of nursing (and life).

Choice X: This reply is nonassertive. It does not respect Jim's right to receive your helpful comments, and it deprives you of the right to communicate effectively. By not picking up on the specific information Jim gives you in his statement, and linking that to the changes you have observed in Jim in the past few weeks, you respond without using half of the data. This reply is superficial, and Jim would likely feel that the weight of his sadness has fully escaped you. He would not likely feel that he can confide any further in you after receiving this insensitive remark.

Choice Y: This response is assertive because it demonstrates your ability to communicate sensitively to Mrs. Urst. Your agreement that her tears are in part due to postnatal blues allows her to feel less embarrassed, yet you do not ignore her real worries about juggling her roles. You do not give her advice that would have been premature, but you give her the option of talking more about her feelings with you if she would like. This invitation allows her to choose if and when she would like to talk and is respectful of her privacy. Your accurate use of empathy lets her know that you understand her confusion and ambivalence. Your style is assertive, and your words are responsible. Mrs. Urst's requests would be met with this response.

Choice Z: This response is only partially assertive and responsible. It comes closer to filling his request for understanding than other options do. You have conveyed understanding of his discomfort at being in a strange place, and you have offered to get the telephone for him. Your attempt at self-disclosure is incomplete and nonspecific, and therefore does not convey the understanding you intend. What is missing is your acknowledgment of his frustration at not being able to function without his glasses, and his strong desire to contact his wife. Mr. James would probably feel somewhat comforted by your attempt to understand him, but he would be left wondering how you could possibly grasp his unique predicament.

References

Ascher BL: *Landscape without gravity: a memoir of grief*, New York, 1994, Penguin Books.

Fuimano J: Acceptance as a management tool, *Nurs Manage* 36(10):8, 2005.

Gallagher-Lepak S, Kubsch S: Transpersonal caring; a nursing practice guideline, *Holist Nurs Pract* 23(3):171, May/June 2009.

Kaufman P, Wetmore C: *The brass tacks manager: getting down to what really counts in the workplace*, New York, 1994, Bantam Doubleday.

Pollock SE, Sands D: Adaptation to suffering, *Clin Nurs Res* 6(1):171, 1997.

Saulter K: Living with Dementia: Discovering what matters most today and for our futures. 8th Lillian & James Portman Conference, Celebrating Direct Care Workers, *Innovations in Dementia Care*, Livonia, Mich, October 12, 2010.

Sheldon LK, Barrett R, Ellington L: Difficult communication in nursing, *J Nurs Scholarship* 38(2):141, 2006.

Sheldon LK, Ellington L, Barrett R, et al: Nurse responsiveness to cancer patient expressions of emotion, *Patient Educ Couns* 76(1):63, July 2009.

Smith-Stoner M, Frost AL: Coping with grief and loss: bringing your shadow self into the light, *Nursing* 28(2):49, 1998.

Vaughn S: Burnout can strike anyone, *The Los Angeles Times*, March 25, 2001.

Viorst J: *Alexander and the terrible, horrible, no good, very bad day*, New York, 2009, Athenaeum.

Watson J: *Nursing: the philosophy of science and caring*, Boulder, Colo, 2008, University Press of Colorado.

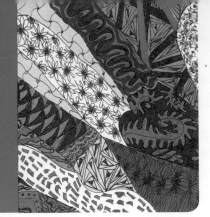

Chapter 26

Communicating Assertively and Responsibly with Aggressive Clients and Colleagues

Objectives

1. Describe the problems presented by aggressive behavior
2. Identify strategies to communicate effectively with aggressive clients and colleagues
3. Formulate an assessment and intervention for given situations involving aggressive behavior
4. Participate in exercises to build skills to communicate with aggressive clients and colleagues

Why Aggressive Behavior Is Problematic for Nurses

Aggressiveness refers to rejecting, hostile, abusive, bullying, and manipulative behaviors. Patient safety is compromised by intimidating communication. In 2008 The Joint Commission introduced new standards, which took effect in January 2009, requiring more than 15,000 accredited healthcare organizations to establish a code of conduct to define acceptable and unacceptable behaviors among healthcare professionals with a formal process to manage unacceptable behavior (Joint Commission, 2008). "The presence of intimidation in the workplace, whether directly experienced or simply witnessed, has an adverse effect on healthcare providers, patients, and their families" (Lamontagne, 2010, p. 63). Verbal abuse is "communication via behavior, tone or words that patronize, demean, isolate, disparage, threaten or accuse, or intend that the individual feel attacked or humiliated" (Christman, 2007, p. 365). Workplace bullying occurs when "the victim is subjected to a series of systematic stigmatizing attacks from a fellow worker or workers which encroach on his or her civil rights" (Quine, 2001, p. 74). Lewis (2006) contends that bullying is a learned behavior in the workplace rather than an individual personality deficit. New employees may be tested, hazed, as a part of the culture, and accepted as "just the way things are" (Lamontagne, 2010). Student nurses and new graduates are often the most vulnerable. It is imperative that nurses learn to deal with aggressive behavior. Aggressive behavior may be a result of anger, an emotion that arises in response to feeling powerless or out of control. The frenzied pace of living, shift work, long hours, perceived harassment from management to "do more with less," increased technology, and "technological stress" set the stage for workplace anxiety and anger. People become irritable and angry, which can lead to a breakdown in communication and aggression (Helge, 2001c; Hollinsworth et al, 2005). Aggressiveness may also indicate another person's lack of respect for our feelings or a violation of our right to be treated with courtesy and consideration. In any case, aggressiveness is unpleasant.

Most of us would like to stand up for our right to be treated with respect in a way that is firm and effective (puts a stop to the aggressive behavior) and embarrasses neither us nor the other person; in other words, we want to handle the aggression assertively and at the same time consider the other person's point of view. Our fears are that we will become enraged and lash out at the other person, fueling the fires of escalating aggression, or that we will remain tight-lipped and slink away, carrying around the smoldering wish that we could more effectively deal with an attacker. "Anger is the most misunderstood emotion in the workplace" (Helge, 2001a). If we understand that anger is based on a sense of powerlessness, frustration, and fear of loss of control, we can understand our own discomfort and the discomfort of others with its expression. Our fears of losing control or embarrassing ourselves, or our insecurity in our ability to communicate assertively and deal with the oppression, keep us from acting effectively.

When we encounter aggressive behavior, our self-esteem and physical safety are threatened. This chapter helps you deal with aggression so that you feel confident and comfortable.

How to Communicate Effectively with Aggressive Clients and Colleagues

Before you deal with aggression or anger remember to breathe deeply and remain calm. Try to separate the problem from the person and avoid taking the behavior personally. Pay attention to people's personal space, do not move in too close, and choose your words carefully to demonstrate respect for the other person (Helge, 2001b). Remember that assertive communication is crucial to dealing effectively with conflict (Antai-Otong, 2001).

Jakubowski and Lange (1978) outline the following ways of dealing with aggression from others.

Get to the Source of the Problem

Asking for more information—so that you are clear about the reason for your aggressor's discontent—demonstrates your interest and opens up a dialogue that can lead to resolution of the problem. Finding out what is causing the aggressor to attack you is a logical place to begin.

For example, you might ask your supervisor, who has just reprimanded you for telephoning the intern on call about one of your seriously ill clients, this question:

Assertive response: "I see that you are angry that I phoned Dr. Jones about our client's unstable vital signs. Could you tell me what upsets you about my calling her?"

This respectful acknowledgment of your aggressor's message allows him or her to clarify the problem. Using an empathic response demonstrates your understanding of the other's feelings and can disarm the aggressor enough to minimize the aggression. The open-ended phrasing of your questions is less threatening than an aggressive approach such as asking "Why are you trying to stop me?"

Increase Your Aggressor's Awareness of Abusive Behavior and Its Negative Effects

Asking questions to determine whether your aggressor is aware of the insulting impact that aggression can have and pointing out the effect of the behavior is a technique to heighten the awareness of an aggressor. Be aware that some people are beyond caring about the effects of their behavior when they are losing control; therefore, when to use this strategy is a judgment call.

For example, after repeated abuse and criticism from the resident on call, you tell him the following:

Assertive response: "Dr. Smith, you may not realize that you are raising your voice and swearing at me. This approach makes working with you unpleasant. I would be glad to talk with you when you can lower your voice and not swear at me." (When someone is repeatedly aggressive, using the "I feel . . . " portion of the assertive statement may give the person more ammunition. Comment, instead, on the results of the behavior and then make your request for a behavior change.)

Remaining calm and controlled in the face of an aggressor provides a contrast that may help that person realize that aggressive behavior is out of line.

Limit the Aggressive Behavior

Using a CARE (Clarify, Articulate, Request, Encourage) confrontation (see Chapter 23) lets your aggressor know, in no uncertain terms, what bothers you about his or her behavior and what changes you would like to see. Sometimes, ignoring or dismissing the aggression and continuing with your own agenda takes the wind out of an aggressor's sails and puts the emphasis on more pressing items.

For example, you are giving the end-of-shift report to the evening staff, and one evening nurse repeatedly interrupts, quizzing you on an irrelevant matter. You curtail her aggression with the following response:

> *Assertive response:* "Sharon, I'd like to finish the report, so please hold your questions and talk to me about it later."

For each aggressor and situation you will have different expected outcomes and will want to use different assertive strategies. What is important is that you develop skills for dealing assertively with aggression so that you can maintain your self-respect while being courteous, and that you have "a constructive impact on the other person" (Jakubowski and Lange, 1978). As a nurse, you must not tolerate continued aggression against yourself if you intend to preserve your self-esteem and credibility with clients and colleagues.

How to Improve Your Communication Skill with Aggressive Clients and Colleagues

The work you do in this chapter provides practice in dealing assertively with aggression so that in real-life situations you will feel and act more confidently. The following examples can help you overcome some of the barriers to relating to aggressive clients and colleagues and generate more effective responses to aggression. You are presented with situations involving aggressive clients and colleagues. Your task is to assess each situation, determine the request being made, and choose the most assertive and responsible communication strategy.

A critique of all the response choices for each situation appears at the end of the chapter, beginning on p. 303.

Communicating with Rejecting Clients

Step 1: Assessment of the Data

1. Review the following situation and formulate your own assessment of the client's thoughts, feelings, and requests.

Mr. Hunter has been a client on your medical burn unit for 6 weeks. He has extensive burns on his arms, upper body, and face as a result of trying to rescue his daughter from a house fire. He has been in isolation for the duration of his hospitalization. Chris, your colleague who has been his primary nurse since his admission, has left for a vacation. As the student having your clinical experience on this unit, you have been assigned to care for Mr. Hunter in Chris's absence. His wounds require extensive debridement and frequent dressing changes.

You are changing a dressing on Mr. Hunter's shoulder when this conversation takes place:

> *You:* "I'm going to let that soak for 5 minutes, Mr. Hunter. Then I'll remove it and do your other shoulder. Your burns are healing nicely."

WIT& *Wisdom*

It's Not Just Nice People Who Get Sick . . .
Some people are nice
And they get sick.
Make them well
And they're nice, real quick.
Some people are mean
And they get sick.
We might make them well,
But nice? There's a trick!
We think with just
The right magic words
We can fix everything.
Oh! How absurd!
Some people's problems
Are bigger than me.
Maybe they'll get well
But nice, they won't be.
Some people's problems
Run deep and wide.
We care for them,
But take it in stride.

Moments of Connection . . .
When Pain Changes Behavior

"In our cancer pain center we had an elderly woman with 'failed back syndrome,' severe scoliosis, and degenerative disc disease. On my first encounter with her, she backed up to the wall and said, 'You're not going to stick me with a needle, are you?' I assured her I was just doing an assessment. Knowing that the doctor wanted to do three epidural blocks, I spent a lot of time explaining the procedure as she paced back and forth in the examination room. She rubbed her hands and was very anxious. On the surface she seemed uncooperative and not very nice. Her daughter confirmed that her behavior had changed with the increasing pain. The whole team spent time explaining the benefits of the procedures. I accompanied her for these procedures and later for implantation of an intrathecal pump. Today she has excellent pain relief and visits our office on holidays to bring treats. She always gives me a hug and thanks me for 'giving me back my life.' We really made a difference."

Mr. Hunter: "That's thanks to Chris. She's a wonderful nurse. You've replaced her on her days off before, and you don't do things like she does. I want you to be careful and do things like they are supposed to be done. You're just a student and I'm going to watch you carefully; if you do anything out of line, I'm going to report you to your instructor."

2. On a separate piece of paper write down your assessment of Mr. Hunter's thoughts and feelings. Indicate what request Mr. Hunter is making of you, his "replacement" nurse.
3. Compare your assessment to the one that follows:

Thoughts: Mr. Hunter is afraid you might do something to undermine Chris's effective nursing care of his burns. He thinks that because you are a student you might not care for his wounds with the same safety and skill that "his" nurse did.

Feelings: He misses the consistent care he had from the daily interaction with his primary nurse, Chris. He feels threatened and at the mercy of your care, in which he does not have confidence. He is afraid that you might do something to set back the progress of his healing.

Request: The aggressiveness of his threat tells you how much Mr. Hunter wants you to take precautions to ensure continued healing of his burns. He wants to be reassured by your actions and words that you will give safe nursing care. His requests are for understanding, comfort, and safe burn treatment.

4. Did your assessment reflect an accurate analysis of the facts as they were presented? If not, return to the original vignette and reassess the cognitive and affective messages. If so, proceed to Step 2.

Step 2: Communication Strategies and Desired Outcomes

5. You have determined that Mr. Hunter needs to be understood and comforted by your actions and your words. Identify which communication behaviors you would use to respond to Mr. Hunter's requests. Indicate the desired outcomes of your strategy. Write your suggestions down on a separate sheet of paper for future reference.
6. Compare your suggested strategy to this one:

Remaining calm is important to avoid escalating his aggression. Relaxation can help you focus and avoid hostility yourself. Visualize responding in a compassionate way and use positive self-talk to remember not to explode at his aggressiveness. Empathic acknowledgment of his respect for Chris's care would reassure him that you understand the importance of safe care to ensure continued healing. Informing him that you will give your best care and explaining what you are doing would dispel his apprehensions about your abilities. Ignoring his threat to report you would likely diminish his hostility.

These interventions would likely let Mr. Hunter know that you understand both his vulnerability as a client and his longing for consistent care from his primary nurse. Your directness, confidence, and calmness would likely make him optimistic and hopeful about the quality of care he will receive from you.

Step 3: Implementation and Evaluation of Your Communication Strategy

7. Now you must reply to Mr. Hunter. Develop your own response to Mr. Hunter and write it on a separate sheet of paper. Keep it handy so that you can refer to it later.
8. At this point you get the chance to compare your suggested response with the following options. Look over each of the response choices and turn to p. 303 at the end of the chapter to read a critique of each. (Notice that the choices are not listed alphabetically. This is to prevent the temptation to quickly scan all the answers without giving yourself the benefit of evaluating each response.)

As you review the following response choices, look for those that are congruent with your assessment of Mr. Hunter's requests and your desire to communicate in an assertive and responsible way.

Choice E: "Report me if you want to, Mr. Hunter. You don't honestly think my clinical instructor would give me the responsibility of caring for you if she didn't think that I could do it, do you? If you'd just give me a chance, you'd see what a good nurse I can be."

Choice A: "If you want a graduate nurse I can arrange a transfer so you can feel safer, Mr. Hunter. It sounds as if you want a fully qualified graduate assigned to you."

Choice M: "You're welcome to watch what I do and ask any questions. I'm sure my way of doing things is a little different from Chris's, but I do guarantee that what I'm doing is safe and in keeping with your physician's orders. It is hard when things are done differently by each nurse, and you are likely missing Chris's style because you worked closely together for the 6 weeks you have been here. Do you want to ask me anything about what I've done so far in changing your dressing?"

Choice Z: "You're just missing Chris, Mr. Hunter, and taking it out on me. I don't want to be compared to another nurse, and I won't have you making threats to report me to my instructor. I am one of the top nurses in my class, and I don't want you to question my care anymore in the future. You had better get used to the idea that I am going to be your nurse."

9. After you have found the most satisfactory strategy and discovered why the other options are not suitable, go back to the suggested response you generated earlier in this exercise. Evaluate your response in terms of how assertive and responsible it was.

Communicating with Rejecting Colleagues

Step 1: Assessment of the Data

1. Review the following situation and formulate your own assessment of your colleague's thoughts, feelings, and requests.

You are a student nurse who has just spent the past 6 weeks of clinical experience in the obstetrical services of the hospital. During that time your clinical instructor has been meticulously thorough in her supervision and teaching of the skills needed for obstetrical nursing.

This area of nursing is one you love and you think you might pursue a career in this field. You believe you are adept at the physical care of both mother and baby, and you have been influential in helping mothers and fathers adjust to caring for their newborns. Your teaching sessions to mothers have been rated as outstanding, and the head nurse in postpartum has indicated that she is pleased with your work.

Despite your certainty that you are doing a good job and the positive feedback from clients and staff, you have never received a word of praise from your clinical instructor. In fact, she takes every opportunity to tell you where you could improve and is petty in her reprimands about your small errors. You are disappointed that your instructor is not more encouraging and enthusiastic about your successes. Today she is meeting with you to give you feedback on the bath class you gave to the fathers. You have had a chance to look over the fathers' evaluation forms, and they clearly state that your manner and content were reassuring in their first experience of bathing their newborns. Your instructor has just listed everything you did wrong and made suggestions about how you could improve such a class in the future.

Instructor: "Overall, you need to polish your professionalism. You are much too casual; you always are, for that matter. How do you expect anyone to treat you like a professional if you are lax and don't have a tight rein on things? You need to shape up in that regard so you'll command a lot more respect."

2. On a separate sheet of paper write down your assessment of your instructor's thoughts and feelings. Indicate what request she is making of you, her nursing student.

3. Compare your assessment to the one that follows:

Thoughts: Your instructor thinks you need to be more professional and that if you could cultivate this demeanor you will gain more respect.

Feelings: She is disappointed in your overall consistent lack of professionalism. It is highly likely that she feels a great responsibility to shape you into her image of a perfectly functioning nurse.

Request: She wants you to change your behavior on a consistent basis to a style of operating that matches her image of professionalism. She expects you to put up with negative feedback in this evaluation, as she has during your complete rotation.

4. Did your assessment reflect an accurate analysis of the facts as they were presented? If not, return to

the original data presented in the vignette and reassess the cognitive and affective messages. If so, proceed to Step 2.

Step 2: Communication Strategies and Desired Outcomes

5. You have determined that your instructor is making an unreasonable request of you. You are disappointed and angry that she continues to be unwilling to give you legitimate praise for the good work you have done. Identify which communication strategies you would use to handle her request. Indicate the desired outcomes of your suggested strategy. Write this information on a separate piece of paper for future reference.
6. Compare your suggested strategy to this one:

It is important to relax and visualize yourself responding assertively in the wave of such rejecting aggression. A request for more specific comments would be in order because the instructor has not really explained what she means by being more "professional." It would be appropriate to express your opinion that the evidence you have received from the two classes indicates that you are performing well as a maternity nurse. A CARE confrontation would be acceptable to let her know that you are disappointed in the absence of positive feedback and that you would like to receive some from her in your final evaluation as a student on the unit.

Strategies such as these would let her clearly know—in a way that respects her as your instructor—that you want to be treated with respect.

Step 3: Implementation and Evaluation of Your Communication Strategy

7. Now you must reply to your instructor. Develop your own response to her and write it down on a separate sheet of paper. Keep it handy so that you can refer to it later.
8. At this point you get the chance to compare your suggested response to the following options. Look over each of the response choices and turn to p. 303 at the end of the chapter to read a critique of each.

As you review the following response choices, look for those that are congruent with your assessment of your instructor's requests and your desire to communicate in an assertive and responsible way.

Choice H: "I can see you are giving me some advice that you believe is very important, but it's not clear

to me. What exactly do you mean by 'professional'? If you explain what you mean it'll be clearer to me so that I will be more likely to improve."

Choice B: "I'm tired of your suggestions for my improvement. You have never once said anything positive in the 6 weeks I have been here. The staff and clients give me more strokes than you do. I need some positive feedback from you, too."

Choice Y: "Well, I'll try to do my best to be more professional in the future."

Choice J: "I know that when you give me all those suggestions about improving you are trying to help me be the best obstetrical nurse I can be. It's disappointing that you haven't also noted some of the good things I've done and some of the ways in which I've acted professionally. I have received enough super evaluations from the clients and encouraging comments from the staff to support my belief that I am doing some things well. Before I leave this rotation, I would like you to give me some positive feedback in addition to your suggestions for improvement. Will you do that for me?"

9. After you have found the most satisfactory strategy and discovered why the other options are not suitable, go back to the response you generated earlier in this exercise. Evaluate your response in terms of how assertive and responsible it was.

Communicating with Hostile Clients

Step 1: Assessment of the Data

1. Review the following situation and formulate your own assessment of the client's thoughts, feelings, and requests.

Debbie is an 18-year-old client on the medical unit where you work. She is a recently diagnosed diabetic and is terrified of receiving her insulin injection. When you try to administer it, she screams and kicks. It requires two staff members to hold her down securely to give her the insulin safely. You know that this situation is unsatisfactory because Debbie will soon be discharged and will have to give herself her own insulin. She will have to overcome her fear and gradually take on more responsibility for her self-care.

You decide to talk with Debbie about your desire for her to be more involved in her diabetic care. You have started the conversation by explaining that you have some ideas about how she can overcome her fear and learn to be more confident in giving herself insulin. Debbie interrupts you with the following:

> *Debbie:* "Hold it! (Raising her voice) I'm not, repeat, not ever going to give myself insulin. Get out, you bloodsucking vampire! You enjoy torturing me every morning. Well, forget it! Get lost! Go find someone else to bug. Just get off my back about this insulin junk." (Debbie comes face to face with you and looks you right in the eye. She is red in the face and has her fists clenched and raised.)

2. On a separate sheet of paper write down your assessment of Debbie's thoughts and feelings. Indicate what request she is making of you, her nurse.
3. Compare your analysis to the following assessment:

> *Thoughts*: Debbie thinks you are cruel to "force" her to get more involved in taking her insulin.
>
> *Feelings*: Debbie is terrified of giving herself insulin and is probably having trouble accepting that she is diabetic. She is enraged and fiercely trying to keep you at bay to protect her denial and fear. Her attack on you comes from her insecurity.
>
> *Request*: Her obvious request is for you to leave her alone. The rational part of her (which is overshadowed by her fear) knows that you are right and that she will have to learn to be calmer about her insulin. Directly, Debbie is requesting to be understood, and she wants you to act by leaving. Indirectly, she is requesting to be comforted.

4. Did your assessment reflect an accurate analysis of the facts as they were presented? If not, return to the original data presented in the vignette and reassess the cognitive and affective messages. If so, proceed to Step 2.

Step 2: Communication Strategies and Desired Outcomes

5. You have determined that Debbie is requesting understanding, action, and comfort. Identify the communication behaviors you would use to show Debbie how you intend to respond to her requests. Indicate the desired outcomes of your suggested strategy. Write down your ideas on a separate sheet of paper.
6. Compare your suggested strategy to this one:

It is reasonable to meet Debbie's request for understanding and her implied request for comfort. She has a great adjustment to make as a diabetic, and you can help her by showing that you understand. It is unreasonable to meet Debbie's request for action by leaving. She is frightened and needs someone to be in control. If you leave by walking away, or become aggressive, her fear and anger will escalate out of control.

Remaining calm will help you think more clearly and might help calm Debbie. Being calm indicates that you are in control. If it is difficult for you to remain calm in the face of such enraged hostility, you need to focus and visualize yourself reacting in a collected way. An empathic response to Debbie's fear and anger about having to take insulin would let her know that you do understand. A firm expression of your opinion—that she needs to learn how to be calmer about receiving her insulin—would indicate that you are in control, want to help her, and will not be put off or reject her because of her angry outburst. A gentle suggestion about how you would like to proceed to help her might make her reconsider your plan and decide that it might not be so terrifying.

This approach would show Debbie that you understand her and that you will stay and help her through her fear and anger; it will also give her hope of regaining self-control. She will not likely feel happy for some time, but this response will help diminish her terror.

Step 3: Implementation and Evaluation of Your Communication Strategy

7. Now you must reply to Debbie. Develop your own response to Debbie and write it down on a separate sheet of paper. Keep it handy so that you can refer to it later.
8. Here is where you have the chance to compare your suggested response to the following options. Look over each of the response choices and turn to p. 303 at the end of the chapter to read a critique of each.

As you review the following response choices, look for those that are congruent with your assessment of Debbie's requests and your desire to communicate in an assertive and responsible way.

> *Choice C: (Reaching out and putting your arm around Debbie's shoulders)* "There, there, Debbie. Don't be so angry. It's just a matter of time before you'll feel OK about taking your insulin. I'm just here to help you. You'll see that you'll be feeling calm about the whole thing in a few weeks."
>
> *Choice K:* "Don't you talk to me like that, young lady. You'd better show a little more respect for me or you'll be in trouble. I know what's best for you.

I've had lots of experience, so if you're smart, you'll cooperate."

Choice Q: "I know it is scary to receive a needle every morning, Debbie. It's a big thing to adjust to, especially for someone as active and as healthy as you. I can help you to feel quite confident, and eventually even comfortable, about taking your insulin. What I'd like you to do is to sit down with me right now and listen to my plan. I want you to hear me out, and then you can ask any questions and consider whether you'd like to try it."

Choice X: "Debbie, I was only trying to help you." *(You leave Debbie's room.)*

9. After you have found the most satisfactory strategy and discovered why the others are not suitable options, go back to the original strategy you generated earlier in this exercise. Evaluate your strategy in terms of how assertive and responsible it was.

Communicating with Hostile Colleagues

Step 1: Assessment of the Data

1. Review the following situation and formulate your own assessment of your colleague's thoughts, feelings, and requests.

You are a nurse working in an outpatient mental health center. There are small interviewing rooms that can be booked for private interviews with clients and their families. As usual, space is an issue and scheduling of rooms is essential. In the past 3 days your interviews have been 5 minutes longer than the half hour that you had booked. By going overtime you have delayed the interviews of others. Your colleague Karen has been annoyed but understanding because you are not usually so inconsiderate.

Today you booked the room for 45 minutes so that you could complete your interview without holding up others. However, your client has just revealed some serious information about her marriage and is upset and crying in the interview room. You know you need about 5 minutes over your time to help your client calm down before vacating the interview room. Karen has booked the room after you. She has knocked on the door twice already to remind you that your time is up. When you come out with your client, she blasts you with the following:

Karen: "It's about time. This is the fourth time this week that I've had to wait for you to leave the room

when I've booked it. This has got to stop. My client's family is here on their lunch hour. You aren't the only one with important things to do, you know." (Karen's voice is raised and her hands are on her hips.)

2. On a separate sheet of paper write down your assessment of Karen's thoughts and feelings. Indicate what request Karen is making of you, her nurse colleague.

3. Compare your analysis to this assessment:

Thoughts: Karen thinks you are rude and inconsiderate to go beyond your allotted time in the shared interview room.

Feelings: Karen is annoyed because you have gone over into the time she had planned to be in the room. She is feeling pressured because the family she wants to interview has only a limited period of time. She is worried about seeming to be rude to them by not being able to get into the only private room available. Karen is frustrated and disappointed that you have behaved in such an inconsiderate way.

Request: Karen wants you to understand how inconvenienced she and her clients were by your thoughtlessness. She wants you to act more responsibly in the future by vacating the room after your time is up.

4. Did your assessment reflect an accurate analysis of the facts as they were presented? If not, return to the original data presented in the vignette and reassess the cognitive and affective messages. If so, proceed to Step 2.

Step 2: Communication Strategies and Desired Outcomes

5. You have determined that Karen wants understanding and action. Identify which communication behaviors you would use to respond to Karen. Indicate the desired outcomes of your strategy. Write your ideas down on a separate sheet of paper so that you can refer to them later.

6. Compare your suggested strategy to this one:

Karen's requests for understanding and future consideration are legitimate. It is reasonable to respond to them with an empathic reply and a promise to be more careful in the future. It is unreasonable to accept Karen's hostile aggressiveness, especially since she embarrassed you in front of both your clients and her clients and any other staff members in the vicinity. It would be important to stay calm and make a CARE confrontation to Karen, asking her to speak more courteously to you about issues that bother her. It would be better to wait until later in the day to speak with Karen, at a time when you both have an opportunity to complete your discussion.

This strategy would assure Karen that you respect her rights and would make her aware of your rights, too.

Step 3: Implementation and Evaluation of Your Communication Strategy

7. Now you must reply to Karen. On a separate sheet of paper develop your own response to Karen and keep it handy.
8. At this point you have the opportunity to compare your suggested response to the following options. Look over each of the response choices and turn to p. 303 at the end of the chapter to read a critique of each.

As you review the following response choices, look for those that are congruent with your assessment of Karen's requests and your desire to communicate in an assertive and responsible way.

Choice D: "I apologize to all of you *(looking at Karen and her clients)* for this inconvenience." *(Later, at a mutually convenient time when you and Karen are alone)* "Karen, I'd like to talk with you about how you handled my overstaying my booking time this morning. Is this a good time or would a little later be better?" *(Proceeding after Karen agrees to do so)* "I will really try not to inconvenience you by going over my booked time in the future. I know I put you in a tough spot, and I was very embarrassed that you scolded me in front of our clients in the middle of the hall where everyone could hear. In the future, I would appreciate it if you would ask to talk about any complaints you have in private. Then no one will be embarrassed and we can keep our staff quarrels away from the clients. Could you do this, Karen?"

Choice L: (At the time) "Just a minute, Karen. What do you mean? I wouldn't deliberately try to annoy you by overstaying my time. You should know there's a very good reason for my delay. I'm not deliberately trying to inconvenience you. The room is yours now."

Choice P: (At the time) Getting red in the face and avoiding eye contact with Karen and her clients, you walk right past them. Later, when you have an opportunity to interact with Karen, you avoid her. You refuse to make eye contact, and you do not initiate conversation with her even though you do with the rest of the staff.

Choice W: (At the time) "I'm sorry, Karen."

9. After you have found the most satisfactory strategy and discovered why the other options are not satisfactory, go back to the suggested response you generated earlier in this exercise. Evaluate your response in terms of how assertive and responsible it was.

Communicating with Abusive Clients

Step 1: Assessment of the Data

1. Review the following situation and formulate your own assessment of your client's thoughts, feelings, and requests.

Mrs. Suit is a 60-year-old client who has been admitted to the coronary care unit with chest pain. She has diabetes, which is poorly managed, and arthritis. She has been very demanding, especially on the days when her husband is unable to get up to visit her. Today she has put her call light on repeatedly, and this time she has asked you to bring her fresh water in a glass with a straw. You start out for the kitchen but are waylaid by the distraught son of another client. He is almost in tears and wants to discuss the news of his father's forthcoming surgery with you. You pause to talk with him before you get Mrs. Suit's drink. When you get back to Mrs. Suit's room she lambastes you as follows:

Mrs. Suit: "Damnation. You could die here before you get a simple glass of water. You're such a smart-ass; you probably think I'm just a sick old lady, but I've got just as much right to service as anybody in this hospital. What in the hell were you doing, melting some ice? Damn it! Just give me the straw; you're slower than molasses in January. I'll open it myself. If I let you do it, you could take all night. You can go now. You smart-assed nurses think you're so damn important, but you can't even get an old lady a drink of water without messing things up."

2. On a separate sheet of paper write down your assessment of Mrs. Suit's thoughts and feelings. Indicate what request Mrs. Suit is making of you, her nurse.

3. Compare your assessment to this one:

Thoughts: Mrs. Suit thinks you took your time bringing her the water because you don't think either she or her request is important.

Feelings: Mrs. Suit's feelings are hurt because of her assumption that your tardiness is associated with lack of respect for her. Her abusiveness is her defense against her feelings of being rejected. It is likely that she is frightened of the monitor and lonely today because she did not receive a visit from her husband. These factors may be compounding her attack on you.

Request: Mrs. Suit is asking you to treat her with more respect by following through on her reasonable requests (like getting a glass of water). Indirectly, she is asking you to understand that she feels insecure and frightened. Obliquely, she is requesting comfort from you and reassurance that you care about her. This request for comfort is for present and future interactions.

4. Did your assessment reflect an accurate analysis of the facts as they were presented? If not, return to the original data presented in the vignette and reassess the cognitive and affective messages. If so, proceed to Step 2.

Step 2: Communication Strategies and Desired Outcomes

5. You have determined that Mrs. Suit needs understanding and comfort. Identify which communication strategy you would use to respond to her requests. Indicate the desired outcomes of your strategy. Write your ideas down so that you can refer to them later.

6. Compare your suggested strategy to this one:

Mrs. Suit's requests are all legitimate. Her way of expressing them is aggressive and irritating, and it would be easy for you to become offended. The best approach is to stay calm and extend warmth to this upset woman. It might be appropriate to explain your delay to prove that you were not acting disrespectfully. Some reassurance of your interest in her would be supportive for her. In the future you could make the effort to ensure that she is made to feel important and cared for by coming in when she has not called and by asking her if there is anything else you could do to make her feel more comfortable before you leave the room.

This strategy would make her feel cared for and respected.

Step 3: Implementation and Evaluation of Your Communication Strategy

7. Now you must reply to Mrs. Suit. On a separate sheet of paper develop your own response to Mrs. Suit and keep it for future reference.

8. At this point you get the chance to compare your suggested strategy to the following options. Look over each of the response choices and turn to p. 303 at the end of the chapter to read a critique of each.

As you review the following choices, look for those that are congruent with your assessment of Mrs. Suit's requests and your desire to communicate in an assertive and responsible way.

Choice AA: "Mrs. Suit, I'm sorry I was so long in coming with your water. It's not that I don't care about you. I was delayed by an upset family member who needed to talk about his seriously ill father. I'm sure you can understand now why I was delayed. I am free for a few minutes now, though, if there's anything you'd like to talk about."

Choice I: "Mrs. Suit, I went out of my way to get you your water. The least you could do is say 'thank you.'" (*You turn and leave.*)

Choice R: "Sorry, Mrs. Suit." (*Your facial expression is flat and you leave after giving her the straw.*)

9. After you have found the most satisfactory strategy and discovered why the other options are not suitable, go back to the original response you generated in this exercise. Evaluate your response in terms of how assertive and responsible it was.

Communicating with Abusive Colleagues

Step 1: Assessment of the Data

1. Review the following situation and formulate your own assessment of your colleague's thoughts, feelings, and requests.

You have been a student nurse on a surgical unit for 3 weeks. For the past 3 days you have been the medication nurse. On this unit the job of giving out medications is particularly difficult and time consuming. Clients are often downstairs having diagnostic tests, having their dressings changed, or working at physical therapy; this makes it difficult to give out the medications smoothly. In addition, there are many intravenous drips (IVs) to be regulated. You find it confusing to keep track of the IVs, the regular medications, and clients' requests for postoperative analgesics.

Your clinical instructor has encouraged you by ensuring you that you are doing a fine job. She has mentioned that you are safe and careful about distributing the medications and has informed you that speed will come with practice. The team leader on the floor has not been so supportive. From the first day you took over as medication nurse, she has been hostile and insulting. She has said destructive things such as: "I know you students have to learn but we've got sick people here who can't wait all day for their medications. You're going to have to speed things up." And "Look out. Here comes Speedy!" (to another nurse at the nursing station). She has undermined you by coming to get the medication keys from you and giving some clients narcotic pain relievers, saying, "If she has to wait for you to get there, her pain will have her on the ceiling."

You are just returning to the nursing station after distributing your morning medications. Your hostile team leader is at the station and confronts you with the following:

Team leader: "Well, what do you know? You're finally here. While you've been poking along out on the floor, I've given three clients their painkillers. I bet you haven't remembered your IVs, have you? Well, Speedy, I've been keeping my eye on them, and you'd better change the bag in room 25. I don't know how you're going to function as a graduate when you don't have someone like me looking over your shoulder."

2. On a separate sheet of paper write down your assessment of your team leader's thoughts and feelings. Indicate what request she is making of you, the student nurse giving medications on this surgical unit.

3. Compare your analysis to this one:

Thoughts: Your team leader thinks you are far too slow as a medication nurse. She believes that you are incapable of taking charge of all the medication nurse's responsibilities at this point.

Feelings: She is concerned about those clients who need their postoperative medications, and she is worried that the IVs will run dry. She is irritated by your slowness and is unwilling to remember that it takes practice to become faster at this complicated task. Her annoyance makes her take out her frustration on you.

Request: Your team leader wants you to be faster as a medication nurse. She wants you to simultaneously keep track of IVs, regular medications, and "as needed" orders for analgesics. She also wants you to develop accurate speed immediately. She is requesting that you understand what she wants and that you comply with it immediately.

4. Did your assessment reflect an accurate analysis of the facts as they were presented? If not, return to the original data presented in the vignette and reassess the cognitive and affective messages. If so, proceed to Step 2.

Step 2: Communication Strategies and Desired Outcomes

5. You have determined that the team leader wants understanding and action. Identify which communication behaviors you would use to respond to her requests. Indicate the desired outcomes of your strategy. Write down your ideas so that you can refer to them later.

6. Compare your suggested strategy to this one:

Your team leader's request for understanding is legitimate, but her request for immediate increased speed as a medication nurse is unreasonable, given your lack of experience. It is important to keep calm and remain calm so as to respond to her in a clear, direct way. If you are out of control, you may be upset for the rest of the day and increase your chances of making an error.

Remain calm, using imagery and positive self-talk to help you stay focused on responding assertively and responsibly to your team leader. It would be appropriate that you thank her for the help she has given you. However, it is also necessary that you ask her to consult you before giving out medications to anybody, to ensure that you, as the person in charge of medications, are kept informed and that no duplications are made. A CARE confrontation to request that she have more patience with your beginning skill would let her know how it would be more helpful for her to relate to you.

This approach will let your team leader know that you do understand the need for speed and accuracy in a medication nurse, but that her request for immediate action is unreasonable. She may not like your assertive response because it will point out to her that she has been aggressive and that you do not intend to tolerate being treated in such a destructive manner. Your strategy may change her behavior in a positive way; however, if she escalates her abusiveness to you, you can confront her again and indicate a more serious consequence (such as reporting her aggressiveness to your clinical instructor).

Step 3: Implementation and Evaluation of Your Communication Strategy

7. Now you must reply to your team leader. On a separate sheet of paper develop your own response to her. Keep it for future reference.

8. At this point you get the chance to compare your suggested response to several options listed below. Look over each of the response choices and turn to p. 303 at the end of the chapter to read a critique of each.

As you review the following response choices, look for those that are congruent with your assessment of your team leader's requests and your desire to communicate in an assertive and responsible way.

> *Choice F:* "I hope that when I am a graduate I am more considerate of students than you are. Don't you remember what it was like when you were learning? Your insults aren't helpful at all."
>
> *Choice N:* "I guess it's hard for you to sit back and have someone less experienced give out the medications. I understand the concerns you have about the clients' receiving their medications on time; however, I have to learn, and it will take a few more days before I am faster at this new job. It would be helpful if you would let me know when clients are asking for, or have received, their analgesics so that I can keep track of who's had what. I appreciate your giving the clients their medications these past days, but I would like to try to do the whole job of being a medication nurse now that I'm getting the hang of it. Will you let me do that?"
>
> *Choice S:* "Oh. I'll go and attend to those IVs right away. Sorry I'm so slow; it must drive you crazy."

9. After you have found the most satisfactory strategy and discovered why the other options are not suitable, go back to the suggested response you generated in this exercise. Evaluate your response in terms of how assertive and responsible it was.

Communicating with Manipulative Clients

Step 1: Assessment of the Data

1. Review the following situation and formulate your own assessment of your client's thoughts, feelings, and requests.

Mr. Gilmour is a 58-year-old gentleman on your rehabilitative stroke unit. He is a heavy smoker, and because he burns holes in his clothing, it is the policy to keep his cigarettes at the nursing station, ensure that he wears a nonflammable smoking jacket, and supervise him when he smokes. Since this is a non-smoking facility, it is necessary for a staff member to take him outside for a cigarette. Mr. Gilmour has a knack of asking for cigarettes at the most inconvenient times. He knows that he is supposed to wait until the report is over before he asks for a smoke, but he invariably bugs the nursing staff at report time. You are the nurse in charge of the day shift, and you want to complete the report to the evening staff so that you can go home. Mr. Gilmour has already interrupted your report three times to ask for a smoke. You gave him a cigarette 30 minutes ago. His fourth manipulative attempt goes like this:

> *Mr. Gilmour:* "Aw, come on. I'll smoke it right here where you can see me. I promise I won't start a fire. (He moves his wheelchair closer and closer to the small area where you are making the report.) It won't hurt you to give me one little smoke. Come on. No one else cares about these stupid hospital rules. I haven't had one all afternoon. Give a guy a break. I had to go for that stupid x-ray, so I missed my after-lunch smoke. Just one and then I won't bother you again."

2. On a separate sheet of paper write down your assessment of Mr. Gilmour's thoughts and feelings. Indicate what request Mr. Gilmour is making of you, the nurse in charge on days.

3. Compare your analysis to the one below:

> *Thoughts*: Mr. Gilmour thinks he deserves a cigarette and believes that if he bugs you enough, he will get what he wants. He knows it is inconvenient for you to take him outside and hopes he can get you to break the rule.
>
> *Feelings*: He is annoyed that you are not giving in to his requests. He feels especially justified in persisting because he thinks that he has not had a cigarette for a few hours.
>
> *Request*: Mr. Gilmour's request is for understanding (about his craving to have a smoke) and action (your giving him a cigarette).

4. Did your assessment reflect an accurate analysis of the facts as they were presented? If not, return to the

original data presented in the vignette and reassess the cognitive and affective messages. If so, proceed to Step 2.

Step 2: Communication Strategies and Desired Outcomes

5. You have determined that Mr. Gilmour wants understanding and action. Identify which communication behaviors you would use to respond to his requests. Indicate the desired outcomes for your suggested strategy. Write your ideas down for future reference.

6. Compare your suggested strategy to this one:

It would be tempting to lash out aggressively at Mr. Gilmour, but this attack would only hurt his feelings, make you feel bad, and embarrass everyone. Even though you are frustrated by Mr. Gilmour's manipulative persistence, it is important to stay calm and handle the situation assertively and responsibly. It would be wise to be consistent with the rule the unit has made of refusing cigarettes during report time. You know that the report will be finished in 5 minutes and that it is not unreasonable for Mr. Gilmour to wait that long. A firm refusal to comply and a request that Mr. Gilmour wait until you complete your nursing report would both be appropriate. It is important to ensure that he does get to smoke a cigarette right after report time.

This strategy would demonstrate to Mr. Gilmour that he cannot break reasonable rules that have been established for good purposes. Your firmness would respect your own right to finish your report without being interrupted and would treat Mr. Gilmour with respect.

Step 3: Implementation and Evaluation of Your Communication Strategy

7. Now you must reply to Mr. Gilmour. On a separate sheet of paper develop your own response to Mr. Gilmour and keep it handy for future reference.

8. At this point you get the chance to compare your suggested response to the following options. Look over each of the response choices and turn to p. 303 at the end of the chapter to read a critique of each.

As you review the following response choices, look for those that are congruent with your assessment of Mr. Gilmour's requests and your desire to communicate in an assertive and responsible way.

Choice G: "Get out of here and leave us alone so that we can finish our report. As soon as we are finished, we will take you out for a cigarette."

Choice U: "Mr. Gilmour, please do not interrupt us while we are doing the report. We will finish in 5 minutes if you stop interrupting us. It's only been 30 minutes since your last cigarette, and when our report is finished one of the evening nurses will take you outside. If you do not leave us alone now, then we will delay giving you a cigarette for another hour."

Choice BB: "Ohhhh! *(exasperated)*. At this point I'd do anything to get this report over so I can leave. Here's a cigarette. Put it out if you see someone coming."

9. After you have found the most satisfactory strategy and discovered why the other options are unsuitable, go back to the suggested response you generated earlier in this exercise. Evaluate your response in terms of how assertive and responsible it was.

It is important to note that manipulation is a method of attempting to get your needs met and is a behavior that can be seen on a continuum from positive and resourceful to negative and destructive. Whenever a nurse feels annoyed with a client, it is useful to examine the interaction and consider whether another issue other than the one at hand is contributing to the annoyance. These issues are explored more thoroughly in psychiatric nursing.

 Moments of Connection . . .
Taking Our Work Professionally Rather Than Personally

"I was busy on my 3:00 to 11:00 shift on a medical surgical unit. One woman was constantly on the call bell and yelling out her needs when we didn't respond as quickly as she expected. By 10:00 PM, things were calmer and her roommate was finally able to get to sleep. We went to the room to do brief evening care. We fluffed her pillow, talked several minutes, and brushed her hair. She looked up at me, patted my hand, touched my cheek, and said, 'You are all my heroes.' Somehow we had given her something. . . . You never know what touches a client or what means a lot; sometimes it's the small things."

Communicating with Manipulative Colleagues

Step 1: Assessment of the Data

1. Review the following situation and formulate your own assessment of your colleague's thoughts, feelings, and requests.

You are a nurse in an outpatient clinic that keeps sample medications on hand to give to clients. It is midway through the day. Your colleague Noreen has suffered a splitting headache all night, and she is concerned that it will develop into one of her immobilizing migraine headaches. You are the only one with the keys to the medication cabinet. She approaches you with this request:

> *Noreen*: "Leslie, I can't take this headache of mine any longer. I feel like my brain has dried up into a hard ball and it's knocking against my skull. On the outside it feels as if a vise was locking in on it. I've already tossed up what little supper I could eat. Leslie, could you give me some of that new analgesic for my head? I've used it in the past, and it stops me from vomiting and somehow eases my head, too. My doctor would agree to it, I swear; so won't you please help me out of my misery? It's not like it's a narcotic I'm asking for. What do you say? I might be of some help to you for the rest of the day if you give me the analgesic."

2. On a separate sheet of paper write down your assessment of Noreen's thoughts and feelings. Indicate what request Noreen is making of you, her colleague on the evening shift.

3. Compare your analysis to the following assessment:

Thoughts: Noreen thinks that the analgesic will help her to feel better. She thinks it is reasonable for you to give her the analgesic without an order from her physician.

Feelings: Noreen is feeling pretty sick with her impending migraine headache and feels hopeful that you will help by giving her the analgesic.

Request: Noreen is asking you to understand that her headache is making her feel violently ill. She is requesting action in the form of your giving her the analgesic.

4. Did your assessment reflect an accurate analysis of the facts as they were presented? If not, return to the original data presented in the vignette and reassess the cognitive and affective messages. If so, proceed to Step 2.

Step 2: Communication Strategies and Desired Outcomes

5. You have determined that Noreen wants understanding and action. Identify which communication strategies you would use to respond to her request. Indicate the desired outcomes of your suggested strategy. Write your ideas down so that you can refer to them later.

6. Compare your suggested strategy to this one:

Warmth and an empathic reply would convey your compassion for Noreen. Her request that you give her prescription medication without a physician's order is unreasonable because it puts you in jeopardy of disciplinary action from your professional nursing association. Furthermore, you would be unwise to administer anything that might be damaging to your colleague because she has not been examined by a physician. A firm refusal to comply with her request would be appropriate, as would be a suggestion that she leave work to attend to her health.

This strategy would show Noreen that you understand and care about how she is feeling and make it clear that you want her to handle her health problems through the correct channels.

Step 3: Implementation and Evaluation of Your Communication Strategy

7. Now you must reply to Noreen. On a separate sheet of paper develop your own response to Noreen and keep it handy for future reference.

8. At this point you can compare your suggested response to the following options. Look over each of the response choices and turn to p. 303 at the end of the chapter to read a critique of each.

As you review the following response choices, look for those that are congruent with your assessment of Noreen's requests and your desire to communicate in an assertive and responsible way.

Choice O: "Are you serious, Noreen? I can't give you anything. If you're that sick, you'd better go home."

Choice T: "Well, I guess that would be OK, Noreen. Do you really think so? You're right, it's a drug you have used before. OK, I'll do it. Do you really think we're doing the right thing?"

Choice V: "Noreen, you sound terrible. I think if you're that uncomfortable, you'd better go home. I will not give you any medications, and I don't think you should take anything until you've checked with your doctor. It's been a slow day, and I know I can manage. Who could we call to come and get you?"

9. After you have found the most satisfactory strategy and discovered why the other options were unsuitable, go back to the suggested response you generated earlier in this example. Evaluate your response in terms of how assertive and responsible it was.

A Final Note

The situations described earlier and others you will face are not so easily handled on the spot. These techniques give you a framework from which to work. You have studied techniques in this book that help you promote your own calm, confident approach to difficult situations. You are equipped to start your own journey to understand the human condition. Perhaps you are reading this book because you've already learned that you need to know more. Do not be fooled; your education just begins when you leave school, but practice helps, so more exercises are included!

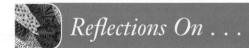

Reflections On . . .

Communicating Assertively and Responsibly with Aggressive Clients and Colleagues

Consider what you read about communicating assertively with aggressive clients and colleagues. Have you already begun to deal with these challenges? Answer the following questions.

What? . . .
Write one thing you learned from this chapter.

So What? . . .
How will this affect your nursing practice?

Now What? . . .
How will you implement this new knowledge or skill?

Think about it . . .

Practicing Communicating Assertively and Responsibly with Aggressive Clients and Colleagues

Exercise 1
Next time you are confronted with someone's aggression, take a few moments later to experiment with the expressive arts to release your emotions. Use your choice of crayons, markers, or colored pencils, and a piece of white paper. Look at the colors and "let a color choose you," perhaps the color that most represents your emotion at the time. Simply begin to lay down color in lines or shapes. Scribble, draw, or color until the piece feels "done" to you. Write a journal entry about what you thought or felt during and after this expressive arts activity. Consider adding doodles or drawings to your journal to add another dimension of self-expression. Nursing students in this author's courses on Expressive Arts in Healing report emotional release and insights and find that they continue this practice of art making for self-care.

Exercise 2
You will need an audio or video recorder for this exercise. Work in groups of three. One of you role-plays an aggressive client or colleague, another acts as the nurse, and the third gives feedback to the nurse. The aggressive client (or colleague) communicates to the nurse in a rejecting, hostile, abusive, or manipulative way. The nurse attempts to respond in an assertive and responsible way. The feedback giver indicates to the nurse how effective he or she was in employing an assertive and responsible style. Record the dialogue between client (or colleague) and nurse so that you can use the recording to complete.

Make sure each member of the group has the chance to play all three roles. After you have completed this exercise in your small group, rejoin your colleagues in the rest of the class. Pool together what you have learned about communicating effectively with aggressive clients and colleagues.

Exercise 3
Review the recording from Exercise 2 by yourself or with the group, taking time to evaluate each situation and come up with an alternative response if you assess that the response to the "client" or "colleague" could be more effective.

Critique: Choices of Responses to Aggressive Clients and Colleagues

Choice A: This is a nonassertive reply. You have acknowledged Mr. Hunter's need for secure, safe nursing care, but you have not given any credit to your ability to provide this care. You have not respected your own skill and abilities. Mr. Hunter may feel reassured that he can get a registered nurse instead of you, a student nurse, but he would not be impressed with your lack of confidence in your own abilities. This response is not responsible because you missed data about his difficulty adjusting to his primary nurse's absence. This strategy might make Mr. Hunter wonder about his safety in your hands, and it might embarrass him that you so easily crumbled under his attack.

Choice B: This response is aggressive and hostile to your instructor. You have harbored resentment about her lack of positive feedback for 5 weeks and have not appropriately brought it up at an earlier time. Today your built-up anger and disappointment have come crashing out against her. Although this response protects your right to speak up, it overrides her right to have her feelings respected. Not only would this response make her feel threatened and angry, but it might result in a discipline case with your school of nursing. This response in no way guarantees that you will receive positive feedback from your instructor in the future.

Choice C: This approach is aggressive in style. There is arrogance in your touching Debbie and telling her not to feel the way she does. Your response is not sensitive of her right to have and express her feelings. This response is irresponsible because it does not pick up on the obvious data that Debbie refuses to be rushed to accept her diabetes and her need for insulin. It may escalate Debbie's fury to touch her at this point. Debbie would likely feel talked down to and disregarded.

Choice D: This strategy is assertive. Your apology to Karen and her clients was timely and respected their legitimate rights. Its brevity and promptness deescalated any further hostility between your two parties. This approach is responsible because it acknowledges your role in inconveniencing others. All concerned would be satisfied with this reply. Waiting until a moment when you and Karen could talk privately and freely about how she embarrassed you was considerate and respected your right to talk about this important issue. Your request to talk to Karen, and your honesty

about the issue, helped to focus on the problem right away. Starting with an apology reassured her of your sincerity. Waiting for her permission to pursue your agenda was respectful. Your CARE confrontation spelled out clearly what bothered you and how you want your colleague to behave in the future. Karen would feel that you understood her irritation with your overstaying in the room, and she would easily be able to receive your feedback about her rudeness.

Choice E: This response is aggressive and almost taunting. It would serve only to escalate the anger building between you. It attacks Mr. Hunter's vulnerability. He has no control over who nurses him, and you have threatened his security by implying that reporting you would be futile. Your sauciness about the decision of your instructor would only make Mr. Hunter feel less secure. This response is irresponsible because it does not attend to the data about Mr. Hunter's feelings of insecurity and his desire to heal without relapse. It shows no sensitivity to his feelings of missing his primary nurse. This response would likely make Mr. Hunter feel insecure and threatened.

Choice F: This response is aggressive. It is a direct, insulting attack on your team leader. It does nothing to respect your right to communicate in a caring way, and it ignores her concerns about your slowness. This style of responding would only make your team leader want to retaliate by being more aggressive with you in the future.

Choice G: You have responsibly acknowledged Mr. Gilmour's need for a cigarette, but your style is aggressive and rude. It does not respect your right to communicate assertively and would likely make everyone a little embarrassed.

Choice H: This response is assertive because it puts the onus on your instructor for more specificity in her suggestion about how you should change. It is her responsibility to clarify her meaning. This strategy is also responsible because it picks up on the data you have been given about her intention to transform you into a professional nurse. This response would likely make your instructor clarify her meaning of "professional" to your satisfaction. With this information you could then decide whether to point out any evidence you have about your professional demeanor. If she cannot be clear in her expectations, then you have the right to ask her to withdraw the accusation that you are unprofessional. The issue of your right to receive some positive feedback from your instructor has not been dealt with in this response. Including such a request would augment the assertiveness of your response.

Choice I: This reply is irresponsible because it does not take into account Mrs. Suit's worry or anxiety. It is aggressive because it sarcastically insults her and does not respect your right to communicate in a caring way. This reply would put down Mrs. Suit and make her feel angry and embarrassed.

Choice J: This is an assertive response. You have pointed out in a CARE confrontation exactly what bothers you and how you want her to change. Your specificity and courteous manner would protect her self-respect while you stand up for your legitimate rights. This strategy is also responsible because your instructor can pick up your hint about giving you feedback in an effort to improve your performance, and you remind her of some data she has overlooked. It is likely that this gentle confrontation will invite your instructor to look at her omissions and try to rectify the situation by being more accepting of your abilities as a maternity nurse.

Choice K: This aggressive approach would likely increase Debbie's anger. At the least, it would dissolve any rapport or trust you had developed. You have not honored her right to be treated with respect and compassion. Irresponsibly, you have not attended to the data about her fear or her need to go slowly in her acceptance. You have not respected your right to communicate in a caring way. Debbie would likely feel even more angry and helpless because you are "pulling rank" on her. It would take a long time to repair the bad feelings generated by this response.

Choice L: This choice is aggressive in style. Your opening phrase attacks Karen and escalates the hostility between the two of you. Your defensiveness embarrasses everyone—staff and clients. This response is irresponsible in its lack of attention to Karen's request for understanding and an apology.

Choice M: This reply is assertive because it confidently assures Mr. Hunter that you know what you are doing and invites him to make any inquiries about your nursing care. Your agreement about differences between nurses might reduce his anxiety over apparent variations in nursing styles. Your acknowledgment of his missing his primary nurse would show him you understand the mutuality that they had developed. Your assurance that your care is safe and congruent with the doctor's orders would reassure him that you understand his urgency to be well cared for. This responsible and assertive response would make Mr. Hunter feel understood and comforted.

Choice N: This reply is assertive and responsible. It stands up for your right to be given a chance to learn, and it shows respect for your team leader. You have acknowledged her legitimate concerns about the clients and requested her help in facilitating your development as a medication nurse. This response would make it clear what behavior you expect in a way that makes it easy for her to comply.

Choice O: This response is aggressive. It blasts Noreen without showing any compassion for how she is feeling; however, it does respect your right to nurse within the limits of the law and your own convictions. Noreen would likely feel attacked, but she would definitely get the message that she should go off duty.

Choice P: This is a nonassertive approach. You have not acknowledged Karen's feelings, nor have you spoken to her about your own anger at her aggressiveness. You have irresponsibly ignored Karen's legitimate requests. By sulking and avoiding her, you are harboring bad feelings instead of dealing with them in a forthright manner. You, Karen, and other staff members would all feel tense if you used this strategy.

Choice Q: This response is assertive because it acknowledges both Debbie's right to be understood and your right to communicate in a caring manner and offer Debbie a way to desensitize herself to the insulin shots. It is responsible because it recognizes her need to have her fear understood. You have comforted her by taking control and offering her a plan that might help her. Leaving or getting angry would have removed your supportive backing from Debbie. This response would make Debbie feel secure that you understand her fear and you have the willingness and interest in her to help her through it.

Choice R: This is an irresponsible and nonassertive response. You have neither attended to Mrs. Suit's request to be treated with respect nor shown that you understand her feelings of helplessness. You have not respected your own rights as a nurse on the unit; you had another important task to accomplish that delayed you, and you have the right and responsibility to communicate in a caring way with all your clients. Mrs. Suit may have felt important because you apologized, but your manner indicated only that you wanted to get out of her presence as soon as possible. Your lack of warmth and genuine respect would let Mrs. Suit know that you did not really care for her.

Choice S: This response is nonassertive. You deserve to be bullied when you encourage it with such a meek reply. You have not respected your right to be treated in a patient manner. Your passivity has invited further putdowns.

Choice T: Clearly you are doubtful about the ethics of giving Noreen the medication, but you nonassertively give in. In so doing you lose your right to act safely and you may do your colleague some unintended harm. You have not acted responsibly because you did not follow-up on the data she provided about her migraines, nor did you show much compassion for her misery.

Choice U: This firm, clear reply is assertive; it respects Mr. Gilmour's dignity and your right to communicate in a respectful way. Your inclusion of a negative consequence demonstrates that you are serious about your request for him to stop bothering you during report time. This reply is responsible because it takes into account that Mr. Gilmour had a smoke recently, that there is a well-established rule about the times and places for his smoking, and that you have a right to finish work on time. Although Mr. Gilmour will likely be displeased by your reply, he will know that you are definite.

Choice V: This reply is assertive and responsible. You acknowledged Noreen's extreme discomfort and wisely suggested that she go home. You protected your right to avoid legal problems and your colleague's right to be properly examined before taking medication by refusing to give her anything. You reassured her that you would manage the shift without her. Noreen might wish to try again to persuade you to give her something for her nausea, but that possibility is unlikely given your firmness.

Choice W: This is a nonassertive response. You have not protected your right to relate to your colleague in a caring way. She requested understanding and a promise that you would not repeat your inconsiderate actions in the future, and you have ignored both of these requests by this nonspecific response. Karen would feel minimally understood. This reply ignores your responsibility to defend your right to be treated respectfully by your colleague Karen.

Choice X: This is a nonassertive response. You respected neither Debbie's right to be understood nor your own right to communicate in a helpful way. Your reply focuses only on your feelings and misses the important data about Debbie's fears and need for guidance. Debbie would likely feel misunderstood and unsupported with this response.

Choice Y: This choice is nonassertive. You have buckled under pressure to accept an unreasonable request. Not only is your instructor's request unclear, but it does not correspond with how you feel about your work and the feedback you have been getting. This response is unlikely to stop any further aggression from your instructor. It is neither assertive nor responsible.

Choice Z: This response is an aggressive overreaction to Mr. Hunter. Returning aggressiveness with aggressiveness only escalates the feud. If Mr. Hunter had been repeatedly comparing your care to Chris's and putting you down, it would then be appropriate to ask him to stop this line of attack. At this point it is irresponsible to do so, because it puts the attention on your feelings rather than his feelings of vulnerability and loss. This is not a helpful response, and it would leave Mr. Hunter embarrassed and discomforted.

Choice AA: This is an assertive response. You calmly and kindly reassured Mrs. Suit that your delay was not out of disrespect for her. The directness and conciseness of your explanation did not make you seem overly apologetic (which would have been nonassertive) or overly defensive (which would have been aggressive). Your reply was responsible because it picked up on her need to be treated with respect. Your offer to stay with her and talk demonstrated that you truly do care about her feelings. The strategy of overlooking her coarse, abusive language was probably appropriate in this situation. Her anger stems from her fear, and if you help her cope with some of her legitimate worries, her abusiveness will likely diminish. If not, you could assertively request that she refrain from using abusive language with you.

Choice BB: This is a nonassertive response. You have given in to Mr. Gilmour's unreasonable request and in the process made it difficult for other staff members to uphold the rule. You have taught Mr. Gilmour that if he persists long enough, you will bend the rules. This reply would make you feel bad that you didn't stick to your decision. It irresponsibly ignores the fact that he had a cigarette recently.

References

Antai-Otong D: Creative stress management techniques for self-renewal, *Dermatol Nurs* 13(1):31, 2001.

Christman K: Workplace abuse: finding solutions, *Nurs Econ* 25(6):365, 2007.

Helge D: Positively channeling workplace anger and anxiety, part I, *AAOHN J* 49(9):445, 2001a.

Helge D: Positively channeling workplace anger and anxiety, part II, *AAOHN J* 49(10):482, 2001b.

Helge D: Turning workplace anger and anxiety into peak performance: strategies for enhancing employee health and productivity, *AAOHN J* 49(8):399, 2001c.

Hollinsworth H, Clark C, Harland R, et al: Understanding the arousal of anger: a patient-centered approach, *Nurs Standard* 19(37):41, 2005.

Jakubowski P, Lange AJ: *The assertive option: your rights and responsibilities*, Champaign, Ill, 1978, Research Press.

Joint Commission: Joint Commission alert: stop bad behavior among health care professionals, July 9, 2008, e, 33(5):219, September/October 2008.

Lamontagne C: Intimidation: a concept analysis, *Nurs Forum* 45(1):54, January-March 2010.

Lewis MA: Nurse bullying: organizational considerations in the maintenance and perpetration of health care bullying cultures, *J Nurs Manage* 14(1):52, 2006.

Quine L: Workplace bullying in nurses, *J Health Psychol* 6(1):73, 2001.

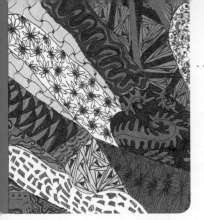

Chapter 27

Communicating Assertively and Responsibly with Unpopular Clients

Objectives

1. Describe characteristics of unpopular clients
2. Identify possible reactions of nurses to unpopular clients
3. Identify strategies to deal with negative attitudes and prevent antagonistic behavior toward unpopular clients
4. Participate in selected exercises to build skills of caring communication with unpopular clients

Who Are the Unpopular Clients?

Consider the distinction between the definition of disease, an interruption or disorder of part of the body, from illness, the state or time of being ill. We must understand disease to treat clients. We must understand the experience of illness to care for them (Cross et al, 2010). Before reading what the literature documents as the most popular and unpopular clients, take a moment to discover and examine your own attitudes toward your clients. Answer the following questions as specifically as possible:

- What are the characteristics of those clients with whom you enjoy working?
- What are the features of clients whom you find unpleasant?

Now, compare your answers with those of your colleagues in your class. Where do your views overlap? In what ways do your preferences and nonpreferences for clients differ? What do your collective opinions suggest to you about the client–nurse relationship?

You might be surprised to learn that all clients are not viewed or treated similarly. All nurses at some time have clients they do not like (Kus, 1990). Although nothing intrinsic makes certain clients likable or not likable, nurses do evaluate some clients as popular and other clients as unpopular. The behavior, appearance, or social status of some clients has an associated stigma. Stigma means both a "societal and self-perception of shame or a flaw" that is seen as irreconcilable and is internalized by the person (Halter, 2002). This chapter helps you become more aware of how your prejudices about clients' behaviors and personalities affect how you relate to them. You become more aware of client characteristics that trigger you to withdraw your caring. This knowledge alerts you to your negative tendencies and reminds you to treat all your clients fairly, safely, and in a way that respects their dignity. Noncaring behaviors may lead to "missed diagnoses and interventions, social isolation, and minimal or negative contact with the nurse" (Maupin, 1995).

In a classic study, Stockwell (1972) set out to determine whether the nursing team enjoyed caring for some clients more than others, and whether there was any measurable difference in the nursing care afforded to the most and least popular clients. Her findings—startling at the time—still have potential impact for nurses. Stockwell reports that foreign clients, those hospitalized longer than 3 months, those with some type of physical defect, and those with a psychiatric diagnosis appear significantly in the unpopular group. Personality factors of clients also play an important part (sometimes the only one) in accounting for whether they are considered unpopular by the nursing team.

Stockwell's research findings reveal that unpopular clients do not generally receive individual holistic care and that nurses withdraw their caring interpersonal communication from these clients. When clients do not fit into our molds, we become annoyed with ourselves and respond to our anger by displacing it onto our clients as dislike. Clients who are estranged from mainstream society may face a wall of fear separating them and the community. The mentally ill have difficulty with clear communication because their perception of reality is impaired. They become alienated in the community and in a healthcare setting because their behavior interferes with treatment. Part of the stigma of mental illness is the misperception that all mentally ill people are violent (Arnold and Hallinan, 2000). Another example of estranged clients is the homeless, who may be referred to as disenfranchised or marginalized and "are defined by their own fear and by the avoidance of others because [other people] are afraid of their behavior or afraid of encountering their intense level of hardship and suffering" (Zerwekh, 2000). Does this also sound like someone with terminal illness? One woman in an "I Can Cope" cancer class said it seemed to her that when she walked down the street in her small town, people acted as if what she had was "catchin'."

In an investigation of the reactions of doctors and nurses to the attitudes and behaviors of surgical clients,

Lorber (1975) found that medical staff label clients who interrupt well-established routines and make extra work for them as "problem" clients. Those who minimize the trouble they cause staff by being cooperative are considered "good."

Characteristics of Unpopular Clients and Their Effects on Nurses

Researchers (Kus, 1990; Lorber, 1975; Stockwell, 1972) report that unpopular clients have the following characteristics:

- They grumble or complain.
- They indicate their lack of enjoyment at being in the hospital.
- They imply that they are suffering more than nurses believe.
- They have conditions nurses feel could be better cared for in other units or in specialized hospitals.
- They require more time and attention than are deemed warranted.
- They are complaining, uncooperative, or argumentative.
- They have severe complications, poor prognoses, or difficult diagnoses.
- They require extensive explanations, reassurance, or encouragement.
- They are of low social value.
- They are of low moral worth.
- They have unchosen stigmata (such as sexual orientation, gender, race, or ethnicity).
- They have illnesses considered to be their "own fault" (such as alcoholism or lung cancer from heavy smoking).
- They have fear-causing conditions (such as highly contagious or incurable diseases or violent tendencies).
- They engender feelings of incompetence in nurses (they have conditions about which nurses know little).

Nurses' Reactions to Unpopular Clients

In reacting to unpopular clients, nurses feel:

- Frustrated and impatient with "grumblers and moaners"
- Afraid of being trapped by complainers
- Irritated that unpopular clients waste their time

- Incompetent to provide the necessary care for complicated cases and psychiatric clients
- Relief when "unmanageable" clients are transferred
- Dissatisfaction with their jobs
- Changes in their health (such as insomnia or anorexia)

Nurses act by:

- Ignoring or avoiding demanding clients
- Indicating to demanding clients that others need their attention more
- Labeling demanding clients as nuisances or hypochondriacs
- Showing a reluctance to provide necessary care if clients are thought to act inappropriately (e.g., repeated lewd behavior or aggressive language)
- Scolding and reprimanding
- Administering tranquilizers and sedatives to control clients' behavior
- Recommending transfer and discharge
- Requesting psychiatric consultation to manage unruly behavior
- Extending minimally adequate care
- Withdrawing from peers
- Becoming critical of the profession or the institution
- Withholding pain medication
- Ignoring clients' call lights or bells
- Being cool, detached, and insensitive
- Feeling guilty

This evidence suggests that nurses and other health professionals have definite ideas of what is acceptable client behavior and what is not. Look at the list you prepared earlier of client characteristics you dislike. How does it compare with the findings from the literature?

In contrast to unpopular clients, popular clients were found to have the following characteristics (Lorber, 1975; Stockwell, 1972):

- They are able to converse readily with nurses.
- They know the nurses' names.
- They are able to joke and laugh with the nurses.
- They are determined to get well again.
- They are cooperative and compliant with the therapeutic regimen.
- They can be managed by routine methods.
- They rarely complain of pain or discomfort.
- They minimize the trouble they cause staff by being cooperative.

Nurses demonstrate the following reactions to popular clients:

- Enjoy interacting with clients who are "fun," have a good sense of humor, are easy to get along with, and are friendly
- Give superior care and do more for popular clients in the long run
- Treat them more leniently
- Give them special favors and readily fill ordinary requests

Look again at your list of appealing client characteristics and compare your reactions to these findings from the literature.

We would all agree that each of our clients deserves to receive courteous care regardless of cultural background, length of illness, personality, and type of illness (including the extent of complications). Is it not surprising to discover that despite the emphasis on compassion in our nursing education, we are unable to consistently extend respectful nursing care to all our clients? It is not humanly possible to like all our clients.

It is, however, a professional expectation and responsibility that we treat all clients with courtesy and provide care that meets standards for nursing practice, regardless of whether we like our clients. Consider one nurse's admonition to consider yourself lucky if the patient does complain because this might give clues to unidentified problems and ways to improve the quality of care. For example, a client afraid of soiling himself may express his fear as rage at the nurse who is delayed in answering the call light (Goldman, 1995).

To ignore or convey dislike to our clients is in direct contrast to the policy of nurturing a therapeutic helping relationship with them. When we show our dislike to clients, they feel unsupported. The message we convey is that they are unimportant and that we do not care about them or their problems. By extending our compassion, administering effective nursing interventions, and minimizing evidence of our dislike, we can be influential in eliminating some of the client behaviors we find problematic.

> *For the sake of the rose, the thorn is watered.*
> **African proverb**
>
> WIT&*Wisdom*

How to Overcome Negative Attitudes and Antagonistic Behavior toward Unpopular Clients

When you become aware of having negative feelings toward your clients, you are in a position to change such behavior. One effective approach is to try to perceive things from the client's point of view. As trite as this sounds, it is difficult to do. Our dislikes and biases blind us from considering things from others' viewpoints. Changing your attitude will not automatically change your nursing behavior, but the effort to view your clients differently may help.

These examples illustrate how to achieve this empathic perspective.

Situation 1

Mrs. White is a 48-year-old accountant who has been diabetic since age 17. In the past 3 years she has been hospitalized for circulatory damage to her feet, which has resulted in amputation of two toes of both feet. She claims that she does not have time for adequate foot care as she is working long hours and is on her feet all day. On this admission she has several lesions on the remaining toes on both feet. If special skin care treatments are ineffective, Mrs. White faces the possibility of further amputations.

Your Possible Negative Attitude and Behavior

Your reaction to Mrs. White's predicament is one of disapproval. You think she is wasting valuable healthcare resources by occupying a hospital bed when she could have avoided the skin breakdown by a few extra minutes of attention to her feet each day. Taking better care of herself would have meant she would be out in the community leading a productive life instead of taking up expensive nursing services that others need. You resent her being on your unit and find yourself taking your time to answer her call bell and leaving her alone for long periods. In the back of your mind you think that if she finds her hospital stay uncomfortable, she might take better precautions to avoid admission in the future.

Your awareness of how you are taking your anger out on Mrs. White by treating her disrespectfully (and possibly unsafely) is the first step in changing your behavior.

Seeing the Situation through the Eyes of Your Client, Mrs. White

To help you change your behavior toward Mrs. White, it helps if you can see things from her point of view. Find a spot where you can think without being interrupted. Mentally put yourself in Mrs. White's position and attempt to understand how she might be thinking and feeling about being in the hospital. Your thoughts might go something like this:

I have to wait so long for the nurse to answer the bell. It's not like I overuse the privilege. I wish they would come sooner, especially when I need the bedpan. I feel so helpless in here; I can't do a thing for myself, it seems. I'm so used to being independent. I'll do anything to get healed and get out of the hospital. The pain I'm having makes me wish I'd been more stringent about my foot care. I hope they don't have to operate. I don't know if I'd be able to walk without a walker if they remove any more toes. How could I work then?

Taking the time to imagine how you would feel in Mrs. White's position is a beginning. Instead of focusing on her neglect, this exercise may help you to pay attention to her distress here and now. Your fresh, empathic viewpoint may help you treat her more respectfully.

You might now respond to her call bell more quickly and extend your warmth to her. You might seek her out when you have a few extra minutes and explore her reactions to her illness and hospitalization. Instead of aggressively taking out your anger on Mrs. White, you might be more direct and confront her about her noncompliant foot care. Your problem-solving ability and empathic listening skills can help you to assess what prevents her from performing more rigorous skin care. From there you can help her work out a plan to overcome these blocks. By making your interventions more positive, you can help her reduce her anxiety about her predicament.

It is responsible to focus your attention on becoming more empathic with this client. Empathy does not always come easily. This fuller vision provides you with more data to complete the nursing process. When you see both sides, it is more likely that you will act assertively, taking into account not only your feelings but also those of your client.

Situation 2

Mr. Evans is a 39-year-old client in the terminal stages of cancer. Although he has only been hospitalized on your unit for the past 4 weeks, he has been in and out of the unit with exacerbations for the past year. He is weak, and most caregivers are certain he will die soon. He is in isolation and requires extensive dressing changes to open areas on his legs. The ulcerated area is draining purulent matter and has a foul odor that is almost suffocating. Mr. Evans has lost 40 pounds over the past year and is emaciated. The darkened areas under his eyes, sagging skin, and low energy level create the impression that he is barely hanging onto life with each breath he takes.

Your Possible Negative Attitude and Behavior

It is painful for you to even enter Mr. Evans's room because you are reminded of the times when he had color in his cheeks and kept you on your toes with his engaging sense of humor. You miss his former self and feel saddened about his impending death. You are distressed because you gag and feel nauseated when you change his dressings. When you go into his room to administer his care, you feel trapped. You are at a loss for what to say, and you just want to finish your physical nursing care so that you can leave. You work at top speed and leave as soon as his dressings are done.

Seeing the Situation through the Eyes of Your Client, Mr. Evans

Find the time and place to quietly contemplate how Mr. Evans thinks and feels. Try to imagine things from his perspective. Your thoughts might go something like this:

> I'm ready to go. I wish I could just die soon. I'm so uncomfortable, I can't sleep, and I'm bored when I'm awake. I'd really like some company. I must be a sight to look at, though. No wonder everyone seems shocked when they see me. It's lonely waiting.

Taking the opportunity to imagine how Mr. Evans is reacting generates several ways you could intervene to be more helpful. This exercise in empathy helps you to focus on how he is here and now as opposed to emphasizing how he used to be.

Even though Mr. Evans does not have much energy to talk, you could arrange to spend time in his room and read to him or arrange for some music he likes. He might be comforted by a back rub. Reading the paper to him, writing letters for him, or updating him on events are several activities that require minimal energy from him, yet allow him contact with you. Ensuring that his analgesics are administered consistently so that he is pain free and reminding him to change his position frequently in the bed are measures that will increase his ability to relax.

Deodorizing the room frequently would make the environment more pleasant for him, his visitors, and staff. Either sweet orange or grapefruit essential oils are used in some hospice settings for odor control. To help you manage the dressing changes, you could wear a mask and increase all the positive stimuli that you can think of (play music, have flowers within view, open the window). It might help distract your attention from the unpleasant odor if you can start telling him a story when you are doing a dressing change. The activity would keep your mind focused on something more positive.

It is assertive to consider the situation from your clients' viewpoints as well as from your own. If we concentrate only on negative aspects, we are likely to act aggressively and attempt to achieve only our own goals. It is responsible to see things from other angles so that we can generate plans that consider the perspectives of our clients. A patient-centered approach transfers your power and authority to the patient. When we learn more about our patients' lives we can offer information that is more relevant to their lifestyle, without labeling clients "difficult" or "noncompliant" (Russell et al, 2003). All our clients have the right to feel cared for.

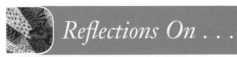

Reflections On . . .

Communicating Assertively and Responsibly with Unpopular Clients

Consider what you read about unpopular clients. Could you identify any of your own problem areas? Answer the following questions.

What? . . .
Write one thing you learned from this chapter.

So What? . . .
How will this affect your nursing practice?

Now What? . . .
How will you implement this new knowledge or skill?

Think about it . . .

Practicing Communicating Assertively and Responsibly with Unpopular Clients

Exercise 1

Identify a client with whom you have worked or are working who is difficult for you. Select one or more expressive writing strategies. 1. Write a poem from this person's point of view, no need to rhyme. One approach is to write a poem in which every line begins with "I am." 2. Write a letter as if the client were writing his or her point of view/requests of you. 3. Write a letter as if writing to the client, expressing your thoughts, feelings, and hopes for the client.

Exercise 2

Meet this challenge. Answer the question of the month in *RN Magazine* (Sindorf et al, 2005): "What is the most creative thing you've ever done to deal with a difficult patient?" Write your brief response to this question as if you were submitting it to the magazine.

Exercise 3

Make a copy of Box 27-1, What Do YOU Think? Cut the sentences apart and put them into a container. Each student draws one and responds to it and facilitates a discussion. If you are working alone, choose random numbers and then reflect upon your reaction to the statements.

Exercise 4

Following are six situations depicting unpopular clients. Possible reactions that you might have to these "problem" clients are suggested. Your task is to put yourself in each client's place and imagine what the situation feels like from his or her perspective. Then your task is to indicate how these insights would free you to interact in a more caring way with your client. Be sure that your new approach in each case is assertive and responsible.

1. A 73-year-old foreign client refuses to eat his hospital food. He is on a special diet, and it is important that he ingest only what the nutritionist and

---

| **Box 27-1** | *What Do YOU Think?* |

1. Addicts are people who just need to try harder to abstain.
2. Suicide is a coward's way out of problems.
3. People who are mentally ill should be institutionalized.
4. Retarded children should be institutionalized.
5. Homeless people are lazy.
6. Obese people eat too much.
7. Clients should be grateful for the nursing care they receive.
8. People should bathe every day.
9. Whiners should be ignored.
10. I don't have to like every client.
11. Everyone has prejudice or bias of some sort.
12. Families should care for the dying at home.
13. Mothers should breast feed their babies to decrease allergies.
14. Clients need to understand a nursing shortage.
15. Depressed clients should be transferred to a psychiatric unit.
16. Family members should get out of the nurse's way so care can be more efficient.
17. People should not use illness to get attention.
18. Nurses deserve to be treated with respect.
19. Assertive communication is useful in dealing with unpopular clients.
20. Finding just the right thing to say will help a client to behave better.

physician have ordered. His wife brings him food that is rich in spices and sauces. Both the client and his wife complain when the ethnic food is withdrawn and hospital food is the only choice.

You feel furious that this client is unwilling to abide by the good judgment of the physician and nutritionist. You feel disdain that he has abused his body for so many years and are amazed that he will not take advantage of the good advice being offered by his caretakers. You avoid eye contact with this client, do not speak to his wife, and spend little time with him. You curtly order him to eat the hospital diet when you deliver his meal tray, and you make a point of picking up his tray so that you can check how much he ate. When his intake has been less than adequate, you tell him you will not remove his tray until he has eaten more.

- Put yourself in this client's place and imagine what things are like from his perspective.
- With your new insight, how would you act assertively and responsibly toward your client?

2. Betty is a 16-year-old girl on your orthopedic unit. She has been in traction for 2 months after a car accident and has multiple fractures and burns. Her parents' home is over a hundred miles away, and they visit Betty only every third weekend. Betty is terribly homesick and cries for hours after her parents leave. She hates being in traction and just wants to go home. She is withdrawn and refuses to do any of the occupational therapy projects her therapist provides. She does not encourage any interaction with the other two teenagers on the unit, despite their extensive efforts to divert her attention away from her unhappy situation. She is curt and stoic with the nursing and physical therapy staff, doing the minimum that is required of her.

You have been Betty's nurse since her admission to the unit. At first you were enthusiastic that you could cheer her up and encourage her to make the best of her situation. When she did not respond positively to your efforts and continued to be morose about being on the unit, you started to withdraw from her. Your once vivacious conversation has become almost nonexistent, and you find yourself talking to the other clients or nurses in the room instead of Betty. When you have a few spare minutes, you refrain from spending them with Betty. After her parents leave one night, you scold her for "acting like a baby" when you find her crying.

- Put yourself in this client's place and imagine what things are like from her perspective.
- With your new insight, how would you act assertively and responsibly toward Betty?

3. Ms. Kerns is a 47-year-old schoolteacher who was transferred to your medical unit from the psychiatric unit upstairs. Over the past 2 years she has been admitted to the psychiatric unit for bouts of depression of unknown origin. Many modalities (medication, psychotherapy, physical therapies) have been employed without success to treat her depression.

She is on your unit for investigation of medical reasons for her low moods. She looks sullen and poorly groomed and mopes around in a housecoat instead of getting dressed. She rarely volunteers to speak to any of the staff, and when you initiate a conversation, it is a tense situation because she is slow to respond and often just nods or sighs.

After some time you begin to realize that you have invested little time in getting to know Ms. Kerns. You have expended almost no effort in finding out about her likes, dislikes, and reaction to being in the hospital. It becomes apparent that you are ignoring her because she is not easy to talk to and because you believe she does not belong on the unit. You are a bit frightened of her flattened affect and the thought that she might be malingering bothers you.

- Put yourself in this client's place and imagine what things are like from her perspective.
- With your new insight, how would you act assertively and responsibly toward Ms. Kerns?

4. Mr. Dire is a 79-year-old client who has just undergone successful cataract surgery in the outpatient surgical center where you work. Preoperatively, he asked many questions and expressed fears about the surgery. You tried to reassure him, but he still kept asking for you and delayed you in your morning schedule. After a successful surgical procedure and patient teaching, he was sent home in the center's van. After he got home, he began to call every 15 minutes with questions. Did he leave his raincoat there? Did you give him an appointment card for a visit to his physician? Was he eligible for a home health nurse? When he sensed impatience in your voice, he snapped at you and said, "Don't get mouthy with me, girlie! I paid good money for this surgery, and you're there to answer my questions. I'm going to report you to the doctor!"

You are angry because you have taken extra time with him and tried to be sensitive, something that is a matter of pride to you. You are embarrassed because you did tell him he should be glad he just had cataract surgery and nothing more serious.

- Put yourself in your client's place and imagine what things are like from his perspective.
- With your new insight, how would you act responsibly and assertively toward Mr. Dire?

Continued

5. Mrs. Gambino delivered a healthy 6-pound boy this morning. Although she is an experienced mother (she has a 12-year-old son and an 11-year-old daughter), she acts otherwise. She asks you to supervise everything she does with her baby. She constantly asks you to repeat all your instructions. Knowing that she, like many other mothers on the unit, is to be discharged within 48 hours, you feel pressured by her demands.

Your attention only temporarily alleviates her anxiety, and you feel overwhelmed by her and the rest of your patient assignment. You find yourself being abrupt with her and trying to get another staff member to answer her calls.

- Put yourself in Mrs. Gambino's place and imagine what things are like from her perspective.
- With your new insight, how would you act assertively and responsibly toward her?

6. A 42-year-old man arrives at the emergency department after taking an overdose of pills. This is his third suicide attempt in 3 months. His wife moved out 6 months ago, leaving a note saying she would not return. She has had no further contact with her husband, who was left with the responsibility of raising their two teenage sons.

You are shocked that a father could be so selfish and irresponsible. You feel resentful that he is using up costly emergency department services when you have other clients who really need you, who couldn't help it that they are in the emergency department. Your first reaction is "Not him again!" You have an urge to tell him that he needs to stop feeling sorry for himself and get on with taking care of his boys. Your anger toward him is smoldering, yet you are uncertain about what to say or how to approach him. Deep down you are frightened by his self-destructiveness.

- Put yourself in this man's place and imagine what things are like from his perspective.
- With your new insight, how would you respond assertively and responsibly toward him?

After you have completed this exercise by yourself, get together with your colleagues in your class and compare your approaches. What similarities and differences were there in your ideas about how the client in each example viewed things? Check to see where your suggestions differ and where they are alike.

Moments of Connection . . .
A Student Nurse Reframes the Day
    I was assigned to a difficult, complex patient that nobody wanted to take care of, always on his call light, asking for pain meds around the clock. I remember telling myself, "You have a mission today to make a difference in this patient's life." He looked very sick, depressed, in pain, and somewhat dirty. He had a bad attitude and was demanding. I listened to his concerns and feelings about his health and family. He always refused to get clean or get out of bed to help his breathing. That day, I gave him a good bath and a back rub. . . . While I was doing this he forgot his pain and joked and laughed. What a rewarding moment.

References

Arnold E, Hallinan K: Mind over matter, *Nursing* 30(10):50, 2000.

Cross SN, Berlin R, Blank DJ, et al: Illness: a collection of poems, *J Med Humanit* 31(2):171, June 2010.

Goldman MC: If we're lucky the patient will complain, *Am J Nurs* 9(2):52, 1995.

Halter MJ: Stigma in psychiatric nursing, *Perspect Psychiatr Care* 38(1):23, 2002.

Kus RF: Nurses and unpopular clients, *Am J Nurs* 90(6):62, 1990.

Lorber J: Good patients and problem patients: conformity and deviance in a general hospital, *J Health Soc Behav* 16(2):213, 1975.

Maupin CR: The potential for noncaring when dealing with difficult patients: strategies for moral decision-making, *J Cardiovasc Nurs* 9(3):11, 1995.

Patterson K, Grenny J, McMillan R, et al: *Crucial conversations: tools for talking when stakes are high*, New York, 2002, McGraw Hill, p 72.

Russell S, Daly J, Hughes E, et al: Nurses and "difficult" patients: negotiating non-compliance, *J Adv Sci* 43(3):281, 2003.

Sindorf C, Wolfer D, Deckard ML, et al: Question of the month: what is the most creative thing you've ever done to deal with a difficult patient? *ModernMedicine* October 1, 2005. http://www.modernmedicine.com/modernmedicine/article/articleDetail.jsp?id=182468. Accessed June 1, 2011.

Stockwell F: *The unpopular patient*, London, 1972, Royal College of Nursing, White Friars Press. (Republished London, 1984, Groom Helm.)

Zerwekh JV: Caring on the ragged edge: nursing persons who are disenfranchised, *Adv Nurs Sci* 22(4):47, 2000.

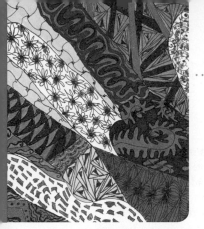

Chapter 28

Managing Team Conflict Assertively and Responsibly

Objectives

1. Define conflict
2. Identify four categories of conflict
3. Identify the steps of win–win conflict resolution
4. Contrast win–win, lose–win, and win–lose methods of handling team conflict
5. Identify the characteristics of multigenerational team members and their impact on the team
6. Participate in selected exercises to build assertive conflict-resolution skills

Definition of Conflict

Conflict can be a source of personal and organizational stress by the very nature of nurses' work (Vivar, 2006). Conflict, often seen as "bad," is a natural part of interactions and, when effectively addressed, improves interpersonal relationships and can promote organizational growth (Chadwick, 2010). A longitudinal study of 53 college student teams indicated that conflict management "has a direct, positive effect on team cohesion and moderates the relationship between relationship conflict and team cohesion as well as that between task conflict and team cohesion" (Tekleab et al, 2009, p. 170). Conflict may be viewed as a feeling, a disagreement, a real or perceived incompatibility of interests, inconsistent worldviews, or a set of behaviors (Mayer, 2000). Conflict arises when interdependency exists, and conflict resolution is necessary to build positive relationships with others as well as to meet our own needs. Whenever two people come together, there is the potential for conflict. Conflict can occupy 30% of a manager's time (Marick and Albright, 2002). Although conflict is inevitable, it can have advantageous outcomes when it is handled in assertive and responsible ways. Conflict resolution can build interdependence and professional collaboration and help team members better address the big-picture issues.

Building positive co-worker relationships, teamwork, and collaboration supports clear communication, which has a direct impact on patient safety. The integration of communication skills and teamwork training in schools of nursing and in the workplace supports this effort (Beckett and Kipnis, 2009; Chapman, 2009; Clark, 2009; Corless et al, 2009; McKeon et al, 2009; Thomas, 2009). The Institute of Medicine's report on medical errors concluded that "as many as 98,000 people die yearly in the United States because of preventable medical errors . . . a startling 70% of these preventable medical errors result from poor communication between healthcare providers" (Kohn et al, 2000, as cited in Lamontagne, 2010, p. 54). The Joint Center for Transforming Healthcare (Zhani, 2010) reports an "estimated 80% of serious medical errors involve miscommunication between caregivers when responsibility for patients is transferred or handed-off." In their Hand-off Communication Project participating hospitals found that more than 37% of hand-offs were defective, preventing the receiver of the information from safely caring for the patient. After implementing targeted solutions to the hand-off communication, the result was a 52% reduction in defective hand-offs.

> *An ounce of prevention is worth a pound of cure.*
>
> **Benjamin Franklin**
>
> **WIT&***Wisdom*

Cushnie (1988) identifies four categories of conflict intensifying in degree of difficulty from first to last: facts, methods, goals, and values.

Facts

Conflicts about facts are differences about data. These disagreements can be resolved by terminating the debate and seeking information from reliable sources.

Methods

Conflicts about methods are differences about how something is done. A conflict about methods occurs when there is no absolute standard shared by all parties affected by the issue. Resolving conflicts of this kind includes acknowledging that there is more than one way to accomplish the same goal or task. A way to minimize this type of conflict is to establish criteria for method selection.

Goals

Goal conflicts are differences about desired outcomes. Discussion often reveals that parties share a common concern. If they are able to identify a common goal, this redefinition opens up new opportunities for problem solving.

Values

Differences in belief systems are the most complex type of conflict, and a high level of motivation is required from involved parties to understand each other's beliefs. If the parties can avoid the divisiveness of allocating others' viewpoints to rigid categories of "right" or "wrong" and find compatible goals, they are on their way to conflict management (Cushnie, 1988).

Several forms of conflict are seen (Kinder, 1981):

- Intrapersonal conflict occurs within an individual.
- Interpersonal conflict occurs between two individuals or among members of a group.
- Intragroup conflict occurs within an established group.
- Intergroup conflict is the struggle between groups.

This chapter focuses on interpersonal conflict in a workplace or school setting.

Healthcare teams are composed of people with many different backgrounds. A variety of professional outlooks are found in a team of nurses, physicians, clergy, nutritionists, occupational and physical therapists, social workers, and others. In addition to the differences in socialization of these professionals, they carry personal views based on sex, age, cultural origin, socioeconomic situation, and life experience. This potpourri is a potential source of conflict in any healthcare team.

This variety results in different perceptions about an issue and the role and obligations each should fulfill. When team members do not agree about a situation or their respective roles, then the potential for conflict is great.

Team members often have different (or opposing) ideological views about a given situation. Their views may come from having different objectives or from endorsing different priorities among the objectives. Conflict results when team members do not agree on what to do, how to do it, and when to do it. Review Chapter 5 for the stages of group behavior. Remember that group conflict is healthy and expected in the storming stage.

Occasionally, conflict resurfaces between team members who have had a long history of disagreement. The level of trust and collaboration has been worn down between these people, and their competitiveness is sharpened. Such a situation fuels conflict.

Conflict-Resolution Approaches

You know you cannot avoid conflict. What you can avoid is feeling impotent or uncomfortable when you encounter situations involving conflict. By now you are familiar with assertive and responsible communication. These approaches can help you resolve conflicts in constructive ways.

Resolving a conflict means acting in such a way that an agreement is reached that is acceptable, and even pleasing, to both parties. If both parties cannot agree on a resolution, the conflict will continue. When conflict drags out and team members do not see a hopeful resolution, then helplessness prevails. Any healthcare team that is stuck in this hopeless situation is not working at its full capacity. Harrington-Mackin (1994) advises dealing with conflicts in a timely way and suggests that most people find it difficult to openly discuss and work through conflicts. Instead, they accumulate grudges and use techniques such as procrastination and sniping to "get even." Client care and morale suffer when conflicts remain unresolved.

You can approach conflict resolution in three ways: win–win, lose–win, or win–lose. Although win–win is preferable, there may be times when a workable compromise is the best solution to avoid having both parties lose. Throughout this book, the point has been made that assertiveness is a matter of choice. There may be times when you feel obligated to insist on your solution to a problem, such as in parenting a small child. There may be times when you choose to allow the other person to win, such as when you recognize that a colleague has been pushed to the limit and your position seems less important than their peace of mind.

The win–win approach to conflict resolution requires you to be assertive and responsible. This approach results in a solution with which you and your colleagues are happy. Not only is the outcome satisfactory, but adopting a win–win approach uses your full creativity and often results in a unique and innovative resolution.

The lose–win approach is one in which you allow your colleagues to resolve the conflict at your expense. Either you are not happy with the outcome or you permit your colleagues to walk all over you. This approach is nonassertive and irresponsible.

The win–lose approach is the opposite of the lose–win approach. You may resolve the conflict in a way that is satisfying to you, but in the process you bulldoze over the rights of your colleagues. This approach is aggressive and irresponsible.

Any win–lose/lose–win approach creates forces that aggravate the struggle and do little to discover constructive solutions acceptable to all involved. A conflict is more constructive when the outcome is satisfying to all the participants than when it is satisfying to only some. Conflict at some point is inevitable, so it helps to know how to use it as an opportunity to be constructive—because the alternatives have unpleasant consequences.

A win–win conflict management strategy covers each of the following steps (Flanagan, 1995):

1. View the problem in terms of needs (what is required) instead of solutions (what should be done) to facilitate a mutual problem-solving approach; detach yourself from biases and stay focused on the actual data.
2. Consider the problem as a mutual one to be solved, requiring the active involvement of all affected persons.
3. Describe the conflict as specifically as possible, using undistorted data.
4. Identify the differences between concerned parties before attempting to resolve the conflict.
5. See the conflict from another point of view.
6. Use brainstorming to arrive at possible solutions instead of adopting the first or most convenient idea.
7. Select the solution that best meets both parties' needs and considers all possible consequences.
8. Reach an agreement about how the conflict is to end and not recur.
9. Plan who will do what and where and when it will be done.
10. After the plan has been implemented, evaluate the problem-solving process and review how well the solution turned out.

Table 28-1 summarizes three different approaches to conflict. The assertive, responsible attitude toward conflict and approach to conflict resolution is contrasted with the nonassertive, irresponsible approaches.

Assertive and Responsible Ways to Overcome Conflict

On healthcare teams, conflict can involve all members or only a few. How to manage conflict using a win–win approach in both these instances is explored.

Table 28-1 *Assertive/Responsible versus Nonassertive/Irresponsible Ways of Handling Team Conflict*

CHARACTERISTIC WIN	WIN–WIN LOSE	LOSE WIN–WIN	WIN–LOSE
Attitude toward conflict	Assumes conflict is inevitable and occurs whenever people work together	Assumes conflicts are sent to try us	Sees conflict as a challenge to be won
	Assumes that conflict can be managed so that creative solutions are achieved	Assumes that in a conflict the other person always wins	Considers that manipulation is needed to win conflicts and that it is never ceasing and thinks fighting is required to get what you want
	Assumes that controversy involves everything in the issue and increases members' commitment	Assume that it is a foregone conclusion that the plan to resolve the conflict will satisfy only others	Believes the other person is trying hard to win
	Assumes that conflict can be resolved in ways that are satisfying to all team members	Wonders why there must be conflict in the workplace	
Approach to conflict resolution	Employs a systematic problem-solving approach	Decides in advance that the other person will win and gives up	Keeps fighting with biased information that supports his or her own viewpoint
Data collection	Examines his or her own thoughts and feelings objectively	Prematurely closes data collection	Seeks, examines, and submits only data that support his or her own desired resolution
	Listen emphatically to colleagues' points of view	Assumes it is hopeless to collect data because of an irrational belief that others will win regardless	
	Seeks relevant information from appropriate resources (literature, consultants)	Dwells on how bad things will be if the conflict is not resolved	
	Shares knowledge of the conflict with all others involved	Passively participates in information sharing	
	Remains objective		
Assessment	Formulates an accurate definition of the conflict	Defines the conflict in terms of how it affects colleagues	Does not seek out colleagues' assessments of the conflict
	Shares assessment with colleagues	Defines conflict from his or her own point of view	Overwhelmingly argues for his or her own assessment of the conflict
	Acknowledges colleagues' perceptions of the conflict		

Table 28-1 *Assertive/Responsible versus Nonassertive/Irresponsible Ways of Handling Team Conflict—cont'd*

CHARACTERISTIC WIN	WIN–WIN LOSE	LOSE WIN–WIN	WIN–LOSE
Resolution generation	Considers resolutions that satisfy all involved	Contributes little to this planning because of the assumption that the winner will tell the loser what to do	Only considers or supports plans that agree with his or her own interpretation of the conflict
	Chooses resolutions that maximize the benefits and minimize the drawbacks		Sabotages plans that oppose his or her own view
Evaluation	Maintains vigilance to ensure that resolution continues to satisfy self and colleagues on the team	Complains that resolution could never be successful; disgruntled	Ignores the fact that others are not satisfied with the resolution

WIT&*Wisdom*

One-Liners to Start a Tough Conversation
I'm puzzled by . . .
    I'm curious about what your thoughts were on . . .
    Could you help me understand . . . ?
    I need your help, (name of person you are addressing) . . .

Conflict Situation Involving the Whole Healthcare Team

1. Before you can do anything to resolve a conflict, you need to fully understand the conflict, including your own thoughts and feelings about the situation as well as the thoughts of your colleagues. If you try to resolve a conflict without completing an assessment, you will probably overlook an important factor that could result in an unsatisfactory resolution.

Example: You believe that clients have the right to be informed about any untoward side effects they might experience when taking a prescribed medication. On your unit, few clients are told in advance of the potential side effects. This omission is incompatible with your beliefs about good nursing care and client rights. You discover that many of your colleagues, including the other nurses and physicians on your team, prefer to keep knowledge of side effects from clients so that they will be more likely to take the medication. Here the conflict is incompatible activities (informing versus not informing) and incompatible beliefs about clients' rights (autonomy versus dependency).

2. To fully understand your side of the conflict, you need to examine your own thoughts and feelings. You cannot complete this step in a hurry. You need to sit down (with paper and pencil if necessary) and discover your answers to the following questions:

What Is It about This Conflict That Bothers Me?
In considering the conflict you might have some of the following thoughts:

- "It bothers me that clients are not warned about side effects that might result from the medications."
- "It's not right that they don't have full knowledge of the treatment and that they are taking the pills without fully understanding the implications."
- "I believe that it is dishonest to withhold information about side effects from clients."
- "I believe that people have the responsibility to decide what they should do about their health. By withholding information, we are keeping the control of clients' health in our hands."

Answering this question makes it clearer what the conflict means to you. You have a strong belief that clients should be given the information they need to make the best decision about what health behavior to adopt.

Our initial reaction to a conflict situation is often influenced more by emotion than by intellect. The tension or anxiety creates a fight-or-flight stress response, and the intensity of the stress response varies in relation to the degree of threat perceived (Cushnie, 1988). Taking time to sort out your emotional reactions as you just did helps you control your emotions and increases your effectiveness in conflict management.

What Resolution to This Conflict Would Be Satisfactory for Me?

In thinking about how you would like to have the conflict resolved, you come up with the following idea:

- "The most satisfactory resolution for me would be to institute a policy that all clients will be informed in advance about any possible side effects of any medication prescribed for them."

It is important to answer this question. Often we know there is a conflict but we are uncertain about how we want it resolved. The clearer you can be in answering these questions, the more articulate you will be to others about your stand on the issue.

3. Discover what your colleagues' responses are to the same two questions you just answered yourself. This step requires you to invest time and energy, but you need this information to have a complete understanding of the conflict. The best approach is to arrange a time to sit down with your colleagues and obtain this information.

What Is It about the Conflict That Bothers Them?

Your colleagues may come up with some of the following ideas:

- "If we told every client about possible side effects, it would take too much time."
- "If clients knew all the possible side effects, they might not take the medications and then they would never benefit from them."
- "I believe that we should not scare clients by telling them everything that can go wrong. After all, they're already sick. Why add to their worries?"

You are learning that your colleagues have their clients' interests at heart when they avoid telling them

about the side effects. They have raised a significant point about the time factor as well. Discovering alternative viewpoints expands your awareness of conflict you encounter.

What Resolution to the Conflict Would Be Satisfactory for Your Colleagues?

These are some examples of what your colleagues might tell you:

- "The only solution I can see is to tell only those clients who ask about the side effects."
- "I think we should give out information only about the most common and significant side effects so that clients will be inclined to take their medications."
- "I think we should continue as usual. I've never known any client who was upset about not knowing the side effects of the medications. They need the medications to get well."

These suggestions from your colleagues tell you that they value something more than client autonomy: they value compliance and recovery from illness. You have learned that some of your colleagues are agreeable to informing clients about side effects under certain circumstances.

Finding the answers to these questions will require your best interpersonal communication skills. When you are invested in an issue, it becomes harder to see other points of view. In a conflict situation it is important to listen actively to what your colleagues have to say and check that you have understood their side of the issue.

4. In addition to information obtained from the thoughts and feelings of the people involved in the conflict, you may need information from other sources. In this example you could seek the counsel of the hospital's legal advisor about the rights of your clients. There may be a clients' rights committee that could advise you.

For example, your legal counsel may advise you that "clients have the right by law to be informed of any likely untoward effects of any treatment regimen, unless such information would be considered by the caregivers to be threatening to the client's well-being."

A guideline such as this is sufficiently nonspecific so that your healthcare team would have to make its own interpretation of its application.

5. Once you have fully explored how you and your colleagues feel about the conflict and you have acquired

any other relevant information, the next step is to search for a resolution that will be satisfactory to all of you. This is no easy feat; the win–win approach takes time and effort.

One creative approach at this stage is to brainstorm. Out of brainstorming is likely to come a creative and original resolution to your conflict. It is important that everyone involved in the conflict have an opportunity to contribute ideas about how to resolve it. In this example, there should be representation from nurses, physicians, and clients.

In the brainstorming process it is important that every idea be considered and that no ideas be ridiculed or eliminated. Using this rule means that team members must acknowledge and respect each other's ideas. This action of listening to one another helps to diffuse any hostility that may have arisen as the conflict grew. In a conflict, competition often reigns, with individuals wanting to get their own way; brainstorming ensures that team members communicate in a cooperative way.

In this situation, the following suggestions for resolution of the conflict were put forward:

- Give information about side effects only to clients who ask for it.
- Before clients start on a medication, require that they be able to recite its benefits and side effects.
- Leave a copy of the drug description manual in the clients' common room so that any clients who wish to check on the side effects of a medication can do so.
- Give clients copies of the telephone numbers of the pharmaceutical companies so that they can call a representative and obtain any information about drugs that are prescribed for them.
- Have the pharmacist prepare information sheets about the side effects of clients' drugs that would be available for them to keep and review.
- Give a card to every client admitted to the unit that defines the right-to-know policy concerning side effects of treatments and medications, and indicates that clients need only ask the staff to receive this information.
- Wait until clients experience side effects and then clearly explain them.
- Initiate a policy of inviting questions from clients about the side effects of a medication.

You can see that the suggestions represent a variety of points of view.

6. The next step is to choose an acceptable resolution from the many suggestions put forth. The most expedient action to take on this unit is to form a committee composed of staff members representing both sides of the conflict, as well as clients and administrators of the unit.

You are selected as a member who favors informed consent. Another nurse—with the point of view that informing clients can cause unnecessary problems—is also selected. The head nurse, one physician, and a representative from the clients' rights committee complete the membership.

This committee has the responsibility to develop a policy about what information to give clients concerning side effects of their medications. The decision it makes must meet certain criteria in a win–win approach to conflict resolution. It must satisfy both points of view, be feasible to carry out on the unit (in terms of cost and staffing abilities), and be legally sound.

7. The next step is to systematically review the pros and cons of the eligible resolutions remaining. At this stage, team members must remain open to others' points of view and give all members a chance to defend or refute points. When a group is trying to reach the best decision, it must create a climate that allows members to speak freely.

Consider the effect that the possibility of territoriality or competition among members might have on communication. Members sabotage each other by providing misleading or biased information that results in mistrust. When the communication breaks down this way, it is unlikely that the best decision will be chosen because the database will be incomplete and inaccurate. It takes a concerted effort by the members and the leader to ensure that all points of view are encouraged and respected.

8. After considerable discussion, the group narrows down the choices for resolution to the following:

- Give a card to clients when they are admitted to the unit that advises them that they have the right to know the side effects of any medications and that they need only ask the staff to receive this information.
- Initiate a policy in which nurses and physicians invite questions from clients about the side effects of their medications at the time clients are started on a new medication.

- Require that before clients start taking a medication, they be able to recite its benefits and side effects.

After much deliberation, the committee decides that distributing cards for clients would be too expensive. The members come up with the idea of adding the following paragraph to the "Permission for Treatment" sheet that all clients must sign on admission:

I am aware that all treatments, including medications, have benefits as well as potential untoward effects. I am aware that I have the right to ask my caregivers about these possible negative effects, and that I can expect to have any information explained to me in language that I am able to understand. I am aware that if after careful consideration I refuse to comply fully with the suggested regimen (treatments and medications), this action will in no way jeopardize the care I receive by the healthcare team in this hospital.

Signature_____ Date_____

Witness_____

This action appeals to all members of the committee. They believe that it would inform clients of their rights at the beginning of their hospital stay and instill the idea that their questions would be welcomed and answered in a clear way.

The second decision made by the committee is to endorse the following suggestion as unit policy:

Each time clients start on a new medication they will be informed of the benefits and untoward effects in a simple, clear way. At this time they will be invited and encouraged to ask any questions.

The committee takes a lot of time to arrive at this decision. None of the committee members has difficulty with the suggestion of telling clients about the benefits of medications, but they are reluctant to explain the potential hazards. After looking at the issue from many angles, all members agree that it is unfair to give clients only half of the picture. A compromise is drawn whereby all concur that only the most likely side effects will be explained to clients and the probability of their occurrence will be specified. Any known corrective action will also be made known to clients (such as taking a laxative for constipation, drinking extra fluids and chewing gum for dryness in the mouth, and avoiding abrupt movements for vertigo).

Committee members agree that the workload for launching this new policy will be shared between physicians and nurses. A physician prescribing a new medication will be responsible for explaining the rationale, benefits, and risks to clients, and will invite questions. This delegation will mean that nurses alone will not incur the extra time that implementing this policy will demand.

In addition, it has been decided that the medication nurse will follow up the physician's explanation when the first dose of the medication is administered. At that time the nurse will find out what the clients understand about the benefits and risks, confirm the facts, correct the errors, and invite any further questions. Sharing the responsibility between physicians and nurses makes the time commitment feasible for both parties.

The committee stresses that no health professional should be expected to remember the side effects of a multitude of medications. Referring to pharmaceutical references and consulting with the hospital pharmacist are encouraged.

The resolutions arrived at by the committee are satisfactory to all team members and are feasible from an administrative point of view.

9. The process does not stop at the point of agreeing on a resolution. Once the plan is implemented, a follow-up evaluation must be carried out to determine if the healthcare team remains satisfied with the implementation of the resolution. Questions to consider in completing this evaluation might include the following:
   - Do those who felt strongly that clients have a right to know about side effects believe that clients are being correctly informed?
   - Do those who objected because it could be time consuming and frightening for clients believe that the new plan avoids these negative consequences?
   - Are clients of the opinion that their rights are being respected?
   - Is the resolution being carried out without undue drawbacks in terms of cost effectiveness and staffing patterns?

In this example the committee decides to meet 6 weeks after the resolution has been adopted to evaluate its effectiveness.

This healthcare team handled its conflict using a win–win conflict-resolution strategy. All sides were asked to contribute their opinions to resolve the conflict. This action was assertive because it prevented any one side from coloring the picture or totally biasing the issue. It was responsible because it considered all the data available in the conflict situation: thoughts and feelings of both parties and objective data from a legal perspective.

Conflict Situation Involving Two Team Members

In contrast to the previous situation, conflict situations can be isolated to a small segment of the healthcare team. An example in which two team members are in conflict is examined next.

Example: You and David are two nursing students on the same medical unit in a general hospital. You are a student in an early stage of your clinical experience and David is in his graduating year. You are studying the concept of loss and its effects on body image. You wish to have Mr. Partain as your client because he has recently had a severe myocardial infarction and it is unlikely that he will be able to resume his former job. Because he has suffered a loss in physical function that affects other areas of his life, he would make an excellent candidate for your assignment.

> David has been assigned as Mr. Partain's nurse and has been caring for him for the past 3 days. When you ask David if he would switch and let you take on Mr. Partain's care, David refuses on the grounds that he needs to learn about postcardiac care for an assignment he is doing.
>
> At the moment, Mr. Partain is the most suitable candidate for both these students. There is a conflict over limited resources in this situation.

1. The first step is to uncover all the information about the conflict. Accomplishing this task involves being open and listening actively. One technique for ensuring that you really understand the conflict from the other's point of view is to reflect with empathy each statement your colleague makes. Here is an example:

David: "I think we have a problem here because I need to continue my care of Mr. Partain to understand how postcardiac clients adjust to the limited activity level and cope with the fear of resuming normal functioning. I can't change with you."

At this point, it would be tempting for you to argue that you too need to study Mr. Partain's recovery to understand his loss. Such a defensive approach would escalate your conflict. Instead, to understand the conflict from David's point of view, all you are allowed to do at this point is to reflect his thoughts and feelings with empathy. You will soon get your turn to state things from your point of view.

You: "You want to continue nursing Mr. Partain for a longer period of time so that you will really understand the reaction of postcardiac patients to changes in their activity levels."

This response allows your colleague to feel understood and encourages him to reveal more of his point of view.

David: "This is one of my last assignments before I graduate and I'm afraid if I give up Mr. Partain now I will not find another postcardiac client with whom to do my assignment."

You: "I can see why you do not wish to switch with me. You're concerned that Mr. Partain may turn out to be the last client with a postcardiac regimen that you encounter before graduation, and you need this experience."

In addition to allowing David to feel understood, reflecting with empathy obliges you to fully understand the conflict from his point of view. Without this information, you could not come up with the most effective resolution.

You are entitled to describe the conflict from your point of view, and you therefore explain to David the importance of Mr. Partain to your own client assignment. You have no control over whether David will listen with empathy to your side of the conflict, but your previous active listening will increase the chances.

2. Once you understand the conflict, the next step is to work out a satisfactory resolution. The resolution most acceptable to both you and David (to be Mr. Partain's primary nurse) is mutually incompatible. You need to generate another suitable resolution. Unlike the situation in the first example, there is limited time in which to do so. You propose the following suggestions to David:
   - When David is off duty, you will take over as the nurse in charge of Mr. Partain's care.
   - You will share with David any information you have on loss, as it applies to the postcardiac client, in return for being able to ask him questions about Mr. Partain's adjustment.

David accepts your suggestions and offers the following ones that might be helpful to you:

- You can be present when he is talking to Mr. Partain (if the client agrees) so that you can apply some of what he gleans to your study of the concepts of loss and body image.
- You can consider the case of Mrs. Tenn, a diabetic client on the unit, who is upset that her diabetes prevents her from becoming pregnant again. Mrs. Tenn might make a suitable client for your study of loss.
- He will give you a copy of his paper when it is completed, since your topics overlap and you might find it helpful.

This brainstorming has generated several possible resolutions that have benefits for both of you. If you and David adopt all the suggestions, both of you will gain more than you could have if you each went your separate ways. In addition to achieving your learning goals, you both will have the opportunity to learn from each other and possibly develop a closer friendship.

3. After adopting any resolution to a conflict, it is important to check to see if the plan continues to meet your expectations. The bottom line in this situation is that both you and David complete your assignments. Any additional happenings will be bonuses.

You can see that two of the important processes in effective conflict resolution are empathy and problem solving. Making these two strategies influential in your conflict-resolution approach ensures that you will be assertive and responsible.

The Multigenerational Team

Nursing involves unique challenges and opportunities in the blend of team members from different generations. Misperceptions about the motivation of nurses older or younger can cause conflict when we expect everyone to have our point of view. Our workforce has traditionalists or veterans, born before 1944; Baby Boomers, born in 1944–1960; Generation X, born in 1961–1980; and the Net Generation or the Millennial Generation, born in 1981–2000 (Anthony, 2006; Kupperschmidt, 2006; Sherman, 2006; Weston, 2006).

Although depending on generalizations about different generations can be problematic, it is helpful to begin to look at some commonalities among these four groups. Traditionalists were raised to value the Protestant work ethic, seeing nursing as a "calling." They pride themselves on doing a good job, believing in discipline and respect. They are team players and realists. Boomers were raised more permissively and were encouraged to be independent, seeing nursing as a "profession." They are idealists, inner-directed, and self-absorbed. The Generation X was raised in two-career families, may have been latch-key children, may have lived in a single parent home, and having seen no evidence of job security in nursing, see themselves as free agents with a responsibility to build skills for their own marketability. They have seen their parents' commitment to work not paying off in their professional or personal life. They want balance and respect for their personal priorities (Kupperschmidt, 2000, 2006). The Millennial Generation has been raised with digital technology and multiculturalism, with their childhood protected and family supported with preschool and after-school programs, seeing nursing as an occupation or job in which there should be cutting-edge technology and a quick response to problems (Kupperschmidt, 2006; Weston, 2006).

Conflict arises when nurses from one generation blame the other for having "an attitude" rather than a different world view based on different life experiences. The framework of CARE (Clarify, Articulate, Request, Encourage) confrontations, discussed in Chapter 23, is a helpful approach to beginning dialogue about differences, perceptions, and expectations. Traditionalists bring attention to details and best use of resources. Boomers can assist with consensus building and mentoring. Nurses from Generation X bring the entrepreneurial spirit and skill with technology. The Millennial Generation is sensitive to different cultures and is comfortable with new technology (Kupperschmidt, 2006). Nurses who begin to see these differences as gifts to round out the skills of the team will be able to broaden their perspective and work better as a team with the goal of quality patient care and high team spirit.

Conflict Resolution and the Nursing Profession

Conflict can be a positive force for nursing if it is used to foster growth-producing change in the profession and in the organizations in which nurses work. In addition to being knowledgeable about managing conflicts, nurses must develop a positive attitude toward conflict by recognizing the potential gains to be realized from it. We need to become more astute at predicting potential conflicts. A study of the complex needs of healthcare teams indicated that team members expect nurses to communicate clearly to ensure quality decisions and to promote team synergy (Propp et al, 2010). People are imperfect communicators, and this imperfection can generate conflict (Mayer, 2000). Misunderstandings, lack of clarity, and discomfort with differences can fuel conflict. Nurses who can keep their perspective and sense of humor will be able to grow through change.

> *Remember: Patience gets short late in any shift.*
>
> **Hammerschmidt and Meador (1993)**
>
> **WIT&***Wisdom*

Moments of Connection . . .
When "Just Listen to the Doctor" Won't Work

"As a pain management nurse, I was concerned about a very sick client who needed a refill for his morphine pump. Our physician said the client had to come into the clinic. Other staff said that since I work full-time, the doctor would not get reimbursement if the client did not make a clinic visit, I should 'just listen to the doctor.' I told the doctor that I could do a home visit and do the refill there. He gave his permission, and I received an orientation from the home health agency staff. I visited the home four times to refill the pump as the dosage was increased. The client and his wife were so happy. He died last month. Yes, it would have been easier to comply without question, but even though everyone anticipated that there would be a problem, there really was no conflict, just a difference of opinion."

Reflections On . . .

Managing Team Conflict Assertively and Responsibly

Consider what you read about team conflict. What conflict have you observed in the clinical setting? How do you assess your own skills at managing conflict? Answer the following questions.

What? . . .
Write one thing you learned from this chapter.

So What? . . .
How will this affect your nursing practice?

Now What? . . .
How will you implement this new knowledge or skill?

Think about it . . .

Practicing Managing Team Conflict Assertively and Responsibly

Exercise 1   **QSEN**

Observe interactions among the multiple team members involved in caring for your client. Describe the interactions concerning how differences of opinion or conflict are handled. Select one example to describe how it was handled.

- How would you describe the interactions and relationships?
- Is there evidence of hierarchy?
- What could be improved?
- What lessons can you learn?
- How did these interactions affect safety?
- What impact will this have on future interactions?

QSEN Competencies: Teamwork and Collaboration; Safety

Exercise 2

Work in groups of three for this exercise. One person takes the "pro" position on the issue, one takes the "con" position on the issue, and the third person acts as coach. You are presented with a conflict situation, and it is the task of "pro" and "con" to resolve the conflict in an assertive and responsible way. The coach will help "pro" and "con" to resolve the issue using a win–win approach.

Guidelines for "Pro" and "Con"

1. Use a systematic problem-solving approach to the conflict you are attempting to resolve.
2. In the data collection phase remember to delve into your own—as well as others'—thoughts and feelings about the conflict.
3. In the resolution-generating phase remember to allow as many suggestions to surface as possible before you make your final decision.
4. The resolution you choose must be one that is agreeable to both. "Pro" and "con" must agree that the resolution satisfies both parties.
5. For the purposes of this exercise you must follow one additional rule: whenever your colleague speaks, you must reflect with empathy on what he or she has said so that your colleague will know you fully understand his or her point of view.

Guidelines for the Coach

1. It is your job to remind "pro" and "con" to use a win–win problem-solving approach in their attempts to resolve the conflict.
2. You have the responsibility to remind "pro" and "con" to use empathic responses with each other after each speaks. Do not let them proceed with their negotiation until the listener has used empathy to show that he or she understands the other's position. (For instance, if "con" has just argued against "pro's" point of view, before "pro" can defend this position, "pro" must acknowledge "con's" perspective.)

Here are three situations involving conflict. So that each of you has the opportunity to play the role of "pro," "con," and the coach, each of you takes a different role in the three conflict situations.

Situation 1. A conflict of values compounded by limited resources. You are two members of the awards selection committee for your school of nursing. You have one task remaining: to select the student in your class who has demonstrated the best clinical practice. You have narrowed the choice to two candidates; however, there is only one prize for this category, and you must agree on one student.

"Pro's" position: You believe the prize should go to Ms. James because she has consistently demonstrated excellent charting and made useful suggestions about the management of her clients' care at case conferences. She is motivated to encourage her clients, and she has given them consistently courteous, caring nursing.

"Con's" position: You disagree with your colleague's choice and would like to see this prize awarded to Mr. Timms, who you believe has gone beyond the call of duty in his nursing care. He has helped clients write letters and has spent time supporting family members of his clients. He is highly regarded by the nurses on the units for his ability to work in a cooperative manner.

Situation 2. A conflict of goals. You work on a surgical unit in your hospital. There is a movement to allow clients to read their own charts. All staff on your unit have been asked to put forth their views on this proposed policy. You and your colleague have opposing opinions.

"Pro's" position: You have a strong belief that clients should be permitted to see anything written on their charts. You are convinced that the charts are really the property of the clients; after all, it is their health that is being charted. You would like to have access to your chart if you were a client.

"Con's" position: You think it is absolutely unreasonable that clients should have access to their charts. You think it would lead to all kinds of problems. For one thing, clients would not understand the medical jargon and might misinterpret information in their charts. Considerable time would be wasted trying to write in a way that clients would understand. In your view nurses and physicians are the experts and clients should have some faith that they will create an accurate document of their care.

Debriefing Questions

1. What was the most difficult aspect of using the win–win conflict-resolution approach?
2. What benefits are there to the win–win approach to resolving conflicts?

Exercise 3

The whole class can participate in this exercise. The goal of this exercise is to resolve a conflict that involves the entire healthcare team.

Your psychiatric unit has been asked to participate in an investigation to study the effects of a newly developed antidepressant. This mood-elevating drug is not yet available on the market because it requires the final phase of testing with human subjects. Your unit has been asked to participate in a study in which half of the depressed clients will be given this new experimental drug and the others will receive a placebo. Researchers will document the effects of the drugs (benefits and untoward reactions) on your client population. Your healthcare team must decide today if it will agree to participate in this study. Six volunteers are needed to role-play the following positions on the healthcare team:

Head nurse: The head nurse is totally against doing research on human subjects. The nurse is adamant that the clients on the unit should not be requested to participate in this study. "We are in the business of helping people, not experimenting on them. Our credibility in the eyes of our consumers will be in question if we get involved in this experiment."

Physician: The physician strongly favors the research. "The only way to achieve new frontiers of excellence in client care is through research."

Staff nurse 1: This nurse is dubious about asking clients to participate in research. "When people are depressed they cannot make the most informed decisions. They might think they have to volunteer to get good healthcare from us."

Staff nurse 2: This nurse supports research in psychiatry and believes your unit should set an example by completing this study. "Wonderful cures have come from clinical research. Psychiatric research has taken a back seat to medical research for too long."

Occupational therapist: The occupational therapist sees so many immobilized depressed clients who take so long to recover from depression that he or she welcomes any research that might discover a more effective treatment for depression. "We should try anything that will help our depressed clients."

Social worker: The social worker is dubious about putting the clients and their families under one more stress at an already stressful time. "We don't know if this new drug will do any good, and it might do harm. Why should our clients and their families have that possibility to worry about?"

This team has opposing points of view about whether to engage in the drug research. This controversy represents a conflict of values.

The task of the team is to resolve the conflict using the win–win approach. As a team you must use the problem-solving approach, and each member must attempt to be assertive in his or her negotiations.

The rest of the class observes the team in its deliberations and is prepared to make comments on their conflict resolution procedure.

The team should take 30 to 40 minutes to complete its resolution.

Debriefing Questions

1. What factors enhanced the team's ability to use a win–win approach to resolve this conflict?
2. What factors made it difficult for the team to use an assertive and responsible approach to resolve this conflict?
3. Was the team able to decide on a resolution that was satisfactory to all team members?
4. If the team did not get to the point of resolving the conflict in the 40 minutes of the role playing, how would you rate its progress in terms of assertiveness and responsible communication?

Exercise 4

In your journal, make a list of people in your professional and personal life who represent each of the four generations discussed. Reflect upon where you fit in the generations and write an entry about differences you have seen in behavior or attitude, assumptions you have made, and what you learn from beginning to understand the four generations.

References

Anthony M: Overview and summary: the multigenerational workforce: boomers and Xers and Nets, oh my! *Online J Issues Nurs* 11(2):11, 2006.

Beckett CD, Kipnis G: Collaborative communication: integrating SBAR to improve quality/patient safety outcomes, *Journal for Healthcare Quality: Promoting Excellence in Healthcare* 31(5):19, 2009.

Chadwick MM: Creating order out of chaos, *AORN J* 91(1):154, January 2010.

Chapman KB: Improving communication among nurses, patients, and physicians, *Am J Nurs* 109(Suppl 11):21, 2009.

Clark PR: Teamwork: building healthier workplaces and providing safer patient care, *Crit Care Nurs Q* 32(3):221, 2009.

Corless IB, Michel TH, Nicolas M, et al: Educating health professions students about issues involved in communicating effectively: a novel approach, *J Nurs Educ* 48(7):367, 2009.

Cushnie P: Conflict: developing resolution skills, *AORN J* 47(3):732, 1988.

Flanagan L: *What you need to know about today's workplace: a survival guide for nurses*, Washington, DC, 1995, American Nurses Association.

Hammerschmidt R, Meador CK: *A little book of nurses' rules*, Philadelphia, 1993, Hanley & Belfus.

Harrington-Mackin D: *The team building tool kit: tips, tactics, and rules for effective workplace teams*, New York, 1994, American Management Association.

Kinder JS: Conflict and diploma nursing education. In *Management of conflict*, New York, 1981, National League for Nursing.

Kohn L, Corrigan J, Donaldson M, editors, for the Committee on Quality Health Care in America, Institute of Medicine: *To err is human: building a safer health care system*, Washington, D.C., 2000, National Academy Press.

Kupperschmidt BR: Multigenerational employees: strategies for effective management, *Health Care Manager* 19(1):65, 2000.

Kupperschmidt BR: Address multigenerational conflict: mutual respect and confronting as strategy, *Online J Issues Nurs* 11(2):14, 2006.

Lamontagne C: Intimidation: a concept analysis, *Nurs Forum* 45(1): 54, January-March, 2010.

Marick MF, Albright RR: *The complete guide to conflict resolution in the workplace*, New York, 2002, AMACOM.

Mayer BS: *The dynamics of conflict resolution: a practitioner's guide*, San Francisco, 2000, Jossey-Bass.

McKeon LM, Cunningham PD, Oswaks JSD: Improving patient safety: patient-focused, high-reliability team training, *J Nurs Care Q* 24(1):76, 2009.

Propp KM, Apker J, Zabava Ford WS, et al: Meeting the complex needs of the health care team: identification of nurse—team communication practices perceived to enhance patient outcomes, *Qual Health Res* 20(1):15, 2010.

Sherman RO: Leading a multigenerational nursing workforce: issues, challenges and strategies, *Online J Nurs* 11(2):13, 2006.

Tekleab AG, Quigley NR, Tesluk PE: A longitudinal study of team conflict, conflict management, cohesion, and team effectiveness, *Group & Organization Management* 34(2):170, April 2009.

Thomas CM, Bertram E, Johnson D: The SBAR communication technique: teaching nursing students professional communication skills. *Nurse Educ* 34(4):176, 2009.

Vivar CG: Putting conflict management into practice: a nursing case study, *J Nurs Admin* 14(3):201, 2006.

Weston MJ: Integrating generational perspectives in nursing, *Online J Nurs Issues* 11(2):12, 2006.

Zhani EE: Joint Commission Center for Transforming Healthcare tackles miscommunication among caregivers: top U.S. hospitals identify causes, develop targeted solutions to save lives, News Release, October 21, 2010. http://www.centerfortransforminghealthcare.org/news/display.aspx?newsid=23. Accessed June 1, 2011.

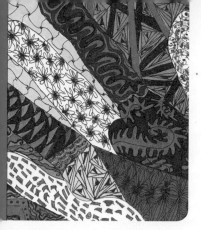

Chapter 29

Communicating at the End of Life

The fear of death follows from the fear of life. A man who lives fully is prepared to die at any moment.

Mark Twain

Objectives

1. Identify fears about communicating with clients near the end of life

2. Discuss strategies for caring communication near the end of life

3. Identify strategies for creative expression for clients at the end of life and their families

4. Discuss the role of self-care for the nurse when working with clients at the end of life and families

5. Participate in exercises to build strategies for caring communication with clients near the end of life and their families

Considerations for the Nurse in End-of-Life Care

In caring for people at the end of life, you will hear two terms you need to understand: *hospice care* and *palliative care*. "Hospice is a program of care provided across a variety of settings and based on the understanding that dying is a part of the normal life cycle. Hospice promotes the idea of 'living until you die'" (American Association of Colleges of Nursing and City of Hope National Medical Center, 2000, p. MI-8). Hospice, considered a philosophy of care, supports families during the dying process and in bereavement (Martens, 2009). Hospice care is provided in the home, residential settings, and designated hospice houses. This movement is credited to Dame Cicely Saunders and is the foundation of the emerging field of palliative care. There can be Medicare and Medicaid support for hospice care, which is usually offered in what is believed to be the last 6 months of life. Palliative care is "the active total care of patients whose disease is not responsive to curative treatment. Control of pain, of other symptoms, and of psychological, social and spiritual problems is paramount. The goal of palliative care is achievement of the best possible quality of life for patients and their families" (World Health Organization, 1990).

Why might you, as a nurse, be uncomfortable or unsure about how to communicate with clients who are approaching the end of their lives? Stop a moment and consider this and then see Box 29-1 and reflect on these ideas.

There are several reasons (see Box 29-1).

Yes, when we work with the dying, we can no longer deny our own mortality. Yet, from becoming clearer about the finite nature of life, we can make better choices about how to live our own lives with

329

From American Association of Colleges of Nursing and City of Hope National Medical Center: *Training program facility guide*, Duarte, Calif, 2000, End-of-Life Nursing Education Consortium (ELNEC); and Matzo ML, Sherman DW, Sheehan DC, et al: Communication skills for end-of-life nursing care, *Nurs Educ Perspect* 24(4):176, 2003.

Box 29-1	*When It Is Hard to Open the Patient's Door . . .*

- We are afraid of facing our own mortality.
- We are afraid that we won't know the "right" thing to say.
- We are afraid that we will say the wrong thing.
- We may have little personal experience with someone who is dying.
- We may have unresolved grief over losses and deaths in our own lives.
- We may be afraid that our emotions will overwhelm us and that we might cry.
- We may be afraid that we will be blamed for the person's death.
- We may be afraid that we will dishonor the family or client because we do not understand the client's culture.
- We may be uncomfortable with just "being" with the client rather than "doing" things.
- We may simply not know what to do and it is the not knowing that frightens us.

more beauty, connection, and meaning. When we accept our own mortality we can be more fully present for our clients. We can listen without fear of being inadequate at this sacred time in life . . . and the listening is enough. We are not called to give answers but to give of ourselves as a companion for the journey (Nouwen, 2005).

Why is it hard to watch someone we love or have come to love die? People we love become a part of us. When they die, it is as if a part of us has died, too. This is the source of the grief, the separation. On holidays or birthdays or the anniversary of the death of a loved one, we are more clearly aware of the loved one's absence. By remembering them, we make them a part of ourselves again, we re-member them. "Remembering them means letting their spirits inspire our daily lives" (Nouwen, 2005, p. 205). Some people experience an even greater closeness after death. Grief counselors may encourage the bereaved to talk to the person who has died and listen to what they think would be the

response and may suggest reflecting on how knowing the person changed his or her life (Loomis, 2009).

Moments of Connection . . .
I Felt Broken and Helpless . . . a Student Nurse Faces Death

On the oncology unit, I cared for a young mother in her 30s whose cancer had metastasized to her bones. She was such a sweet wife and mother. All the prayers I could pray just kept coming to my mind because I did not want her to die. Up until that point, she had been a very strong person and accepted what was going on as God's will. When I came into her room, she burst into tears. I felt so broken and helpless. I sat at the end of her bed, held her hand, and rubbed her leg for comfort. She cried and cried as I remained silent for about 20 minutes. She talked about her fears of dying and leaving her three little girls and her husband. We cried together and I had the opportunity to educate her about hospice. She was discharged to hospice the next day. We hugged each other as we said goodbye and I felt as if I had been a part of something so special. I will never forget her.

Caring Communication Near the End of Life

The Process

Communication at the end of life is a process of interactions through which a relationship is created. These interactions are an exchange of thoughts and ideas and feelings, communicated verbally and nonverbally. "Dying is more than a medical event; it is a spiritual event" (Young and Koopsen, 2005, p. 175). Staff and family can help create an environment in which personal transformation, reconciliation, and the expression of love can occur. Essential qualities of being with the dying are acceptance, being calm and open-minded, listening deeply, and proactive intervention, advocacy, on behalf of clients and their families (Norlander, 2008; Seno, 2010). Consider the following:

1. Be present for the person, relating to the person and not the illness.

2. Pay attention by listening, without judgment, to the needs, wishes, and personal wisdom of the dying person. Compassionate listening means setting aside your own discomfort and those automatic, reassuring responses that help the listener more than the person who is dying. Compassionate listening is letting the person talk in whatever way they need to talk (Davis et al, 2004). It is OK to laugh with your client or just sit silently.

3. Show compassion by gentle touch, using lotion on your hands, or giving a backrub. Offer a cool cloth when your client is perspiring.

4. Create a peaceful environment, perhaps lowering the lights or opening the blinds to let in the light if desired. These considerations create a climate in which thoughts and feelings can be shared openly (Box 29-2) (Corr et al, 2003; Young and Koopsen, 2005).

It is interesting and, perhaps, comforting to know that research confirms the existence of deathbed visions and deathbed coincidences, involving the appearance or apparition of a dying person to someone close to them at the time of death, or a strong feeling that the person has died and is "all right." This supports what appears to be a need for "spiritual connection and meaning, requiring compassionate understanding and respect from those who provide end-of-life care" (Fenwick and Brayne, 2011, p. 7).

Wisdom from a Hospice Nurse

As a nurse author, I have had the added privilege of the experience of working part-time as an expressive arts facilitator with hospice clients, their family, and staff. As are other nurses, I am in awe of the ability to do this work as our mission in nursing. After 5 years of experience of contact with one nurse whose comfort with dying and touching support of patients are remarkable, I asked her to share her observations, experience, and beliefs with you. This is the demonstration of how one hospice nurse sees her work and makes sense of it. Elizabeth Labatte shares her experiences throughout this chapter where noted (Boxes 29-3 and 29-4). When you understand more about the dying process, you can better reassure the client and inform the family, who value sensitive, specific presentation of what to expect at the end of life (Boucher et al, 2010; Zomorodi and Lynn, 2010).

Box 29-2	*My Commitment to You and Your Family When I Care for You at the End of Life*

- I will be truthful.
- I will not abandon you.
- I will ask you what is important to you.
- I will do my best to help you meet these goals.
- I will respond to your questions in a timely manner.
- I will ask you what you need and what I can do for you.
- I will be an active part of your healthcare team.
- I will seek help when I don't know what to do.
- I will reflect on how I would want a beloved family member to be treated.
- I will listen to you with compassion.
- I will work on my own issues with grief to better serve you.
- I will pay attention to my own self-care so I can pay full attention to you.
- I will bring my best self to you, including my tears and my laughter.

Modified from End-of-Life Nursing Education Consortium (ELNEC): *Training program facility guide*, Duarte, Calif, 2000, Consortium American Association of Colleges of Nursing and City of Hope National Medical Center.

The bitterest tears shed over graves are for words left unsaid and deeds left undone.

Harriett Beecher Stowe

WIT&*Wisdom*

Wisdom Sharing from One Hospice Client

People at the end of life or dealing with life-threatening illness may want to share their wisdom. Cancer survivors benefit from exchanging support, wisdom, and coping strategies. One client, in fourth-stage ovarian cancer, used her storytelling and writing skills in a newsletter to her Cancer Connection Prayer Group. She collected stories of answered prayer in her life as part of her legacy, a way to inspire others. I met this client in her home; she had vomited seven times the night before, but she got out of bed to give me copies

Box 29-3 — When Death Is Near: A Hospice Nurse's Observations for the Nurse, Client, and Family

Some know for months that the end is coming, but don't talk about it. Some believe that to speak of it is to hasten it. They may see death negatively, not be ready for it, or not have spiritual beliefs and may be afraid. Some people may withdraw as they become aware of their impending death. They may be quieter as they process and evaluate their life and have less interest in worldly things such as television, and then family and friends. They may nap more and then may sleep most of the day. Family may not recognize this process. Now touch and facial expression become important. Nutrition is less important as the body shuts down. At this time feeding a person more than they desire causes more pain and suffering. Teach the family that this is a natural process. Offer liquids and soft food.

Early on, the person can't hold his or her eyes open, but can still be awakened. Some professionals believe seeing departed family members is a hallucination. I believe the person is more easily confused as he or she wanders from this world to the next. The person often speaks to deceased loved ones, reaches with hands, picks items in the air, and talks about unfamiliar places and events. Blood pressure may lower the pulse and respirations may increase or decrease dramatically. Perspiration increases, skin may be cool and moist, and its color may change from normal to flushed, or cool and blue, or yellow. Nail beds may be blue. Breathing may stop only to restart with abdominal breaths and pursed lips. With congestion comes the "death rattle," fluid that the person may be unable to clear, sounding more upsetting than it is to the client.

There may be restlessness from less oxygen and a sense that the end is near. Just before the active dying process, a brief energy surge may occur, giving family false hope. Some believe this is spiritual energy expressed as physical energy. Now eyes may be open but unseeing. Consciousness may decrease until the person is unresponsive. The sense of hearing may be acute and the person may feel your touch. Continue to communicate with the person until death. Treat a person with respect and dignity up until and even past the very last breath.

© Elizabeth Labbate, MS, RN, LMT, CHPN. Used with permission.

Box 29-4 — This I Believe about Death and Dying: A Gift from One Hospice Nurse's Experience of the Mystery of Death

As patients enter the final hours, some need direction to leave this world. They talk about "wanting to go," believe that they have accomplished all that they need to in this lifetime, and are ready for "God" to take them; they feel frustrated that they do not die just then. When their bodies are shutting down, if the person believes in a life after death, tell them to look for their deceased loved ones and to take their hands. I remember a patient telling me that his sister was visiting. He told her to lose weight. She had been dead a year. He was so intent on telling her what to do that he missed seeing the hand she extended. We were able to redirect him to take her hand. He passed quickly and peacefully. Many patients live until all issues are resolved and then pass peacefully. Others, after a life review, make remarkable transitions in resolving conflict. Some stop years of fighting and decide that "all is forgiven." Often, the patient is given an understanding of why situations happened that they were not privy to during their lifetime. Some fight until the last moment, saying, "I'm not going," as if talking with someone. Patients who have not decided that it is their time to leave may have a difficult time leaving. This is especially true of younger people. The person may fight until the body cannot sustain life, lapse into a coma, or collapse and die.

Personal choices become evident. Some die with their family present. Others die alone. Having the personal choice of time determines who is present at our death. Some tell me it is too painful for family to be present. Family members might sit vigil for 72 hours nonstop, leave the room for a few minutes, and the loved one dies. Or the patient will hold on longer than expected, until family finally arrives and greets them, and then may die within a few minutes.

© Elizabeth Labbate, MS, RN, LMT, CHPN. Used with permission.

Having recounted other times when her prayers had been answered, she wrote: "I had begun to talk out loud to God and sing, too. What is the proper response when God shows up in your life to be your Companion and Friend? I wasn't alone. My silent witness was my little boy, Evan, who was 3 years old and absorbing everything that was going on. One day Evan and I were going for a walk when he remarked that he would really like some peanut butter when we got home. I told him we were out of peanut butter and tried to explain about money on payday; every Mom knows the kind of convoluted discussions it is possible to have with a 3 year old. Evan was silent for a moment and then said, 'But God could put money in the mailbox, couldn't he, Mom?' 'Oh yes,' I said. 'That would be no problem for God at all.'

We were gone several hours and when we returned, Evan said, 'Lift me up to the mailbox and see if God put any money in there.' I was thinking that Grandma would sometimes send a check for $30 and I thought that could possibly be there. Instead, Evan pulled out a blank envelope with four twenty-dollar bills.

'Hey,' Evan said, 'God gave us four dollars! Is that enough for peanut butter?' 'Yes,' I said, 'We have plenty for peanut butter and more besides. God didn't give us four dollars, but lots more.'

I took him across the street to the bank and asked the cashier to change the bills to ones. Then I handed the pile of cash to Evan. 'See, Doll . . . THAT is how much God gave us."

the client select words or images that are appealing and glue them to the background, helping whenever needed. Then, ask the client if a story comes to mind from the art. Families can be offered a time to create a memory box about their loved one. Cigar boxes serve as a surface for collage and a keepsake box for mementos.

You have been introduced to mandalas in the introduction of this text and on the front cover. Coloring mandala designs can be relaxing. Mandala coloring books are available. Find mandalas online to print at www.free-mandalas.com or by searching the images files on www.google.com. Offer colored pencils or colored markers.

Offer watercolors and watercolor paper. Having your client or family member simply paint lines of blue and green and purple can be self-soothing. Suggest that even imaging this process can help when you have difficulty sleeping (Hayes, 2006).

Before the client is actively dying, favorite music may assist with reminiscence and storytelling. When you don't know the client well, you can try using the client's age to calculate in what year the patient was 20 years old and introduce music of that era. Closer to the time of death, music that has been found to be helpful comes from the field of music thanatology, a subspecialty of palliative care, such as *Rosa Mystica*, a CD from the Chalice of Repose Project (Schroeder-Sheker, 2006).

Encourage clients and family to keep a journal or write poetry if that appeals to them. If you decide to give a journal to a patient or family member, have them write something on the first page to take away the fear of getting started or "messing it up." Poetry magnets can help. Have the person just choose words that appeal to them and arrange them into a poem, assuring the person that there is no right way to make a poem and that rhyme is unnecessary.

of her writing that had not been published and chose this story to share (see Box 29-5).

Strategies for Creative Expression

The expressive arts offer creative ways for clients and families to access emotion. Offering materials for collage from magazines can evoke personal stories and create legacy pieces for the family. Bring a few magazines that might be of interest to your client as well as scissors, glue, and colored paper or mat board. Have

 Moments of Connection . . .
A psychiatrist working with clients for over 30 years talks about helping them deal with their fears about dying, saying this was not taught in his medical training. When asked, "where will I go when I die?" a response he gives is that when we die we return to the place we were before we are born (Yalom, 2009).

Moments of Connection . . .

Sarah, a 77-year-old woman with lung cancer, was a patient in a hospice house. I offered her art materials for card-making and as she painted she began to talk about her life. She seemed sad and we talked about to whom she might send the card. I asked her if there was anyone in her life with whom there were things left unsaid. She teared up and said she wished she could just tell her daughter that she loved her and that she knew her daughter always felt criticized by her. We talked about how she might be able to do that. Later she arranged for her daughter to visit and afterward talked about how much better she felt.

Moments of Connection . . .

Suzanne, a 71-year-old hospice patient, had just been admitted to an assisted living facility and spoke little. She answered questions vaguely due to memory loss. Her affect was bland and she seldom made eye contact. The expressive arts facilitator from hospice talked with her about what music she liked from the 1950s and brought a CD. Suzanne brightened and was able to sing all the lyrics to her favorite, "Chantilly Lace," by the Big Bopper. She began to talk about how much she loved the opera Carmen and that living near New York City, she had been taught about opera in junior high school and had taken field trips to the opera in the city. The facilitator was able to find a CD with selections from the opera. Suzanne became animated and related the story of the opera.

Self-Care for Nurses Working with Clients at the End of Life

Holistic self-care is the foundation of holistic nursing. As you care for yourself, so you care for your clients. As you care for yourself, so you care for your colleagues. When we work with clients and their families at the end of life, the experience touches us at a very deep level and calls upon us to give of ourselves in new ways. We stretch to grow. We ponder and reflect upon our own life and its meaning. We sigh a breath of relief that it is not our time or the time of our loved ones. We go home and tuck our children into bed more tightly. We look at our family and friends with softened eyes. We experience gratitude. All this takes energy and although, like all of nursing, this is noble work, we are not the only nurse who can be present. When we are off duty physically, we need to find ways to maintain healthy boundaries from our work. We do work hard and now we need to play hard. We need time for respite and activities with no social value, that are just *fun*.

Now, reread the strategies for creative expression and substitute nurse for client; creative expression is a valuable tool for self-care for the nurse. Nurses at international meetings of Sigma Theta Tau, the nursing honor society, were given an opportunity to submit examples of their own art making, including submissions such as visual arts, fabric art, prose, and poetry (Wendler, 2005). See Chapter 30 for more information on self-care.

Dame Cicely Saunders wrote, "How people die remains in the memories of those who live on." Let this theme guide you as you work with clients near the end of life. Ask yourself how you can contribute to a positive experience for the family, creating memories that can be carried into the bereavement period and beyond (Kuebler et al, 2002, p. 49).

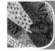

Reflections On . . .

Caring Communication in End-of-Life Care

Consider what you read about working with clients and families at the end of life. Answer the following questions.

What? . . .
Write one thing you learned from this chapter.

So What? . . .
How will this affect your nursing practice?

Now What? . . .
How will you implement this new knowledge or skill?

Think about it . . .

Practicing Caring Communication in End-of-Life Care

Exercise 1

In your journal, make a list of the people and activities that are important to you. Take a few moments to reflect on your thoughts and feelings concerning any of these that have been lost to you. Write a reflective journal entry in response of your thoughts and feelings to help you better understand clients at the end of life.

Exercise 2

Rent the movie *Tuesdays with Morrie*, the story of a man who wants to relate his experience at the end of life as a legacy. Watch the movie with several other students or colleagues and then discuss its implications for your work with clients at the end of life.

Exercise 3

Read the book *The Fall of Freddie the Leaf* by Leo Buscaglia, an allegory about life and death through the format of a children's book on the life of a leaf throughout the seasons. Write a reflective journal entry on what you learned in this comparison of the life of a person through the story of a leaf.

References

American Association of Colleges of Nursing and City of Hope National Medical Center: *Training program facility guide*, Duarte, Calif, 2000, End-of-Life Nursing Education Consortium (ELNEC).

Boucher J, Bova C, Sullivan-Bolyai S, et al: Next-of-kin's perspectives of end-of-life care, *J Hosp Palliat Nurs* 12(1):41, January/February 2010.

Corr CA, Nabe CM, Corr DM: *Death and dying, life and living*, ed 4, Belmont, Calif, 2003, Thomson/Wadsworth.

Davis M, Paleg K, Fanning P: *How to communicate workbook: powerful strategies for effective communication at work and home*, New York, 2004, MJF Books.

Fenwick P, Brayne S: End-of-life experiences: reaching out for compassion, communication, and connection—meaning of deathbed visions and coincidences, *Am J Hosp Palliat Care* 28(1):7, 2011.

Hayes PM: Art therapy and anxiety: healing through imagery, Cross Country Education seminar, Tampa, Fla, March 2006.

Kuebler KK, Berry PH, Heidrich DE: *End-of-life care: clinical practice guidelines*, Philadelphia, 2002, WB Saunders.

Loomis B: End-of-life issues: Difficult decisions and dealing with grief, *Nurs Clin North Am* 44(2):223, 2009.

Matzo ML, Sherman DW, Sheehan DC, et al: Communication skills for the end-of life nursing care, *Nurs Educ Perspect* 24(4):176, 2003.

Martens ML: A comparison of stress factors in home and inpatient hospice nurses, *J Hosp Palliat Care* 11(3):144, May/June 2009.

Norlander L: *To comfort always: a nurse's guide to end-of-life care*, Indianapolis, Ind, 2008, Sigma Theta Tau International.

Nouwen HJM: *The dance of life: weaving sorrows and blessings into one joyful step*, Notre Dame, Ind, 2005, Ave Maria Press.

Schroeder-Sheker T: *The Chalice of Repose Project* (website). http://www.chaliceofrepose.org/history.htm. Accessed June 1, 2011.

Seno VL: Being with dying: authenticity in end-of-life encounters, *Am J Hosp Palliat Care* 27:377, 2010. (Originally published online May 3, 2010.)

Wendler C, editor: *The heART of nursing: expressions of creative art in nursing*, New York, 2005, Sigma Theta Tau International.

World Health Organization: Cancer pain relief and palliative care. Report of a WHO Expert Committee, *World Health Organ Tech Rep Ser* 804:1, 1990.

Yalom ID: *Staring at the sun: overcoming the terror of death*, San Francisco, 2009, Jossey-Bass.

Young C, Koopsen C: *Spirituality, health, and healing*, Thorofare, N.J., 2005, SLACK Incorporated.

Zomorodi M, Lynn MR: Critical care nurses' behaviors with end-of-life-care, *J Hosp Palliat Care Nurs* 12(2):89, March/April 2010.

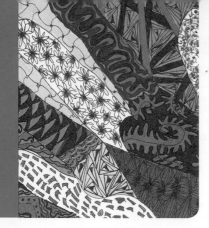

Chapter 30

Continuing the Commitment

Objectives

1. Examine proactive approaches to reality shock, the transition from student to graduate
2. Identify three competencies for achieving life balance
3. Identify strategies for renewal
4. Discuss the importance of commitment to nursing to continue to build communication skills

Putting It All Together

Take a deep breath and imagine yourself in the nursing role of which you dream. What will you be doing? How will you look? What will you feel? Where will you be? This chapter invites you to be proud of your accomplishments and to be confident about the contribution you are and will continue to be making. It encourages you to respect the challenge of making your way in the work world, to pay attention to specific, successful strategies that have helped those who have gone before you, and to continue your commitment to learning and growing through your day-to-day experiences.

As you become more comfortable with your ability to communicate, you will soon become increasingly aware of how complex a venture it is. Beyond the technique comes the art, the intuitive application of what you know. This concluding chapter asks you to consider the commitments necessary to move on in your chosen profession: to remain open and sensitive to the human condition, to renew your energy, and to embrace change. To do these, you must find balance in life as you explore the challenges of moving from the role of student to graduate: from transitioning from the clear expectations of school to the ambiguity of nursing practice; from a low nurse-to-client ratio to the conflicting needs of many patients; from, perhaps, a focused role as student to stressors from additional life changes such as marriage, having children, moving, and adjusting to a new, perhaps first, job (Tingle, 2001).

Reality Shock: the Transition to Nursing Practice

Marlene Kramer conducted a classic study of the problem of "reality shock," when young graduates find themselves in a work situation, thinking they were going to be prepared and finding that they were not (Kramer, 1974). Understanding these findings provides you with an opportunity to be more proactive in your approach to the work world, although it may not make it easier to deal with the emotions encountered in this transition toward personal and professional development. Although this may not be the exact situation in which you will find yourself, it is useful to examine her findings and the research that has followed.

As a student you learn how to be successful in the role of student, moving from novice to expert in that role by the time you graduate. In a new work setting, you again become the novice. Kramer describes the development of the professional–bureaucratic conflict, in which the nurse faces the challenge of not being able to give the desired amount of time to an individual client. Kramer identified four phases of this culture shock (Box 30-1).

Emotions you may experience during this transition include "exhilaration, anger, grief, excitement, resentment, nervousness, euphoria, self-doubt, or satisfaction" (Tingle, 2001). Understand that a range of feelings is normal. To deal with stress at this time, self-care is important. For example, take a break during your shift and eat your meal off the unit if possible, making sure that your clients' immediate needs are met before you leave them in someone else's care. Your confidence will grow over time. Be patient with yourself. Tingle (2001) summarizes transition strategies through the mnemonic, NURSES:

Never fail to ask for help!
Use available facility resources!
Reenergize with professional associations!
Stay in contact with friends!
Evaluate your own growth realistically!
Stay focused on your goals!

A study of 612 newly licensed registered nurses in New York identified several themes in these nurses' experience: colliding expectations between nurses' personal view of nursing and their lived experience; the need for speed and not enough time to get everything done and get to know the patients; high expectations and too much work and responsibility; mistreatment by physicians, rudeness, and criticism; and yet, a theme of hope, that after the first 6 months of difficult transition, things were better and the nurses were more resilient (Pellico et al, 2009). A study in Norway of job satisfaction and job values among new nurses found that the transition from school to work was less dramatic than initially assumed (Daehlen, 2008).

Box 30-1 | *Phases of Reality Shock*

1. *Honeymoon phase*: Enthusiasm, excitement, high energy
2. *Shock phase*: The realization that nursing is not what you expected: anger, frustration, disappointment, fatigue, being critical, having a negative life view
3. *Recovery phase*: A realization that there is more than one perspective in the work situation, returning sense of humor
4. *Resolution phase*: Choosing a way to resolve the conflict between the subcultures of school and work, with different values and emphasis. (Behaviors in this phase may include frequent job changes; fleeing work by returning to school; quitting nursing; burnout, the result of unresolved work conflict with chronic complaining; or Bicultural Adaptation, a constructive form of resolution that integrates both value systems.)

WIT&*Wisdom*

Employers want to recruit and retain high performers. Consider each new clinical rotation in school as a job audition. Pay attention to your appearance, integration of your knowledge and clinical skills, communication, and engagement in your work. Begin to build networks with nurse professionals and organizations. Consider working in unlicensed assistive positions if you work while in school or in the summers. Employers often give preference to candidates with such experience (Sherman and Dyess, 2010).

Proactive Approaches to Reality Shock: The Transition from Student to Nurse

Communication is important at this time of transition. When you have questions, be clear about what you are asking and take time to decide who is the most appropriate person to ask. More experienced staff may assume you know steps you do not, so don't hesitate to keep asking until you get the information you need. If a situation is urgent, communicate this. Listen carefully to answers you receive and repeat the answer to make sure your anxiety has not prevented you from listening.

Kramer (1974) offers the following suggestions to achieve Bicultural Adaptation: evaluate situations in the workplace by looking at all sides to the issue, consider how your behavior will affect other colleagues, and identify appropriate and attainable goals.

Other proactive strategies include the following: when interviewing for a job, inquire about the length of the orientation and internships or preceptor programs for new graduates (Dyess and Sherman, 2009); do your homework about the organization's philosophy and mission statement, available online; when you accept a position, ask questions about the history of the organization; focus on gaining a reputation for competence in skills and interpersonal relationships; identify someone who will understand what you are experiencing, and let you express your feelings, not someone with whom you work, and someone you trust to keep a confidence; expect to be tested as the "new kid on the block," and avoid being defensive; understand that other staff members also feel pressure and experience stress; keep a journal to record the thoughts, feelings, reflections, and ideas you have about how things could be changed, ideas you might share when you have earned the respect of your colleagues.

> *Stay the course. Light a star. Change the world where'er you are.*
>
> **Richard Le Gallienne**
>
> **WIT&** *Wisdom*

Achieving Generative Balance

Guterman (1994) proposes a model he calls *generative balancing*, which focuses on three competencies: "creating success, finding meaning, and renewal." "All three competencies are necessary for balancing, and the real thrill, the excitement of the ride—just as in life— comes from the movement, not from finding a steady-point" but from balance.

In a classic column, Ann Landers relates an essay that compares life to a journey on a train. The essay advises that the focus of life should not be the station, or the destination, but rather the journey itself.

Creating Success

To create success is to set goals, to see the station or the destination. Guzzetta (1998) compares her own journey toward holistic nursing practice to the weaving of a tapestry: "master weavers of a tapestry have described the weaving of a tapestry as a calling, as transformation, as healing, or as a sacred work." What would your tapestry of success as a nurse contain? How would you embellish and color it to reflect your unique contribution?

Achievement of success, however, is often not enough in itself. Balance comes from a life view that provides joy along the way, says Rabbi Harold Kushner. Consider his well known quotation "Nobody on his deathbed ever said, 'I wish I had spent more time on my business' (2002). Nursing provides many opportunities for success—clinical practice, administration, teaching, research, advanced practice—and many emerging roles for the nurse entrepreneur. Balance comes from attention to all three components of the model and setting the intention to care for yourself, knowing that the foundation of holistic nursing is self-care for the nurse.

Finding Meaning

Meaning for the Nurse

To find meaning is essential for the nurse. Arnold (1989) sees this process as crucial for the nurse to prevent burnout, which she proposes is an existential crisis, and for the patient, who needs the nurse in the role of "meaning maker." Arnold's work confirms what many career nurses have come to view as the essence of nursing.

Arnold (1989) suggests that many nursing students grow up with a set of values and beliefs that translate into rules and regulations. Faith may be seen as a gift that is tied to good behavior. Do the right things and all will be well. When nurses are faced with seemingly meaningless tragedies, "or an accumulation of stressors, the nurse's spiritual perspective is thrown off balance. Beliefs previously used no longer provide an accurate internal guide on which to base decisions." It may become hard to pray or attend religious services. Traditional passive beliefs in a higher power may "not necessarily lend any understandable meaning to life experience. If one thinks of spirituality in such narrow terms, the essence of spirituality as a relationship with a higher power is lost." Through the resolution of this existential crisis comes "a total acceptance and commitment to stewardship, anchored by a reasoned loyalty and trust in a higher purpose. What is needed is a broader perspective, a transcendent level of meaning that reorders the incomprehensible circumstances of pain and suffering that a nurse experiences on a daily basis." An examination of nurses' stories from their work with disenfranchised people, clients who frighten us or who are afraid, revealed four dimensions of meaning: the reward of meaning as overcoming challenges through facing our own fears and prejudices, the reward of meaning from a sense of having been called to the work, the reward of meaning as a legacy of caring connected with family experience or tragedy, and the reward of meaning from the experience of common humanity, the belief that each person has a right to care and respect (Zerwekh, 2000).

Kushner (2001) faced just such an existential crisis when his own child died of progeria, a disease of premature aging. He questioned his own beliefs: how could he, a rabbi, a good person, have such a senseless tragedy occur in his life? In his book *When Bad Things Happen to Good People*, he concludes that you cannot control the events in your life, only the attitude that you take toward life. Kushner discusses three ways that he found to give meaning to life: belong to people, accept pain as a part of life, and know that you have made a difference. These are all a part of your life as a nurse if you remain open and sensitive to the human condition (Kushner, 2002).

To belong to people is to have a few people who are a permanent part of your life, people with whom you share yourself. Nurses sometimes lament their poor relationships with family members. Until you can work through these relationships, claim close friends as new relatives.

To accept pain as a part of life is also to be able to experience the contrasting joy. To be fully present with a client or family member is to be open to sharing suffering but also to be open to rejoicing in the triumph of coping and changing in the face of crisis.

To know you have made a difference can be a comfort when you are unable to control the course of life's events. Savor the thank-you's you get. Save the notes and cards you receive and place them in a book. Later, these notes will bring you renewed joy and pride.

The Nurse as Meaning Maker

The ability to develop a belief system, an inner process, as a way of understanding or explaining events that seem beyond human understanding is reflected in interpersonal communication with clients and family. A nurse who isn't exactly sure what she believes reports that when a client's family was distressed, she spontaneously said, "There are some things that are beyond our understanding, but I believe that life has a purpose." Listen to colleagues as they comfort family and clients and you will experience a demonstration of their belief systems.

Moments of Connection...
Nursing ... Days of Wonder

"I worked in the intensive care unit and took care of an elderly man who was dying. He was a brilliant philosopher and teacher. We spent many evenings talking, and he touched me in ways I did not think were possible. He died one evening when I was not working. I was sad for days. One morning I saw his surgeon, who asked me if I would like to see the autopsy results. When I went with him, I was shocked to see we were in the actual autopsy. When I saw the body, I realized for the first time what death was all about. This body was just a shell, and his eyes were vacant. I knew all his experiences and stories and brilliant knowledge were with me and everyone else with whom he had come into contact. The experience allowed me to accept my father's death a few years later and to help me in my work with the dying."

Arnold (1989) advocates involvement as a part of life, but recognizes that detachment and renewal of energy are necessary to maintain personal wellness and the continued ability to nurture our own interpersonal relationships. Loss of meaning can cause spiritual distress, but setting impossible standards of perfection in your professional and personal life can be overwhelming and exhausting. The level of intimacy in communication in nursing can take its toll on energy reserves; thus attention to renewal is essential.

Renewing Energy

Now that the inevitable stressors facing nurses today have been discussed, it is time to actively consider how you can add energy, fun, and laughter to your life. Consider a body–mind–spirit approach.

The Body

Find a physical activity you like and do it on a regular basis, but not obsessively. Dance, play tennis, walk, or run; the list is endless. Start with 10 minutes twice a day—just move. Look in the mirror. Do you like what you see? Are you a role model for health and wellness? Do you see your body as sacred?

The Mind

As with a computer, the functioning of the mind is only as good as the data taken in. Choose music or movies or reading material that renew your energy. Add play and laughter and humor to your life (see Chapter 15). Embellish your world with beauty in your home. In a workshop for healthcare givers and volunteers in hospice and palliative care, three creative self-care strategies were introduced. Here are the strategies and a participant's comment regarding each: journal writing—"What I can do with words! I just needed to know where to start"; expressive art—"Being able to express myself in art puts me in touch with feelings I wasn't aware of"; music therapy—"Music gave me a sense of freedom I had forgotten I ever had" (Murant, 2000). Journal, play with art, and listen to music to suit or shift your mood.

Moments of Connection . . .
Daring to Be Yourself

A staff nurse recalls a patient with whom she had had deep conversations when the patient was very ill. She had used the crisis intervention strategy of asking the woman if anything like this had happened before and how she had handled it. The patient had been able to identify coping resources that had helped earlier in her life: "A former patient came up to me in a restaurant and thanked me for helping her to remember what she had considered important in her life and what had worked for her in the past. After leaving the hospital where I had cared for her, she had started back to church. She remembered me years later."

Moments of Connection . . .
Pass It On!

"I was able to speak to a group of high school students about careers in healthcare and talk about my job responsibilities and education. I shared the path I had taken and how good nursing had been to me and the rewards it has brought. Later that week, I received a note from one of the students thanking me for helping her to solidify her decision to become a nurse."

The Spirit

Nourish your spirit by taking time to read inspirational material or stories. Take time to be silent and to just be and not do. Set aside a regular time to contemplate life. Review the chapters on imagery and relaxation. Write your own mission statement for your personal and professional life (Kenney, 1998). Mine is to "respirit, reinspire, and revitalize nurses to provide sensitive care and find humor and joy and meaning along the journey." See Jones's *The Path* (1998) for specific directions to help you write your mission statement.

> *I like to think of men and women as artists of their own lives, working with what comes to hand though accident or talent to compose and recompose a pattern in time that expresses who they are and what they believe in—making meaning even as they are studying and working and raising children, creating and recreating themselves*
>
> **Bateson (2010, p. 24)**
>
> **WIT&*Wisdom***

Continuing Connections

Read and think about Box 30-2, reflections from each of the 30 chapters in this book.

A few final points demonstrate continuing the commitment and the risks and joy it entails.

One nurse concludes that although nurses may wear many hats, they all maintain the "commitment to the art of nursing" (Schettle, 1998). Nurses are taking on

Box 30-2 *Putting it All Together . . . upon Reflection*

Chapter 1: Practice assertive communication, which does not guarantee that you will get what you want but increases the probability that you will.

Chapter 2: Take a breath and listen, letting go of having to have answers, being willing to not know.

Chapter 3: Offer your support and information when appropriate and remember that people make their own decisions.

Chapter 4: Focus on things we have in common rather than on differences.

Chapter 5: When working in a group, claim your value by sharing your knowledge and ideas.

Chapter 6: Remember, electronic communication is a convenience, but a hand-written note is a legacy.

Chapter 7: Smile from your eyes and your heart, a valuable demonstration of warmth.

Chapter 8: Shared respect is a good foundation for health caring.

Chapter 9: Share your authentic self. Authenticity is the absence of self-deception.

Chapter 10: Be clear that we can try to put ourselves in another's place but true empathy is expressed with humility, knowing we can never succeed.

Chapter 11: Use self-disclosure in the service of the client, family, or colleague.

Chapter 12: Pay attention. Details do matter and being specific can save lives.

Chapter 13: Ask questions for what you need to know. Be aware that clients are vulnerable and trust you not to ask for more information than you need.

Chapter 14: Remember that expressing an opinion and giving advice are not the same.

Chapter 15: Learn to laugh at yourself, to not take yourself so seriously.

Chapter 16: Work on meeting your own spiritual needs to be able to offer support for another to express theirs.

Chapter 17: Remember that if you refuse to ask for support and help from others when you need it, you deny them the good feeling you get when you are able to help another.

Chapter 18: Understand that a small amount of anxiety helps you focus and learn and grow.

Chapter 19: Remember Ashleigh Brilliant's adage: "I may not be totally perfect, but parts of me are excellent."

Chapter 20: When you must stop at a traffic light or wait in a store, reframe this as a time to practice deep breathing and relaxation.

Chapter 21: Consider that your neurophysiology doesn't know the difference between your being in Hawaii and imagining you are there. Take an instant vacation.

Chapter 22: Remember the *Little Engine That Could*: I think I can, I think I can, I think I can,

Chapter 23: Consider that sometimes when you confront a person, you grow the relationship and become closer.

Chapter 24: You get to choose when to turn down an unreasonable request and when to choose to fulfill it. It is a matter of choice as long as you know you can say no. Sometimes yes is the right answer.

Chapter 25: Remember that today someone else may be distressed; tomorrow it might be you.

Chapter 26: Remember that you deserve to be treated with respect. Sometimes you must teach others that.

Chapter 27: Remember that you cannot be all things to all people but you can grow in understanding of yourself, stretching sometimes and maintaining boundaries at other times.

Chapter 28: Consider that conflict and differing opinions can generate better solutions.

Chapter 29: Reflect on this quote: "He not busy being born is busy dying" (Bob Dylan). We are all in this together.

Chapter 30: Consider this thought: As I care for myself, so I care for others.

---

many expanded clinical and administrative roles to make an impact on healthcare delivery in complex integrated delivery systems, and yet they maintain the commitment to quality care for clients and families and to the promotion of wellness for individuals and communities; through electronic communication they move on to global concerns for healthcare. Nurses are asked to develop education for house-wide hospital education. Nurses are moving into industry to design corporate wellness programs. These new roles demand new skills and a commitment to the goal of being a lifelong learner.

The examples in this text deal with one issue at a time. Clinical situations present the complex lives of real people struggling with many of life's challenges at once. To face this complexity and what may seem like impossible situations, nurses must grow with their clients and families. Honest, clear communication takes a commitment to continue to grow, to deal with change, and to stay connected with people. The rewards are substantial. Work can bring joy, but the cost is too great if you lose the joy that comes from having a rich personal life, interests to pursue, and people to whom you are connected. Consider these final exercises to help you along the journey.

Good-bye and blessings for your journey.

> *Happiness is not a goal. It is a by-product of something you do.*
>
> **Author unknown**

WIT&*Wisdom*

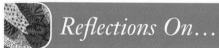

Reflections On...

Continuing the Commitment

Consider what you read about continuing the commitment. What have you learned about the importance of life balance strategies for renewal?

What? . . .
Write one thing you learned from this chapter.

So what? . . .
How will this affect your nursing practice?

Now what? . . .
How will you implement this new knowledge or skill?

Think about it . . .

Practicing Continuing the Commitment

Exercise 1
List all the roles you play in your life, such as nurse or student, daughter or son, spouse, parent, community volunteer, and so on. Then draw two circles 4 inches in diameter. Divide the first circle into portions like a pie, with as many pieces as you have roles, with each portion sized in proportion to the amount of time you spend in each role. When you are finished, consider if your use of time reflects your values. After this reflection, divide the second circle into portions according to how you would prefer to spend your time. If there are discrepancies between the two distributions of your time, consider alterations you might choose to make.

Exercise 2
Begin a journal to record the ups and downs in your daily nursing practice. Make daily entries for 2 weeks. Review your journal to regain perspective. Continue your journal if this is helpful or try it again when times are tough. To start, answer just one question: "What brought me a sense of wonder, a sense of awe today?"

Exercise 3
Begin a "joy book" in which you write the joyful things that happen in your life. Review your joy book when you do not feel joyful. If you do not see how you make a difference, choose a worthwhile cause or activity and volunteer your services.

Exercise 4
Begin a "joy box," an "antidepression kit," to collect mementos, motivational clippings, thank-you notes, small toys, and things that lift your spirits. Encourage a child in your life to do the same thing; call it a treasure box.

Exercise 5

Create a collage of your own healing journey. Glue pictures cut from magazines, greeting cards, copies of special photographs, and bits of memorabilia to a heavy piece of cardboard or mat board. Take time to reflect on the meanings of your selections. Write about what you learned. If you are in a class, share your thoughts briefly with others doing the collage. This activity can be used with clients and family members for a variety of purposes. To tap the power of your inner wisdom, using your dominant hand (your writing hand), write three questions about the collage for yourself, such as, "What lessons do I need to learn?" Using your nondominant hand, answer the questions. Reflect on your responses.

Exercise 6

Define a goal you have for yourself. Write it in positive terms, such as "to pass my examination for licensure." Envision yourself having successfully completed the goal. Write a journal entry about your future self. How do you look? How do you sound? Do you carry yourself in a different way? Hold this vision of yourself (Bolton et al, 2006).

Exercise 7

As a self-care practice, go outside and sit in a beautiful spot in nature such as park, a garden, or the woods. Pay attention to what you experience. Write a haiku poem about what you experience. This short 17-syllable poem is a traditional Japanese poetry form from the eighth century. "The philosophy behind haiku says that in losing oneself in involvement in the natural world, the writer becomes open to learning everything of importance, thereby open to gaining peace and acceptance of life's vicissitudes" (Bolton et al, 2006, p. 126). The first line of a haiku has five syllables, the second line has seven syllables, and the third line has five syllables. Example: Breeze blowing through trees. In and out and up and down. Some leaves cling, some fall.

References

Arnold E: Burnout as a spiritual issue: rediscovering meaning in nursing practice. In Carson VB, editor: *Spiritual dimensions of nursing practice*, Philadelphia, 1989, WB Saunders.

Bateson MC: *Composing a further life: the age of active wisdom*, New York, 2010, Knopf.

Bolton G, Field V, Thompson K: *Writing works: a resource book for therapeutic writing workshops and activities*, London, 2006, Jessica Kingsley Publishers.

Daehlen M: Job satisfaction and job values among beginning nurses: a questionnaire survey, *Int J Nurs Stud* 45(12):1789, 2008.

Dyess SM, Sherman RO: The first year of practice: new graduate nurses' transition and learning needs, *J Cont Educ Nurs* 40(9):403, September 2009.

Guterman MS: *Common sense for uncommon times: the power of balance in work, family, and personal life*, Palo Alto, Calif, 1994, CPP Books.

Guzzetta CE: Weaving a tapestry of holism, *J Cardiovasc Nurs* 12(2):18, 1998.

Jones LB: *The path: creating your mission statement for work and for life*, New York, 1998, Hyperion.

Kenney EG: Creating fulfillment in today's workplace: a guide for nurses, *Am J Nurs* 98(5):44, 1998.

Kramer ML: *Reality shock: why nurses leave nursing*, St. Louis, 1974, The C.V. Mosby Co.

Kushner H: *When bad things happen to good people*, New York, 2001, Schocken Books.

Kushner H: *When all you've ever wanted isn't enough: a search for a life that matters*, New York, 2002, Fireside.

Murant GM: Creativity and self-care for caregivers, *J Palliat Care* 16(2):44, 2000.

Pellico LH, Brewer CS, Kovner CT: What newly licensed registered nurses have to say about their new experiences, *Nurs Outlook* 57(4):194, 2009.

Schettle S: A nurse's reflection: nursing in the 90s—old hats, new ways. *Am J Nurs* 98(5):16J, 1998.

Sherman RO, Dyess S: New graduate transition into practice during turbulent economic times (guest editorial), *J Nurs Educ* 49(7):367, 2010.

Tingle CA: Workplace advocacy as a transition tool, *The Student Nurse Advisor* 1(16):July 15, 2001.

Zerwekh JV: Caring on the ragged edge: nursing persons who are disenfranchised, *Adv Nurs Sci* 22(4):47, 2000.

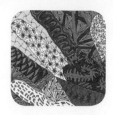

Index